Biliary Tract and Primary Liver Tumors

Editor

TIMOTHY M. PAWLIK

SURGICAL ONCOLOGY
CLINICS OF NORTH AMERICA

www.surgonc.theclinics.com

Consulting Editor
NICHOLAS J. PETRELLI

April 2014 • Volume 23 • Number 2

ELSEVIER

1600 John F. Kennedy Boulevard ● Suite 1800 ● Philadelphia, Pennsylvania, 19103-2899

http://www.theclinics.com

SURGICAL ONCOLOGY CLINICS OF NORTH AMERICA Volume 23, Number 2
April 2014 ISSN 1055-3207, ISBN-13: 978-0-323-29018-0

Editor: Jessica McCool
Developmental Editor: Stephanie Carter

Surgical Oncology Clinics of North America (ISSN 1055-3207) is published quarterly by Elsevier Inc., 360 Park Avenue South, New York, NY 10010-1710. Months of publication are January, April, July, and October. Business and Editorial Offices: 1600 John F. Kennedy Blvd., Ste. 1800, Philadelphia, PA 19103-2899. Customer Service Office: 3251 Riverport Lane, Maryland Heights, MO 63043. Periodicals postage paid at New York, NY and additional mailing offices. Subscription prices are $290.00 per year (US individuals), $421.00 (US institutions) $140.00 (US student/resident), $330.00 (Canadian individuals), $533.00 (Canadian institutions), $205.00 (Canadian student/resident), $410.00 (foreign individuals), $533.00 (foreign institutions), and $205.00 (foreign student/resident). Foreign air speed delivery is included in all *Clinics* subscription prices. All prices are subject to change without notice. **POSTMASTER**: Send address changes to *Surgical Oncology Clinics of North America*, Elsevier Health Science Division, Subscription Customer Service, 3251 Riverport Lane, Maryland Heights, MO 63043. **Customer Service: 1-800-654-2452 (US and Canada). 314-447-8871 (outside US and Canada). Fax: 314-447-8029. E-mail: journalscustomerservice-usa@elsevier.com** (for print support); **journalsonline support-usa@elsevier.com** (for online support).

Reprints. For copies of 100 or more, of articles in this publication, please contact the Commercial Reprints Department, Elsevier Inc., 360 Park Avenue South, New York, New York 10010-1710. Tel. 212-633-3874; Fax: 212-633-3820; E-mail: reprints@elsevier.com.

Surgical Oncology Clinics of North America is covered in *MEDLINE/PubMed (Index Medicus)* and *EMBASE/ Excerpta Medica, Current Contents/Clinical Medicine,* and *ISI/BIOMED.*

Printed and bound by CPI Group (UK) Ltd, Croydon, CR0 4YY

Contributors

CONSULTING EDITOR

NICHOLAS J. PETRELLI, MD, FACS
Bank of America Endowed Medical Director, Helen F. Graham Cancer Center at Christiana Care, Newark, Delaware; Professor of Surgery, Thomas Jefferson University, Philadelphia, Pennsylvania

EDITOR

TIMOTHY M. PAWLIK, MD, MPH, PhD
Professor of Surgery and Oncology, John L. Cameron MD Professor of Alimentary Tract Diseases; Chief, Division of Surgical Oncology; Director, Johns Hopkins Medicine Liver Tumor Center Multi-Disciplinary Clinic, Johns Hopkins Hospital, Baltimore, Maryland

AUTHORS

ALBERT AMINI, MD
Clinical Instructor, Hepatobiliary Fellow, Division of Surgical Oncology, Department of Surgery, Medical College of Wisconsin, Milwaukee, Wisconsin

MATHEW M. AUGUSTINE, MD
Surgical Oncology Fellow, Hepatobiliary Service, Department of Surgery, Memorial Sloan-Kettering Cancer Center, New York, New York

KIMBERLY M. BROWN, MD, FACS
Department of Surgery, University of Texas Medical Branch, Galveston, Texas

BRYAN M. CLARY, MD
Division of Surgical Oncology, Duke University Medical Center, Durham, North Carolina

CELIA P. CORONA-VILLALOBOS, MD
The Russell H. Morgan Department of Radiology and Radiological Sciences, The Johns Hopkins School of Medicine, Baltimore, Maryland

DAVID C. COSGROVE, MD
Department of Medical Oncology, Johns Hopkins Hospital, Baltimore, Maryland

LAURA A. DAWSON, MD
Professor, Department of Radiation Oncology, Princess Margaret Cancer Centre, University of Toronto, Toronto, Ontario, Canada

YUMAN FONG, MD
Attending Surgeon, Hepatobiliary Service, Department of Surgery, Memorial Sloan-Kettering Cancer Center, New York, New York

T. CLARK GAMBLIN, MD, MS
Associate Professor, Chief of Surgical Oncology, Division of Surgical Oncology, Department of Surgery, Medical College of Wisconsin, Milwaukee, Wisconsin

DAVID A. GELLER, MD, FACS
Richard L. Simmons Professor of Surgery, Liver Cancer Center, University of Pittsburgh School of Medicine, Pittsburgh, Pennsylvania

THEODORE S. HONG, MD
Associate Professor, Department of Radiation Oncology, Massachusetts General Hospital, Boston, Massachusetts

IHAB R. KAMEL, MD, PhD
The Russell H. Morgan Department of Radiology and Radiological Sciences, The Johns Hopkins School of Medicine, Baltimore, Maryland

DAVID A. KOOBY, MD, FACS
Director of Surgical Oncology, Emory/Saint Joseph's Hospital; Associate Professor, Division of Surgical Oncology, Department of Surgery, Winship Cancer Institute, Emory University School of Medicine, Atlanta, Georgia

NEHA LAD, MD
Research Fellow, Division of Surgical Oncology, Department of Surgery, Winship Cancer Institute, Emory University School of Medicine, Atlanta, Georgia

DAVID C. MADOFF, MD
Professor of Radiology, Chief, Division of Interventional Radiology, Department of Radiology, New York-Presbyterian Hospital/Weill Cornell Medical Center, New York, New York

DAVID M. NAGORNEY, MD
Professor, Department of Surgery, Mayo Clinic, Rochester, Minnesota

ANDREW J. PAGE, MD
Department of Surgery, Johns Hopkins Hospital, Baltimore, Maryland

ABHISHEK D. PARMAR, MD
Department of Surgery, University of Texas Medical Branch, Galveston, Texas; Department of Surgery, University of California San Francisco-East Bay, Oakland, California

TIMOTHY M. PAWLIK, MD, MPH, PhD
Professor of Surgery and Oncology, John L. Cameron MD Professor of Alimentary Tract Diseases; Chief, Division of Surgical Oncology; Director, Johns Hopkins Medicine Liver Tumor Center Multi-Disciplinary Clinic, Johns Hopkins Hospital, Baltimore, Maryland

BENJAMIN PHILOSOPHE, MD
Department of Surgery, Johns Hopkins Hospital, Baltimore, Maryland

CHARLES B. ROSEN, MD
Professor of Surgery, Chair, Division of Transplantation Surgery, Mayo Clinic, Rochester, Minnesota

KEVIN N. SHAH, MD
Division of Surgical Oncology, Duke University Medical Center, Durham, North Carolina

JUNICHI SHINDOH, MD, PhD
Department of Surgical Oncology, The University of Texas MD Anderson Cancer Center, Houston, Texas

AKHILESH K. SISTA, MD
Assistant Professor, Division of Interventional Radiology, Department of Radiology, New York-Presbyterian Hospital/Weill Cornell Medical Center, New York, New York

ADAM D. TALENFELD, MD
Assistant Professor, Division of Interventional Radiology, Department of Radiology, New York-Presbyterian Hospital/Weill Cornell Medical Center, New York, New York

MELANIE BYRNE THOMAS, MD, FACP
Grace E. DeWolff Chair of Medical Oncology, Associate Director of Clinical Investigations, Hollings Cancer Center, Associate Professor of Medicine, College of Medicine, Medical University of South Carolina, Charleston, South Carolina

JEAN-NICOLAS VAUTHEY, MD
Department of Surgical Oncology, The University of Texas MD Anderson Cancer Center, Houston, Texas

JENNIFER Y. WO, MD
Assistant Professor, Department of Radiation Oncology, Massachusetts General Hospital, Boston, Massachusetts

VICTOR M. ZAYDFUDIM, MD, MPH
Assistant Professor, Department of Surgery, University of Virginia, Charlottesville, Virginia

ANDREW X. ZHU, MD, PhD
Associate Professor, Department of Medical Oncology, Massachusetts General Hospital, Boston, Massachusetts

Contents

> Primary liver and biliary tract tumors encompass a range of benign and
> malignant neoplasms. They consist of histologically distinct types of tu-
> mors that arise from and are influenced by hepatocytes, biliary epithelial
> cells, and mesenchymal cells. Improvements in imaging have allowed
> the detection and diagnosis of these neoplasms to be refined. Investiga-
> tion at the histologic, molecular, and genetic levels has allowed neoplasms
> to be categorized and treated. Epidemiology has improved understanding
> of geographic, ethnic, gender, and cultural differences that link exposures
> with cancer risk. This article focuses on the epidemiology of major primary
> adult liver and biliary tract tumors.

> Cross-sectional imaging can be useful in the diagnosis of biliary tract and
> primary liver tumors. Hepatobiliary tumors are diverse in growth patterns,
> histologic types and tumor location. A fundamental understanding of the
> imaging features of hepatobiliary tumors is critical for diagnosis, staging
> and treatment. Knowledge about various manifestations and mimickers
> of biliary and primary liver tumors is essential for tumor diagnosis and suit-
> able management. Magnetic resonance imaging and computed tomogra-
> phy technology continues to rapidly evolve and these tools not only aid in
> evaluation and treatment, but also can potentially define response to ther-
> apy and overall patient prognosis.

> Advances in percutaneous and endoscopic techniques have improved
> preoperative selection and optimization in patients with biliary and liver tu-
> mors, but are not without their own controversies. Selective rather than
> routine preoperative biliary drainage (PBD) should be employed, as PBD
> may be associated with increased infectious complications. Endoscopic
> ampullectomy (EA) offers advantages in morbidity and mortality over sur-
> gical approaches and should be the first line therapy for benign ampullary
> lesions. Ampullary cancers require pancreaticoduodenectomy. Effective-
> ness of percutaneous ablative techniques is dependent on tumor size

and can be used as palliative therapy, as a bridge to transplantation, or, in select situations, as definitive therapy.

strategies for HCC have become more methodical and more successful. This article focuses on some of the most critical advances relating to carcinogenesis, surveillance, and management.

Junichi Shindoh and Jean-Nicolas Vauthey

For patients with hepatobiliary malignancies, various therapeutic options are currently available. To optimize the selection of these treatment options, adequate stratification of patients according to their prognosis is practically important. Various staging systems have been introduced and used for hepatobiliary malignancies. However, current staging systems have strengths and limitations, and none have addressed both patient prognosis and the best treatment strategy for individual patients. Hepatic function is also a potent prognostic factor for patients with hepatobiliary malignancies. Therefore, interpretation of tumor staging and selection of treatment should be done with care, understanding individual characteristics of each staging system.

Adam D. Talenfeld, Akhilesh K. Sista, and David C. Madoff

Over the last decade, transarterial therapies have gained worldwide acceptance as standard of care for inoperable primary liver cancer. Survival times after transarterial chemoembolization (TACE) continue to improve as the technique and selection criteria are refined. Transarterial treatments, frequently provided in an outpatient setting, are now safely and effectively being applied to patients with even advanced malignancy or partially decompensated cirrhosis. In the coming years, newer transarterial therapies such as radiation segmentectomy, boosted-transarterial radioembolzation, combined TACE-ablation, TACE-portal vein embolization, and transarterial infusion of cancer-specific metabolic inhibitors promise to continue improving survival and quality of life.

Jennifer Y. Wo, Laura A. Dawson, Andrew X. Zhu, and Theodore S. Hong

Radiation therapy is emerging as a potentially effective treatment of locally advanced, unresectable hepatocellular carcinoma (HCC). Outcomes from early prospective studies seem promising, with improved survival compared with historical controls. Cure of early stage and unresectable HCC may be possible with high-quality radiation therapy. Many questions remain, including determination of the ideal radiation dose and fractionation schema, optimal patient selection criteria based on tumor size, tumor location, extent of vascular invasion, and baseline liver function, and the role of radiation therapy compared with other localized standard treatments including radiofrequency ablation or transarterial chemoembolization.

Melanie Byrne Thomas

Tumors of the biliary tract and hepatocellular carcinoma (HCC) are complex tumors with heterogeneous carcinogenic mechanisms. Patients with hepatobiliary cancer have advanced disease and need systemic therapy to palliate symptoms and extend survival. Development of effective systemic therapy is a significant unmet medical need. It is hoped that current and future clinical trials will identify additional effective systemic agents, combination systemic therapies, and combined modality options. The HCC community needs validated biomarkers to help identify the patients who will benefit most from emerging treatment options.

This article summarizes the current literature in treatment of unresectable biliary tract and primary liver tumors. Locoregional therapies including radiofrequency ablation, percutaneous ethanol injection, cryoablation, microwave ablation, transarterial chemoembolization, hepatic artery infusion, radioembolization (^{90}Y), and bland embolization are discussed and clinical trials compared. Palliative strategies including surgical, percutaneous, and endoscopic techniques to decompress the biliary system and improve symptoms are also summarized. Systemic chemotherapy and sorafenib used in conjunction with locoregional therapies or as sole therapeutic options are discussed.

SURGICAL ONCOLOGY
CLINICS OF NORTH AMERICA

DOWNLOAD Free App!

Review Articles
THE CLINICS

NOW AVAILABLE FOR YOUR iPhone and iPad

Foreword

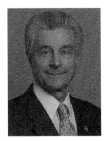

Nicholas J. Petrelli, MD, FACS
Consulting Editor

This issue of the *Surgical Oncology Clinics of North America* takes on the subject matter of biliary tract tumors and primary liver tumors. The editor is Timothy M. Pawlik, MD, MPH, PhD, Chief of the Division of Surgical Oncology and Professor of Surgery at Johns Hopkins University. Dr Pawlik's interests are in experimental therapeutics of hepatic malignancies and clinical trials in gastrointestinal malignancies. He has brought together an outstanding group of researchers and clinicians for this issue.

In the United States, there are approximately 30,600 new cases of liver and intrahepatic bile duct cancers every year with an estimated 21,000 deaths. Gallbladder and other biliary tract cancers account for another 10,000 cases annually with an estimated 3,200 deaths. The article entitled, "Imaging of the Patient with a Biliary Tract or Primary Liver Tumor," by Drs Corona-Villalobos and Kamel, coauthored by Dr Pawlik, is an excellent example of the quality of articles in this issue of *Surgical Oncology Clinics of North America*. This article has excellent discussions on imaging with associated figures describing ultrasound and magnetic resonance imaging of hepatocellular carcinoma. There is also an excellent discussion of treatment response of hepatocellular carcinoma asssessed by functional magnetic resonance imaging and a detailed discussion of imaging in gallbladder carcinoma including lymphoma of the gallbladder.

Additional articles include staging of biliary tract and primary liver tumors and intra-arterial therapies for primary liver tumors.

The last issue of *Surgical Oncology Clinics of North America* covering biliary tract tumors was published in 2009 under guest editor, Joseph Bennett, MD. Hence, five years later it is important to update this especially challenging topic. I congratulate Dr Pawlik and his colleagues for an outstanding issue of the *Surgical Oncology*

Surg Oncol Clin N Am 23 (2014) xiii–xiv
http://dx.doi.org/10.1016/j.soc.2013.11.006
1055-3207/14/$ – see front matter © 2014 Published by Elsevier Inc.

Clinics of North America and encourage the readers of this issue to share it with their residents and surgical oncology fellows.

Nicholas J. Petrelli, MD, FACS
Helen F. Graham Cancer Center at Christiana Care
4701 Ogletown-Stanton Road, Suite 1213
Newark, DE 19713, USA

E-mail address:
npetrelli@christianacare.org

Preface

Biliary Tract and Primary Liver Tumors

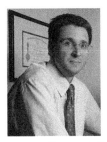

Timothy M. Pawlik, MD, MPH, PhD
Editor

This issue of the *Surgical Oncology Clinics of North America* brings together experts in the field of biliary tract and primary liver tumors. Biliary and primary liver tumors require the surgeon to have excellent clinical judgment, superb operative skills, and a deep understanding of the available therapeutic options. To this end, the authors of this issue have contributed a series of articles that defines the wide array of topics that range from epidemiology and risk factors, to imaging and workup, to the treatment of patients with biliary and primary liver tumors. The authors were asked to critically review and place into a contemporary, practical clinical context the "state-of-the-art" data on the management of these challenging diseases. Over the past decade, the body of knowledge around biliary and primary liver tumors has expanded greatly. For the practicing surgeon, it can be challenging to remain well-informed about a field that has become highly specialized and nuanced. In this issue, the participating authors have done an exemplary job synthesizing the available data, providing their own unique clinical insights, and presenting the salient, most relevant information on biliary and primary tumors for the practicing hepatobiliary surgeon.

The issue provides an overview of important topics such as the epidemiology and risk factors associated with biliary and primary liver tumors. In addition, an article is devoted to recent advances in imaging with an emphasis on cross-sectional imaging and MRI in particular. A separate article examines percutaneous and endoscopic approaches to patients with biliary and primary liver tumors, while another discusses staging. Other articles focus on important nonsurgical options such as intra-arterial therapy and radiation therapy. Most articles, however, are disease-specific and provide an opportunity for each author to review thoroughly the management and therapeutic options for intrahepatic, hilar, and distal cholangiocarcinoma, as well as hepatocellular carcinoma. In this way, the reader can obtain an in-depth perspective

Surg Oncol Clin N Am 23 (2014) xv–xvi
http://dx.doi.org/10.1016/j.soc.2013.11.005
surgonc.theclinics.com

of the management of each of these diseases, which have unique tumor biologies, natural histories, as well as clinical management options.

I believe that readers of this issue of *Surgical Oncology Clinics of North America* will gain a contemporary understanding of the current data on the diagnosis, management, and prognosis of patients with biliary and primary liver tumors. It is also my hope and belief that readers of this issue will find the information as a practical means to help improve the care of patients with these challenging diseases.

Timothy M. Pawlik, MD, MPH, PhD
Division of Surgical Oncology
Department of Surgery
Johns Hopkins Hospital
600 North Wolfe Street, Blalock 688
Baltimore, MD 21287, USA

E-mail address:
tpawlik1@jhmi.edu

Epidemiology and Risk Factors of Biliary Tract and Primary Liver Tumors

Mathew M. Augustine, MD, Yuman Fong, MD*

KEYWORDS

- Hepatocelluar cancer • Gallbladder cancer • Cholangiocarcinoma • Viral hepatitis
- Benign liver tumor

KEY POINTS

- Primary liver and biliary tumors are a significant health threat globally.
- These tumors have wide geographic, ethnic, and gender variation.
- Research investigating the epidemiology and risk factors associated with these tumors has resulted in significant global public health measures to reduce incidence rates.
- Recently identified risk factors, such as metabolic disorders, show the important role that epidemiology will continue to have in the understanding and treatment of these tumors.

HEPATOCELLULAR CANCER

Hepatocellular cancer (HCC) is the most common form of primary liver cancer, accounting for 85% to 90% of all primary liver cancers, with the burden of disease expected to increase in coming years, especially in the developing world.[1] It is the fifth most common cancer worldwide and the third most common cause of cancer mortality, accounting for more than 600,000 deaths annually.[2] HCC was one of the first cancers to be linked epidemiologically to a defined risk factor (hepatitis B virus [HBV] in Taiwan). Approximately 80% of HCC worldwide is caused by chronic infection with HBV or hepatitis C virus (HCV). Chronic hepatitis B infection remains the most common risk factor for HCC worldwide. There are an estimated 450 million carriers of HBV worldwide. However, chronic hepatitis C has become an important cause of chronic liver disease around the world, with an estimated 200 million people infected with HCV. HCC has several interesting epidemiologic features, including dynamic temporal trends; marked variations among geographic regions and racial, ethnic,

The author has nothing to disclose.

Hepatobiliary Service, Department of Surgery, Memorial Sloan Kettering Cancer Center, 353 East 68th Street, New York, NY 10065, USA

* Corresponding author.

E-mail address: fongy@mskcc.org

and gender groups; and the presence of several well-documented, preventable environmental risk factors.

Global Incidence of HCC

The incidence of HCC is not evenly distributed throughout the world. It is broadly divided into 3 major geographic subgroups: (1) sub-Saharan Africa; (2) eastern Asia; and (3) North and South America, northern Europe, and Oceania. Most cases occur in sub-Saharan Africa or in eastern Asia. Recent estimates published in the GLOBO-CAN analysis indicate that 82% of liver cancer cases occur in developing countries, with more than 50% of cases in China (male, 35.2 per 100,000; female, 13.3 per 100,000). Other areas of high incidence include South Korea (male, 48.8 per 100,000; female, 11.6 per 100,000), Gambia (male, 39.7 per 100,000; female, 14.6 per 100,000), and Senegal (male, 28.5 per 100,000; female, 12.2 per 100,000). The rates of HCC in North America, South America, and northern Europe are lower compared with the geographic regions mentioned earlier, typically with incidence rates of less than 5 per 100,000. Southern European countries tend to have incidence levels between these 2 geographic extremes.

Although the incidence of HCC remains high, several regions are experiencing a decrease in overall rate, accounted for by public health measures including vaccination and environmental exposure restriction. The world's first nationwide hepatitis B vaccination program was implemented in Taiwan in 1984 and resulted in a decrease in the average annual incidence of hepatocellular carcinoma from 0.7 per 100,000 children between 1981 and 1986 to 0.36 per 100,000 children between 1990 and 1994.[3–5] The mortality from HCC also decreased during this period. Aflatoxin contaminants in corn and peanuts infected with *Aspergillus flavus* correlated with HCC mortality and the presence of aflatoxin-albumin adducts is higher in hyperendemic HCC areas.[6] A Chinese government program started in the late 1980s to shift the diet of the Jiangsu Province from corn to rice may have limited exposure to known hepatocarcinogen aflatoxin B1 in this area.[6] However, registries in several low-rate areas, including the United States, United Kingdom, and Australia, have shown an increase in HCC incidence. It is thought that the increased incidence in low-rate areas has resulted from the later introduction of HCV infection through intravenous drug abuse within these areas.

HCC is the fastest growing cause of cancer-related mortality in the United States. Between 1985 and 2002, age-adjusted HCC incidence doubled.[7,8] The increase in HCC started in the mid-1980s, with the greatest proportional increase occurring in Hispanic and non-Hispanic white people.[9] In the United States, the mean age of diagnosis is approximately 65 years, with 75% of cases in men. The racial distribution is 48% white, 15% Hispanic, 13% African American, and 24% other (predominantly Asian).[1] The greatest proportional increase occurred in HCV-related HCC, whereas HBV-related HCC had the lowest rate.

Gender

Liver cancer is the fifth most common cancer in men worldwide and the seventh most common cancer in women. In almost all populations, the rate of HCC is higher among men than among women, with the male/female ratio usually averaging between 2:1 and 4:1. According to GLOBOCAN estimates for 2002, the overall male/female incidence ratio was 2.4.[2] The most discrepant ratios are found in Europe where registries have reported male/female ratios of greater than 5:1. Some of the lowest differences are found in Central and South America. In Colombia and Costa Rica, male/female ratios have been as low as 1.2:1.[1] It is thought that the discrepancy in the ratio of

HCC rates between men and women is related to differences in environmental risk factor exposure. Men are more likely to be exposed to HBV and HCV, to consume alcohol, and to smoke cigarettes. However, environmental exposure may be only part of the explanation. Gender difference in hormone levels may also alter the virulence of these risk factors. A positive association between increased circulating testosterone levels and HCC in men infected with HBV has been found even when accounting for the effects of other hepatocellular carcinoma risk factors.[10]

Age

HCC is rarely seen during the first 4 decades of life, except in populations in which HBV infection is hyperendemic. The mean age of diagnosis of HCC is 55 to 59 years in China and 63 to 65 years in Europe and North America, reflecting high-risk and low-risk populations. In Qidong, China, where the HBV and HCC burden is among the world's highest, the age-specific incidence rate of HCC in men peaks at around 45 years of age.[11] HBV tends to be acquired at a younger age with a longer incubation period than HCV, with mother-to-child transmission being the main route of transfer. The differences in age of onset of HCC vary based on gender, with male rates peaking earlier by 5 to 10 years. These differences in age-specific incidence are related to the type of virus that is dominant within a population as well as age at infection.

Distribution of Risk Factors

The distribution of risk factors varies by geographic location. In most developing countries, which tend to be the high-risk areas, HBV infection is the dominant risk factor. In Asia, excluding Japan, HBV infection is usually acquired through mother-to-child transmission. However, in Africa, sibling-to-sibling transmission is also common. Exposure to AFB1-contaminated foodstuffs is the other major HCC risk factor in high-risk areas. In Japan, HCV is the predominant virus causing HCC and it has been documented that the older the age in Japan, the higher the prevalence. Shortly after World War II, HCV began to circulate in Japan.[12] It is thought that this occurred because of illicit intravenous amphetamine abuse. As a result, HCC rates began to increase in the mid-1970s, and the incidence is expected to peak around 2015.

In low-rate HCC regions, cirrhosis from chronic alcohol consumption and the increasing metabolic syndrome epidemic are the leading causes of HCC development. The predominant causal factors include HCV and, to a lesser extent, HBV infection. Infection by HCV and HBV began in the 1960s and 1970s and spread as a result of intravenous drug abuse. The presence of the virus in the national blood supply further enhanced its spread. With the advent of a screening test in the 1990s, the rates of new infection decreased greatly. It is thought that, in low-rate areas, peak incidence of HCV-related HCC occurred around 2010.

Risk Factors for HCC

HBV

Worldwide, HBV is the most frequent underlying cause of HCC. HBV is a member of the Hepadnaviridae family, which are small, partially double-stranded DNA viruses containing 4 overlapping genes that encode for the nucleocapsid, envelope, polymerase with reverse transcriptase activity, and X proteins. It is thought that HBV can contribute to the development of HCC through at least 4 mechanisms. HBV DNA can integrate into the host chromosome resulting in nonselective, insertional mutagenic events. The hepatitis Bx gene product can function as a transcriptional transactivator of various cellular genes associated with growth control. Chronic HBV infection causes hepatocyte injury, inflammation, and cell turnover, increasing the risk for malignant transformation. In addition, a high HBV replication phenotype and mutations in the core promoter region have been identified as viral risk factors for the development of HCC.

Approximately 350 million to 400 million people are infected with this HBV. Carriers of HBV have a 5-foldto 15-fold increased risk of HCC compared with the general population. Approximately 8% of the population of Asia and sub-Saharan Africa are carriers of HBV surface antigen, whereas only 2% carry it in North America and northern and western Europe.[13] Although 70% to 90% of carriers of HBV who develop HCC do so in the context of cirrhosis, HCC develops in the absence of cirrhosis. HBV infection is most commonly passed from mother to child (vertical transmission). Up to 90% of these transmissions result in chronic infection. However, HBV infection is also passed on through sexual and parenteral routes (horizontal transmission). In these instances, more than 90% of acute infections resolve spontaneously. The annual rate of HCC incidence in chronic HBV carriers ranges between 0.4% and 0.6%. Risk factors associated with increased rate of HCC in HBV carriers include male sex; older age, because of the longer time course of infection; exposure to alcohol, tobacco, or aflatoxin B1; Asian or African race; or coinfection with HCV or hepatitis D viral infection. Higher levels of HBV replication, as shown by increased presence of hepatitis B e antigen and high HBV DNA levels, also increase the HCC rate.

Hepatitis B vaccination is the most effective measure of prevention from HBV infection and HCC formation. The results from the Taiwanese vaccination program show that, 10 years after the initiation of immunization, the incidence of HCC among children 6 to 14 years old had declined from 0.7 per 100,000 to 0.36 per 100,000.

HCV

HCV is a single-stranded RNA virus. Unlike HBV, it does not integrate into the host genome so insertional mutagenesis does not play a role in malignant transformation. It is thought that HCV infection results in HCC by one of 2 mechanisms. The first involves inflammation from chronic HCV infection leading to subsequent regeneration, fibrosis, and cirrhosis. It is within these cirrhotic foci that HCC develops, possibly from adenomatous hyperplastic or dysplastic nodules. The other mechanism may involve HCV proteins that influence cellular genes, resulting in the malignant phenotype.

Chronic HCV infection that promotes inflammation, fibrosis, and cirrhosis is a significant risk factor for the development of HCC. HCC risk is increased approximately 17-fold in patients infected with HCV compared with HCV-negative controls.[14] The annual rate of HCC development is about 1% to 5% once HCV-related cirrhosis has developed, which is 10 times that in HBV. Various risk factors are associated with the progression to cirrhosis. These factors include older age, older age at the time of acquisition of infection, male sex, heavy alcohol intake (>50 g/d), diabetes, obesity, and coinfection with human immunodeficiency virus or HBV.

Alcohol

Heavy alcohol intake, defined as greater than 50 to 70 g/d for prolonged periods, is a well-established risk factor for hepatocellular cancer. Despite the association between heavy alcohol intake and HCC, there is little evidence of a direct carcinogenic effect of alcohol. There is evidence of a synergistic effect of heavy alcohol ingestion with HCV or HBV. It is thought that the combination of these factors increases HCC risk by promoting cirrhosis. One report indicated that, with the concomitant presence of HCV infection among alcohol drinkers, there was an additional 2-fold increase in HCC risk compared with that observed with alcohol alone.

Aflatoxin

AFB1 is a mycotoxin produced by the Aspergillus fungus (A flavus and Aspergillus parasiticus). This fungus grows on foodstuffs such as corn and peanuts stored in warm, damp conditions. Animal experiments have shown that AFB1 is a hepatocarcinogen. Once ingested, AFB1 is metabolized to an active epoxide intermediate that can bind to DNA and cause damage. It can produce a mutation in the p53 tumor-suppressor gene.[15] This mutation has been observed in 30% to 60% of HCC tumors in aflatoxin-endemic areas.[15] Regions that have AFB1 exposure also have high rates of HBV infection. Prospective studies in Shanghai, China, showed that urinary excretion of aflatoxin metabolites increased the risk of HCC 4-fold.[15] HBV infection increased the risk 7-fold. However, individuals who excreted AFB1 metabolites and had HBV infection had as much as a 60-fold increased risk in HCC.

Nonalcoholic fatty liver disease

Studies in the United States evaluating risk factors for chronic liver disease or HCC failed to identify HCV, HBV, or heavy alcohol intake in approximately 30% to 40% of patients. Several clinic-based, case-control studies have indicated that patients with HCC with cryptogenic cirrhosis tend to have clinical and demographic features that suggest non-alcoholic steatohepatitis (NASH) compared with age-matched and sex-matched patients with HCC of well-defined viral or alcoholic cause.[16] In one study of 210 patients who underwent resection for HCC, patients with no identifiable cause for chronic liver disease had higher rates of obesity and diabetes compared with patients with alcohol and viral hepatitis. A systematic review and meta-analysis found a significant association between HCC and diabetes that was independent of alcohol and viral hepatitis.[17] Longer duration of diabetes has been reported to increase the risk of HCC.[18] A prospective cohort study of more than 900,000 individuals that spanned a 16-year period showed that liver cancer mortality was 5 times greater among men with the highest body mass index (range, 35–40) compared with those with a normal body mass index.[19] Two other population-based cohort studies from Sweden and Denmark found 2-fold to 3-fold increased risk of HCC in obese men and women compared with those with a normal body mass index.[20,21] Insulin resistance is associated with obesity and is known to contribute to hepatic steatosis. There is a growing metabolic syndrome epidemic in the United States. The contribution of this disorder to future trends in cirrhosis and liver cancer will be watched closely.[22]

HEMANGIOMA

Hepatic hemangioma is the most common benign lesion of the liver, with an estimated prevalence of 5% to 20% in the general population.[23] Hepatic hemangiomas are vascular abnormalities characterized by blood-filled, sinusoidal spaces lined with endothelium. It is thought that dilatation of these spaces, and not angiogenesis, causes enlargement over time. These lesions are incidentally found on abdominal exploration and on imaging studies. Most hepatic hemangiomas are identified in patients between the ages of 30 and 50 years. They are seen more commonly in women than in men, with a female/male ratio of 6:1.[24] They are typically seen as solitary lesions but in more than 10% of cases they are found as multiple hemangiomas.[25] These lesions are benign with no malignant potential, but can cause symptoms. Symptomatic lesions are more frequently found in women and can cause abdominal discomfort, pain from capsular stretch, spontaneous rupture, or thrombocytopenia and hypofibrinogenemia from consumption (Kasabach-Merritt syndrome).

FOCAL NODULAR HYPERPLASIA

Focal nodular hyperplasia (FNH) is a benign, indolent tumor of the liver with no known malignant potential. It is the second most common benign liver tumor after hepatic hemangiomas. FNH is reported to occur with a frequency between 0.31% and 3%.[26,27] It is more commonly identified incidentally in young women between the ages of 30 and 50 years.[27,28] The female/male ratio has been reported to be between 8:1 and 12:1.[27,29] FNH is rarely found in the pediatric population and the elderly. The higher risk of FNH in women raises the possibility that these benign tumors are under hormonal influence (pregnancy or oral contraceptive pills). In most cases, FNH is asymptomatic and is commonly seen as an incidental finding on imaging studies. It is thought to arise as a hyperplastic lesion from a preexisting arterial malformation. There are reports in the literature of rupture as well as bleeding caused by FNH.[30,31]

HEPATOCELLULAR ADENOMA

Hepatocellular adenoma is a noncancerous neoplasm of the liver, but, unlike liver hemangiomas and FNH, it has malignant potential. Hepatic adenoma is usually a solitary lesion that on histologic analysis consists of normal to slightly enlarged hepatocytes arranged in a trabecular pattern. The pathogenesis is strongly associated with oral contraceptive use.[32] In North America and Europe, the incidence is about 0.1 per 100,000 in non–oral contraceptive users and 3 to 4 per 100,000 in oral contraceptive users.[33] This neoplasm is discovered more frequently in women than in men, with a female/male ratio of 11:1.[23] However, exposure to modern contraceptives did not reveal an increased risk for hepatocellular adenoma.[34] It is seen most commonly in women in their third and fourth decades of life. There is an increased trend in hepatocellular adenomas in men, which is thought to arise from the increasing prevalence of obesity and the metabolic syndrome in this gender.[35,36] The prevalence of malignancy is 10 times higher in men than in women and is the reason for a more aggressive surgical approach in men.[36] Hepatocellular adenoma is rare in Asia because of the lower prevalence in women and because of oral contraceptive use.[37]

GALLBLADDER CANCER

Gallbladder cancer is the fifth most common cancer involving the gastrointestinal tract, but the most common malignant tumor of the biliary tract worldwide. When diagnosed, it is typically found incidentally during cholecystectomy. However, gallbladder cancer frequently presents with vague symptoms and, as a result, its diagnosis occurs at an advanced stage. The late stage of presentation results in patients showing both locally advanced as well as metastatic spread. The overall mean survival rate for patients with advanced gallbladder cancer is 6 months, with a survival rate of 5% at 5 years. Although the cause of gallbladder cancer is unclear and most likely multifactorial, it is thought that chronic irritation and inflammation of the mucosa may play a central role in adenocarcinoma development.

Carcinoma of the gallbladder is predominantly a disease of elderly women, with a peak incidence in the seventh decade of life. The incidence is reported to be up to 3 times higher among women than among men in all populations.[38] The incidence of gallbladder cancer varies by geographic location and racial groups. The highest incidence rate of gallbladder cancer is found among populations in the Andean region, in North American Indians, and in Mexican Americans.[39,40] Intermediate rates of 3.7 to 9.1 per 100,000 are reported from Peru, Ecuador, Colombia, and Brazil. The highest mortalities are also found in South America: 3.5 to 15.5 per 100,000 among Chilean

Mapuche Indians, Bolivians, and Chilean Hispanics. In Europe, the rates are highest in Poland, the Czech Republic, and Slovakia.[41] The mortality is lower in North America but is selectively higher within the American Indian population (11.3 per 100,000) and among Mexican Americans. Women from Delhi (21.5 per 100,000) and South Karachi, Pakistan (13.8 per 100,000), also show high incidence rates.[41] Gallbladder cancer is rare in developed countries. For example, in the United States, it accounts for 0.5% of all gastrointestinal malignancies (approximately 5000 cases per year).[42] There is no consistent global trend in the incidence of gallbladder cancer because there are regions and countries where the incidence is increasing and decreasing.

Risk Factors

Cholelithiasis
Multiple risk factors are associated with the development of gallbladder cancer. Most patients who have gallbladder cancer have cholelithiasis; however, gallstones are a common problem, especially in the developing world, and most patients with cholelithiasis do not go on to develop gallbladder cancer.[43,44] Moreover, 20% to 40% of patients with gallbladder cancer never form gallstones.[38] Nevertheless, a history of gallstone disease is associated with the highest risk of gallbladder cancer. The reported relative risk of gallbladder cancer associated with gallstone disease is 5.[41] Increasing stone size, volume, number, and weight have all been implicated in an increased risk of gallbladder cancer.[45] The odds ratio for gallbladder cancer in individuals with gallstone diameters of 2 to 2.9 cm compared with stone size less than 1 cm was 2.4.[46] This ratio was 10.1 for stones 3 cm or larger. The chemical composition of gallstones has also been implicated in cancer risk. In patients with gallbladder cancer, chronic cholecystitis, and xanthogranulomatous cholecystitis, calcium and magnesium were significantly higher in gallbladder cancer than in benign disease. Cholesterol stones are more commonly associated with gallbladder cancer than pigmented stones.[47] However, there is less cholesterol in stones from patients with gallbladder cancer than in stones from patients with benign gallbladder disease. Patients with gallbladder cancer were more likely to have multiple stones and larger stones than patients with asymptomatic gallstones. However, patients with gallbladder cancer tend to be older and the number and size of the stones may be related to chronic cumulative changes associated with age. One study reported that the incidence of gallbladder cancer decreases when the cholecystectomy rate increases, and this is related to decrease in cholelithiasis prevalence.[48] Despite this finding, routine cholecystectomy is not considered standard of care because the rate of gallstones is high in relation to the rare occurrence of gallbladder cancer.

Calcification and inflammation
Chronic inflammation from infection and autoimmune disease, and chronic irritation from cholelithiasis have been associated with the development of gallbladder cancer. Inflammation is thought to result in deposition of calcium within the gallbladder mucosa, resulting in a fragile, bluish discolored gallbladder universally known as the porcelain gallbladder. Calcification associated with gallbladder cancer was reported in the 1960s.[49] In addition to diffuse calcium layering, gallbladder calcification can also been seen as a selective, punctate mucosal calcification, and in one report it was associated with increased risk of cancer.[50] The incidence of gallbladder cancer associated with calcification is reported to be between 12% and 61%.[50,51] However, recent studies have reported that this association is lower or not seen at all.[52,53]

Primary sclerosing cholangitis (PSC), an autoimmune condition resulting in inflammation and stricturing of the biliary system more commonly associated with cholangiocarcinoma, results in an increased likelihood of gallbladder malignancy.[54] In one study from Sweden of 286 patients with PSC, a gallbladder mass lesion was identified in 18 (6%) of the patients, of whom 56% had gallbladder cancer. In 9 patients without evidence of a gallbladder mass lesion, histology showed gallbladder epithelial dysplasia.[55] It is difficult to determine whether symptoms associated with gallbladder disease are caused by incidental polyps or stones because many patients with gallbladder polyps also have gallstones. Over a 7-year period of follow-up in 34 patients with gallbladder polyps little change was seen in the diameter of the polyp, with no evidence of malignant disease in any individual.[56]

Infection

Inflammation from chronic infection has also been linked to malignant transformation. Infection accelerates the turnover of primary bile acids to secondary bile acids that may act as tumor initiators and promoters.[57] *Salmonella typhi* infestation has been implicated as a risk factor in the development of gallbladder cancer. Chronic typhoid and paratyphoid carriers have increased risk of cancer of the gallbladder, pancreas, colorectum, and lung.[58] In a case-control study performed in India of patients with and without gallbladder cancer, typhoid carrier state was one of 3 independent risk factors for the development of gallbladder cancer among patients with gallstones.[59] In addition to salmonella infestation, *Helicobacter* species have also been investigated as possible infectious risk factors for gallbladder cancer. In polymerase chain reaction analysis of bile samples from Japanese and Thai patients, approximately 80% of patients with bile duct and gallbladder cancer tested positive for *Helicobacter bilis* in their bile, whereas only 40% of patients with gallstone and/or cholecystitis tested positive.[60] However, a recent study comparing patients with gallbladder cancer and cholelithiasis did not show an increase risk of *H bilis* in patients with cancer.[61]

Anomalous pancreaticobiliary duct junction

Anomalous pancreaticobiliary duct junction (APBDJ), a congenital condition caused by the abnormal communication of the bile duct and pancreatic duct outside the duodenal wall and beyond the regulation of the sphincter of Oddi, is associated with various pancreatic and biliary disorders including choledochal cysts, pancreatitis, and malignancy. It is thought that reflux of pancreatic juice into the biliary tract in patients with APBDJ may cause the development of biliary tract cancers because of chronic inflammation. In one report, 23 of 126 patients with gallbladder cancer had anomalous pancreaticobiliary junctions.[62] Patients with this anomaly and gallbladder cancer tended to be young women with less to no cholelithiasis.[63] A separate study evaluating patients with gallbladder cancer in China who underwent endoscopic retrograde cholangiopancreatography also found an increased frequency of anomalous pancreaticobiliary ductal junction with malignancy.[64]

Gallbladder polyps

Polypoid lesions of the gallbladder affect approximately 5% of the adult population.[65] A prospective study of 3647 Chinese patients determined that approximately 7% of patients possessed polypoid lesions of the gallbladder.[66] In an investigation of healthy Japanese subjects who underwent abdominal ultrasound, gallbladder polyps were more common in men and obese patients, and increased with increase in the obesity index.[67] Gallbladder polyps are most commonly found in middle-aged men.[67,68] In a study of 194,767 asymptomatic patients undergoing health screening examinations in Japan, gallbladder polyps were found in 5.6% of the population. Nineteen individuals were diagnosed with gallbladder cancer, with most in the sixth or seventh decades of life. In another report, approximately 4.5% of a random population had gallbladder polyps by ultrasound.[69] The prevalence of polyps was not significantly associated with age, sex, social factors, weight, or metabolic conditions. Although most gallbladder polyps are benign, there is always a concern from malignant transformation. Most of these polyps are detected incidentally during ultrasound examination. However, distinguishing benign from malignant polyps is difficult, even with current radiologic imaging modalities. Multiple features, including symptoms, age, size and number of polyps, and growth rate, have been described to help differentiate benign from malignant polyps. Although there are no clear discriminatory elements that identify malignant transformation, symptoms, age greater than 50 years, size greater than 1 cm, and growing polyps are considered reasons to remove the gallbladder. In a recent study of 213 patients with questionable gallbladder neoplasm on ultrasound who underwent surgery, significant predictors of malignancy were age greater than 52 years, gallstones on ultrasound, size greater than 9 mm, invasion of the liver interface, and wall thickening.[70]

Other risk factors

In addition to the risk factors mentioned earlier, other risk factors have been postulated to be associated with gallbladder malignancy. A meta-analysis found an association between obesity and the risk of gallbladder cancer. The relative risk of gallbladder cancer in obese patients was 1.66 (95% confidence interval, 1.47–1.88) and the association with obesity was stronger for women than for men (relative risk, 1.88 vs 1.35).[71] Genetic factors associated with cholesterol metabolism have also been evaluated. The D allele of LRPAP1 (low density lipoprotein receptor related protein-associated protein), a receptor-associated protein that serves as a molecular chaperone, has been associated with gallbladder cancer in female patients.[72,73]

CHOLANGIOCARCINOMA

Cholangiocarcinoma, or malignant strictures of the biliary tract, arises from the ductal epithelium of the biliary tree, either within the liver substance (intrahepatic) or outside the liver (extrahepatic). It is a disease that, when detected early, is amenable to surgical resection. However, in many instances, it is discovered at a locally advanced or widely disseminated stage and as a result portends a poor prognosis. The molecular mechanisms involved in malignant transformation of biliary epithelium are not well known. As a result, therapy directed uniquely at cholangiocarcinoma is currently not available. Instead, the therapy is similar to that for pancreatic adenocarcinoma, with modest to little efficacy.

Cholangiocarcinoma accounts for 3% of all gastrointestinal malignancies.[74–76] It is the second most common primary hepatic malignancy. Intrahepatic and extrahepatic cholangiocarcinoma are rare diseases. As a result, little is known about the risk factors and the molecular mechanisms associated with this commonly fatal disease. However, the incidence rate and mortality are similar. The peak age for cholangiocarcinoma is in the seventh decade and it has a higher incidence in men than in women. The incidence in the United States is 1 to 2 per 100,000.[77] In the United States, there are approximately 6000 cases of cholangiocarcinoma yearly, equally divided between intrahepatic and extrahepatic origins.[78] Epidemiologic data indicate that the rate of cholangiocarcinoma, especially intrahepatic cholangiocarcinoma, seems to be increasing worldwide.[79,80] This increase, evident across both genders, is occurring in both the developed and developing worlds. The average estimated annual change in mortality for men was 6.9% ± 1.5% and 5.1% ± 1.0% for women.[79,80] In a report from the United Kingdom, mortality statistics showed a selective increase in intrahepatic cholangiocarcinoma.[81] A study of trends in the epidemiology of intrahepatic cholangiocarcinoma in the United States indicated an increase in incidence and mortality as well.[82] The increase in mortality was seen in both white people and black people. However, one study argued that classification has affected the reported shifts in incidence rates of intrahepatic and extrahepatic cholangiocarcinoma.[83,84] It is thought that the increased incidence is related to improvements in detection through modern imaging modalities. However, there is no conclusive evidence that this is the case because of the lack of evidence identifying earlier stage cholangiocarcinoma.

Risk Factors

PSC

Chronic inflammation seems to be a common risk factor in the development of bile duct cancer. PSC is thought to be an autoimmune disease of unknown cause, causing chronic cholestasis resulting in inflammatory injury of the intrahepatic and extrahepatic biliary epithelium, and resulting in destruction and stricturing of the biliary system. PSC can result in biliary stasis, hepatocellular injury, cirrhosis, and liver failure. It is also the most common predisposing cause of cholangiocarcinoma in the West. Unlike most autoimmune diseases, PSC is most commonly found in men (2:1 predominance) and presents most commonly in the fourth decade of life.[85,86] An evaluation of patients in Olmsted County, Minnesota, revealed that the incidence of PSC in men was 1.25 per 100,000 person-years and 0.54 per 100,000 person-years in women, with prevalences of 20.9 and 6.3 per 100,000, respectively.[87] Reports from Scandinavia and northern Europe show an increasing incidence and prevalence of this disease.[88,89] Patients with PSC live shorter lives than comparable populations without the disease.[87] This is thought to be caused by its chronic, progressive impact on the liver, its association with inflammatory bowel disease (73% of cases of PSC), and the increased risk of cancer. There is a known association between PSC and cholangiocarcinoma. In a population-based study of 199 patients with PSC from 1992 to 2005, PSC was associated with a 4-fold increase in mortality and an increased risk of cholangiocarcinoma.[90] In a cohort study of 604 patients with PSC identified between 1970 and 1988, the frequency of cholangiocarcinoma was 13%.[91] A study from the Mayo Clinic reported that approximately 7% of patients with PSC later developed cholangiocarcinoma over a mean follow-up of 11.5 years.[92] The relative risk of cholangiocarcinoma in patients with PSC was significantly increased (relative risk, 1560) compared with the general population. No association was found between the duration of PSC and the incidence of cholangiocarcinoma.

Liver fluke

PSC is rare in Asia and therefore is not a common clinical risk factor for the development of cholangiocarcinoma. However, in the East, cholangiocarcinoma is a significant problem as a result of endemic infection with liver flukes. The consumption of undercooked fish results in worm infestation within the liver where the flukes produce eggs that are released through the biliary system into the intestinal tract. Infection within the biliary system results in chronic inflammation. It is this chronic inflammation and oxidative stress that is thought to stimulate malignant transformation. Liver flukes, including Clonorchis sinensis and Opisthorchis viverrini, members of the family Opistorchiidae, are both classified as carcinogenic to humans by the International Agency for Research on Cancer.[93] Liver fluke infestation is more common in men than in women in this region, which is thought to result from the more common consumption of alcohol with raw fish among men than among women. The prevalence of these infectious agents correlates with increased cholangiocarcinoma.[94–99] A meta-analysis of the published literature indicates a relative risk of cholangiocarcinoma of

4.98 with liver fluke infection. The number of people infected with *Clonorchis* in China is estimated to be around 12.5 million.[100] Thailand, where *Opisthorchis* is common, has a prevalence of 6 million infected.[100] Implementation of control measures including health promotion, education, environmental reconstruction, and chemotherapy has resulted in significant reductions in infection rate.[101]

Viral hepatitis

Chronic HCV and HBV infection have been implicated as risk factors for cholangiocarcinoma development. In a report of examined explanted livers, biliary ductal dysplasia was more common in livers from chronic HCV cirrhotic patients than in controls.[102] In a study comparing cases of cholangiocarcinoma with controls, patients with intrahepatic cholangiocarcinoma had a significantly higher prevalence of anti-HCV antibodies.[103] This association was not seen in patients with extrahepatic cholangiocarcinoma. Pathologic examination of resected HBV-associated intrahepatic cholangiocarcinoma revealed the selective presence of a mass-forming growth pattern with a more favorable prognosis than in patients without chronic HBV infection.[104] This finding was supported by reports showing that patients with intrahepatic cholangiocarcinoma and HBV infection have a more favorable outcome after surgery than patients not infected with HBV.[105,106]

Bile duct cysts

Bile duct cysts are rare congenital disorders characterized by cystic dilatation of a portion of the intrahepatic or extrahepatic biliary ductal system. They are known risk factors for cholangiocarcinoma. It is thought that these cysts arise as a result of abnormal communication between the pancreaticobiliary junction, resulting in reflux of pancreatic enzymes into the biliary tree. Increases in pancreatic enzymes, bile stasis, and increased concentration of biliary acids are thought to result in malignant transformation. Between 10% and 30% of adults with bile duct cysts develop cholangiocarcinoma.[107–114] Patients with biliary ductal cysts have a 20-fold to 30-fold increased risk of developing cholangiocarcinoma. The risk of development of cholangiocarcinoma extends beyond the point of surgical resection. The mean age of malignancy development is 30 years, which is decades earlier than that seen in the general population.[115] It is most commonly seen in patients with type I and IV cysts.

Hepatolithiasis

Primary hepatolithiasis is a disease endemic to East Asia with a reported incidence of up to 20%.[116,117] It is rare in the West, occurring in 0.6% to 1.3% of the population.[116,117] Cholangiocarcinoma is the most serious consequence of this disease entity. It is thought to arise from bile stasis leading to chronic infection and inflammation, and resulting in malignant transformation. Especially in the East, it is common to find concomitant infection with parasites such as *C sinensis* and *Ascaris lumbricoides* in patients with hepatolithiasis.[118] Hepatolithiasis is also associated with combined hepatocellular cancer and cholangiocarcinoma.[119] Previous studies have suggested that the mean interval from the treatment of stones to the diagnosis of cholangiocarcinoma is approximately 3 to 8 years. Smoking, family history of cancer, and symptoms lasting more than 10 years have been identified as risk factors in cholangiocarcinoma development.[120]

Thorotrast

Exposure to thorotrast, a radiographic contrast agent in use before the 1960s, is strongly associated with increased risk of cholangiocarcinoma. Once injected, thorotrast is taken up by the reticuloendothelial system, with 70% captured in the liver.

Thorium has a half-life of 400 years, resulting in prolonged tissue exposure to low-level alpha radiation from thorium decay, which is thought to be the agent of carcinogenesis.[121] In a study following 241 war-wounded military personnel in Japan, patients exposed to thorotrast had 47 times the risk of liver cancer and 20 times the risk of liver cirrhosis. Patients exposed to thorotrast had a statistically significant increase in hemangiosarcoma and cholangiosarcoma, and their estimated risk of cholangiocarcinoma was 303 times that of the general population.[122]

REFERENCES

1. El-Serag HB, Rudolph KL. Hepatocellular carcinoma: epidemiology and molecular carcinogenesis. Gastroenterology 2007;132(7):2557–76. PubMed PMID: 17570226.
2. Parkin DM. Global cancer statistics in the year 2000. Lancet Oncol 2001;2(9): 533–43. PubMed PMID: 11905707.
3. Chang MH, Chen CJ, Lai MS, et al. Universal hepatitis B vaccination in Taiwan and the incidence of hepatocellular carcinoma in children. Taiwan Childhood Hepatoma Study Group. N Engl J Med 1997;336(26):1855–9. PubMed PMID: 9197213.
4. Chang MH, You SL, Chen CJ, et al. Decreased incidence of hepatocellular carcinoma in hepatitis B vaccinees: a 20-year follow-up study. J Natl Cancer Inst 2009;101(19):1348–55. PubMed PMID: 19759364.
5. Ni YH, Chen DS. Hepatitis B vaccination in children: the Taiwan experience. Pathol Biol 2010;58(4):296–300. PubMed PMID: 20116181.
6. Yu SZ. Primary prevention of hepatocellular carcinoma. J Gastroenterol Hepatol 1995;10(6):674–82. PubMed PMID: 8580413.
7. El-Serag HB. Epidemiology of hepatocellular carcinoma in USA. Hepatol Res 2007;37(Suppl 2):S88–94. PubMed PMID: 17877502.
8. El-Serag HB, Mason AC. Rising incidence of hepatocellular carcinoma in the United States. N Engl J Med 1999;340(10):745–50. PubMed PMID: 10072408.
9. El-Serag HB, Lau M, Eschbach K, et al. Epidemiology of hepatocellular carcinoma in Hispanics in the United States. Arch Intern Med 2007;167(18): 1983–9. PubMed PMID: 17923599.
10. Yu MW, Chen CJ. Elevated serum testosterone levels and risk of hepatocellular carcinoma. Cancer Res 1993;53(4):790–4. PubMed PMID: 8381328.
11. Chen JG, Zhu J, Parkin DM, et al. Trends in the incidence of cancer in Qidong, China, 1978-2002. Int J Cancer 2006;119(6):1447–54. PubMed PMID: 16596645.
12. Moriya T, Koyama T, Tanaka J, et al. Epidemiology of hepatitis C virus in Japan. Intervirology 1999;42(2–3):153–8. PubMed PMID: 10516469.
13. Seeff LB, Hoofnagle JH. Epidemiology of hepatocellular carcinoma in areas of low hepatitis B and hepatitis C endemicity. Oncogene 2006;25(27):3771–7. PubMed PMID: 16799618.
14. Donato F, Tagger A, Gelatti U, et al. Alcohol and hepatocellular carcinoma: the effect of lifetime intake and hepatitis virus infections in men and women. Am J Epidemiol 2002;155(4):323–31. PubMed PMID: 11836196.
15. Bressac B, Kew M, Wands J, et al. Selective G to T mutations of p53 gene in hepatocellular carcinoma from southern Africa. Nature 1991;350(6317): 429–31. PubMed PMID: 1672732.
16. Stickel F, Hellerbrand C. Non-alcoholic fatty liver disease as a risk factor for hepatocellular carcinoma: mechanisms and implications. Gut 2010;59(10):1303–7. PubMed PMID: 20650925.

17. El-Serag HB, Hampel H, Javadi F. The association between diabetes and hepatocellular carcinoma: a systematic review of epidemiologic evidence. Clin Gastroenterol Hepatol 2006;4(3):369–80.

18. Hassan MM, Curley SA, Li D, et al. Association of diabetes duration and diabetes treatment with the risk of hepatocellular carcinoma. Cancer 2010; 116(8):1938–46. PubMed PMID: 20166205.

19. Calle EE, Rodriguez C, Walker-Thurmond K, et al. Overweight, obesity, and mortality from cancer in a prospectively studied cohort of U.S. adults. N Engl J Med 2003;348(17):1625–38. PubMed PMID: 12711737.

20. Moller H, Mellemgaard A, Lindvig K, et al. Obesity and cancer risk: a Danish record-linkage study. Eur J Cancer 1994;30A(3):344–50. PubMed PMID: 8204357.

21. Wolk A, Gridley G, Svensson M, et al. A prospective study of obesity and cancer risk (Sweden). Cancer Causes Control 2001;12(1):13–21. PubMed PMID: 11227921.

22. Siegel AB, Zhu AX. Metabolic syndrome and hepatocellular carcinoma: two growing epidemics with a potential link. Cancer 2009;115(24):5651–61. PubMed PMID: 19834957. PubMed Central PMCID: PMC3397779.

23. Reddy KR, Kligerman S, Levi J, et al. Benign and solid tumors of the liver: relationship to sex, age, size of tumors, and outcome. Am Surg 2001;67(2):173–8. PubMed PMID: 11243545.

24. Mergo PJ, Ros PR. Benign lesions of the liver. Radiol Clin North Am 1998;36(2): 319–31. PubMed PMID: 9520985.

25. Trotter JF, Everson GT. Benign focal lesions of the liver. Clin Liver Dis 2001;5(1): 17–42. v. PubMed PMID: 11218914.

26. Pain JA, Gimson AE, Williams R, et al. Focal nodular hyperplasia of the liver: results of treatment and options in management. Gut 1991;32(5):524–7. PubMed PMID: 2040476. PubMed Central PMCID: 1378930.

27. Wanless IR, Mawdsley C, Adams R. On the pathogenesis of focal nodular hyperplasia of the liver. Hepatology 1985;5(6):1194–200. PubMed PMID: 4065824.

28. Luciani A, Kobeiter H, Maison P, et al. Focal nodular hyperplasia of the liver in men: is presentation the same in men and women? Gut 2002;50(6):877–80. PubMed PMID: 12010893. PubMed Central PMCID: 1773241.

29. Nguyen BN, Flejou JF, Terris B, et al. Focal nodular hyperplasia of the liver: a comprehensive pathologic study of 305 lesions and recognition of new histologic forms. Am J Surg Pathol 1999;23(12):1441–54. PubMed PMID: 10584697.

30. Koch N, Gintzburger D, Seelentag W, et al. Rupture of hepatic focal nodular hyperplasia. About two cases. [Rupture d'une hyperplasie nodulaire focale. A propos de deux cas. fre]. Ann Chir 2006;131(4):279–82. PubMed PMID: 16443188. Epub 2006/01/31 [in French].

31. Machida T, Hirayama M, Horita S, et al. Telangiectatic focal nodular hyperplasia accompanied with hemorrhage and necrosis during the course: report of a case. Nihon Shokakibyo Gakkai Zasshi 2008;105(6):847–53. PubMed PMID: 18525192 [in Japanese].

32. Edmondson HA, Henderson B, Benton B. Liver-cell adenomas associated with use of oral contraceptives. N Engl J Med 1976;294(9):470–2. PubMed PMID: 173996.

33. Rooks JB, Ory HW, Ishak KG, et al. Epidemiology of hepatocellular adenoma. The role of oral contraceptive use. JAMA 1979;242(7):644–8. PubMed PMID: 221698.

34. Heinemann LA, Weimann A, Gerken G, et al. Modern oral contraceptive use and benign liver tumors: the German Benign Liver Tumor Case-Control Study. Eur J Contracept Reprod Health Care 1998;3(4):194–200. PubMed PMID: 10036602.

35. Chang CY, Hernandez-Prera JC, Roayaie S, et al. Changing epidemiology of hepatocellular adenoma in the United States: review of the literature. Int J Hepatol 2013;2013:604860. PubMed PMID: 23509632. PubMed Central PMCID: PMC3595661.

36. Farges O, Ferreira N, Dokmak S, et al. Changing trends in malignant transformation of hepatocellular adenoma. Gut 2011;60(1):85–9. PubMed PMID: 21148580.

37. Sasaki M, Nakanuma Y. Overview of hepatocellular adenoma in Japan. Int J Hepatol 2012;2012:648131. PubMed PMID: 22973519. PubMed Central PMCID: PMC3438775.

38. Lazcano-Ponce EC, Miquel JF, Munoz N, et al. Epidemiology and molecular pathology of gallbladder cancer. CA Cancer J Clin 2001;51(6):349–64. PubMed PMID: 11760569.

39. Andia ME, Hsing AW, Andreotti G, et al. Geographic variation of gallbladder cancer mortality and risk factors in Chile: a population-based ecologic study. Int J Cancer 2008;123(6):1411–6. PubMed PMID: 18566990. PubMed Central PMCID: 2864002.

40. Serra I, Calvo A, Csendes A, et al. Gastric and gallbladder carcinoma in Chile: epidemiological changes and control programs. [Cancer gastrico y cancer de la vesicula biliar en Chile: cambios epidemiologicos y programas de control]. Rev Med Chil 1989;117(7):834–6. PubMed PMID: 2519441 [in Spanish].

41. Randi G, Franceschi S, La Vecchia C. Gallbladder cancer worldwide: geographical distribution and risk factors. Int J Cancer 2006;118(7):1591–602. PubMed PMID: 16397865.

42. Pandey M. Risk factors for gallbladder cancer: a reappraisal. Eur J Cancer Prev 2003;12(1):15–24. PubMed PMID: 12548106.

43. Kratzer W, Kron M, Hay B, et al. Prevalence of cholecystolithiasis in South Germany–an ultrasound study of 2,498 persons of a rural population. [Pravalenz der Cholezystolithiasis in Suddeutschland–eine sonographische Untersuchung an 2.498 Personen einer landlichen Bevolkerung]. Z Gastroenterol 1999;37(12): 1157–62. PubMed PMID: 10666839 [in German].

44. Kratzer W, Mason RA, Kachele V. Prevalence of gallstones in sonographic surveys worldwide. J Clin Ultrasound 1999;27(1):1–7. PubMed PMID: 9888092.

45. Stinton LM, Shaffer EA. Epidemiology of gallbladder disease: cholelithiasis and cancer. Gut Liver 2012;6(2):172–87. PubMed PMID: 22570746. PubMed Central PMCID: PMC3343155.

46. Shrikhande SV, Barreto SG, Singh S, et al. Cholelithiasis in gallbladder cancer: coincidence, cofactor, or cause! Eur J Surg Oncol 2010;36(6):514–9. PubMed PMID: 20537839.

47. Kimura W, Shimada H, Kuroda A, et al. Carcinoma of the gallbladder and extrahepatic bile duct in autopsy cases of the aged, with special reference to its relationship to gallstones. Am J Gastroenterol 1989;84(4):386–90. PubMed PMID: 2929559.

48. Diehl AK, Beral V. Cholecystectomy and changing mortality from gallbladder cancer. Lancet 1981;2(8239):187–9. PubMed PMID: 6114251.

49. Polk HC Jr. Carcinoma and the calcified gall bladder. Gastroenterology 1966; 50(4):582–5. PubMed PMID: 4286335.

50. Stephen AE, Berger DL. Carcinoma in the porcelain gallbladder: a relationship revisited. Surgery 2001;129(6):699–703. PubMed PMID: 11391368.

51. Cunningham SC, Alexander HR. Porcelain gallbladder and cancer: ethnicity explains a discrepant literature? Am J Med 2007;120(4):e17–8. PubMed PMID: 17398213.

52. Kim JH, Kim WH, Yoo BM, et al. Should we perform surgical management in all patients with suspected porcelain gallbladder? Hepatogastroenterology 2009; 56(93):943–5. PubMed PMID: 19760916.

53. Towfigh S, McFadden DW, Cortina GR, et al. Porcelain gallbladder is not associated with gallbladder carcinoma. Am Surg 2001;67(1):7–10. PubMed PMID: 11206901.

54. Lewis JT, Talwalkar JA, Rosen CB, et al. Prevalence and risk factors for gallbladder neoplasia in patients with primary sclerosing cholangitis: evidence for a metaplasia-dysplasia-carcinoma sequence. Am J Surg Pathol 2007;31(6): 907–13. PubMed PMID: 17527079.

55. Said K, Glaumann H, Bergquist A. Gallbladder disease in patients with primary sclerosing cholangitis. J Hepatol 2008;48(4):598–605. PubMed PMID: 18222013.

56. Kratzer W, Haenle MM, Voegtle A, et al. Ultrasonographically detected gallbladder polyps: a reason for concern? A seven-year follow-up study. BMC Gastroenterol 2008;8:41. PubMed PMID: 18793401. PubMed Central PMCID: PMC2553794.

57. Kumar S, Kumar S, Kumar S. Infection as a risk factor for gallbladder cancer. J Surg Oncol 2006;93(8):633–9. PubMed PMID: 16724347.

58. Caygill CP, Hill MJ, Braddick M, et al. Cancer mortality in chronic typhoid and paratyphoid carriers. Lancet 1994;343(8889):83–4. PubMed PMID: 7903779.

59. Dutta U, Garg PK, Kumar R, et al. Typhoid carriers among patients with gallstones are at increased risk for carcinoma of the gallbladder. Am J Gastroenterol 2000;95(3):784–7. PubMed PMID: 10710075.

60. Matsukura N, Yokomuro S, Yamada S, et al. Association between *Helicobacter bilis* in bile and biliary tract malignancies: *H. bilis* in bile from Japanese and Thai patients with benign and malignant diseases in the biliary tract. Jpn J Cancer Res 2002;93(7):842–7. PubMed PMID: 12149151.

61. Pandey M, Mishra RR, Dixit R, et al. *Helicobacter bilis* in human gallbladder cancer: results of a case-control study and a meta-analysis. Asian Pac J Cancer Prev 2010;11(2):343–7. PubMed PMID: 20843113.

62. Elnemr A, Ohta T, Kayahara M, et al. Anomalous pancreaticobiliary ductal junction without bile duct dilatation in gallbladder cancer. Hepatogastroenterology 2001;48(38):382–6. PubMed PMID: 11379314.

63. Keswani RN, Mahvi DM. Education and imaging. Hepatobiliary and pancreatic: anomalous pancreaticobiliary junction and gallbladder cancer. J Gastroenterol Hepatol 2012;27(10):1644. PubMed PMID: 22994436.

64. Hu B, Gong B, Zhou DY. Association of anomalous pancreaticobiliary ductal junction with gallbladder carcinoma in Chinese patients: an ERCP study. Gastrointest Endosc 2003;57(4):541–5. PubMed PMID: 12665766.

65. Myers RP, Shaffer EA, Beck PL. Gallbladder polyps: epidemiology, natural history and management. Can J Gastroenterol 2002;16(3):187–94. PubMed PMID: 11930198.

66. Chen CY, Lu CL, Chang FY, et al. Risk factors for gallbladder polyps in the Chinese population. Am J Gastroenterol 1997;92(11):2066–8. PubMed PMID: 9362194.

67. Segawa K, Arisawa T, Niwa Y, et al. Prevalence of gallbladder polyps among apparently healthy Japanese: ultrasonographic study. Am J Gastroenterol 1992;87(5):630–3. PubMed PMID: 1595653.

68. Lin WR, Lin DY, Tai DI, et al. Prevalence of and risk factors for gallbladder polyps detected by ultrasonography among healthy Chinese: analysis of 34 669 cases. J Gastroenterol Hepatol 2008;23(6):965–9. PubMed PMID: 17725602.

69. Jorgensen T, Jensen KH. Polyps in the gallbladder. A prevalence study. Scand J Gastroenterol 1990;25(3):281–6. PubMed PMID: 2320947.
70. Konstantinidis IT, Bajpai S, Kambadakone AR, et al. Gallbladder lesions identified on ultrasound. Lessons from the last 10 years. J Gastrointest Surg 2012; 16(3):549–53. PubMed PMID: 22108768.
71. Larsson SC, Wolk A. Obesity and the risk of gallbladder cancer: a meta-analysis. Br J Cancer 2007;96(9):1457–61. PubMed PMID: 17375043. PubMed Central PMCID: PMC2360167.
72. Pandey SN, Dixit M, Choudhuri G, et al. Lipoprotein receptor associated protein (LRPAP1) insertion/deletion polymorphism: association with gallbladder cancer susceptibility. Int J Gastrointest Cancer 2006;37(4):124–8. PubMed PMID: 17987404.
73. Xu HL, Cheng JR, Andreotti G, et al. Cholesterol metabolism gene polymorphisms and the risk of biliary tract cancers and stones: a population-based case-control study in Shanghai, China. Carcinogenesis 2011;32(1):58–62. PubMed PMID: 21062971.
74. Gatto M, Bragazzi MC, Semeraro R, et al. Cholangiocarcinoma: update and future perspectives. Dig Liver Dis 2010;42(4):253–60. PubMed PMID: 20097142.
75. Patel T. Cholangiocarcinoma. Nat Clin Pract Gastroenterol Hepatol 2006;3(1): 33–42. PubMed PMID: 16397610.
76. Shaib Y, El-Serag HB. The epidemiology of cholangiocarcinoma. Semin Liver Dis 2004;24(2):115–25. PubMed PMID: 15192785.
77. Greenlee RT, Hill-Harmon MB, Murray T, et al. Cancer statistics, 2001. CA Cancer J Clin 2001;51(1):15–36. PubMed PMID: 11577478.
78. Jemal A, Siegel R, Ward E, et al. Cancer statistics, 2009. CA Cancer J Clin 2009; 59(4):225–49. PubMed PMID: 19474385.
79. Khan SA, Taylor-Robinson SD, Toledano MB, et al. Changing international trends in mortality rates for liver, biliary and pancreatic tumours. J Hepatol 2002;37(6): 806–13. PubMed PMID: 12445422.
80. Patel T. Worldwide trends in mortality from biliary tract malignancies. BMC Cancer 2002;2:10. PubMed PMID: 11991810. PubMed Central PMCID: 113759.
81. Taylor-Robinson SD, Toledano MB, Arora S, et al. Increase in mortality rates from intrahepatic cholangiocarcinoma in England and Wales 1968-1998. Gut 2001; 48(6):816–20. PubMed PMID: 11358902. PubMed Central PMCID: 1728314.
82. Patel T. Increasing incidence and mortality of primary intrahepatic cholangiocarcinoma in the United States. Hepatology 2001;33(6):1353–7. PubMed PMID: 11391522.
83. Khan SA, Emadossadaty S, Ladep NG, et al. Rising trends in cholangiocarcinoma: is the ICD classification system misleading us? J Hepatol 2012;56(4): 848–54. PubMed PMID: 22173164.
84. Welzel TM, McGlynn KA, Hsing AW, et al. Impact of classification of hilar cholangiocarcinomas (Klatskin tumors) on the incidence of intra- and extrahepatic cholangiocarcinoma in the United States. J Natl Cancer Inst 2006;98(12): 873–5. PubMed PMID: 16788161.
85. Angulo P, Lindor KD. Primary sclerosing cholangitis. Hepatology 1999;30(1): 325–32. PubMed PMID: 10385674.
86. Chapman RW. The management of primary sclerosing cholangitis. Curr Gastroenterol Rep 2003;5(1):9–17. PubMed PMID: 12530943.
87. Bambha K, Kim WR, Talwalkar J, et al. Incidence, clinical spectrum, and outcomes of primary sclerosing cholangitis in a United States community. Gastroenterology 2003;125(5):1364–9. PubMed PMID: 14598252.

88. Boonstra K, Beuers U, Ponsioen CY. Epidemiology of primary sclerosing cholangitis and primary biliary cirrhosis: a systematic review. J Hepatol 2012;56(5): 1181–8. PubMed PMID: 22245904.
89. Lindkvist B, Benito de Valle M, Gullberg B, et al. Incidence and prevalence of primary sclerosing cholangitis in a defined adult population in Sweden. Hepatology 2010;52(2):571–7. PubMed PMID: 20683956.
90. de Valle MB, Bjornsson E, Lindkvist B. Mortality and cancer risk related to primary sclerosing cholangitis in a Swedish population-based cohort. Liver Int 2012;32(3):441–8. PubMed PMID: 22098097.
91. Bergquist A, Ekbom A, Olsson R, et al. Hepatic and extrahepatic malignancies in primary sclerosing cholangitis. J Hepatol 2002;36(3):321–7. PubMed PMID: 11867174.
92. Burak K, Angulo P, Pasha TM, et al. Incidence and risk factors for cholangiocarcinoma in primary sclerosing cholangitis. Am J Gastroenterol 2004;99(3):523–6. PubMed PMID: 15056096.
93. Bouvard V, Baan R, Straif K, et al. A review of human carcinogens–Part B: biological agents. Lancet Oncol 2009;10(4):321–2. PubMed PMID: 19350698.
94. Lim MK, Ju YH, Franceschi S, et al. *Clonorchis sinensis* infection and increasing risk of cholangiocarcinoma in the Republic of Korea. Am J Trop Med Hyg 2006; 75(1):93–6. PubMed PMID: 16837714.
95. Sriamporn S, Pisani P, Pipitgool V, et al. Prevalence of *Opisthorchis viverrini* infection and incidence of cholangiocarcinoma in Khon Kaen, northeast Thailand. Trop Med Int Health 2004;9(5):588–94. PubMed PMID: 15117303.
96. Choi D, Lim JH, Lee KT, et al. Cholangiocarcinoma and *Clonorchis sinensis* infection: a case-control study in Korea. J Hepatol 2006;44(6):1066–73. PubMed PMID: 16480786.
97. Honjo S, Srivatanakul P, Sriplung H, et al. Genetic and environmental determinants of risk for cholangiocarcinoma via *Opisthorchis viverrini* in a densely infested area in Nakhon Phanom, northeast Thailand. Int J Cancer 2005;117(5): 854–60. PubMed PMID: 15957169.
98. Shin HR, Lee CU, Park HJ, et al. Hepatitis B and C virus, *Clonorchis sinensis* for the risk of liver cancer: a case-control study in Pusan, Korea. Int J Epidemiol 1996;25(5):933–40. PubMed PMID: 8921477.
99. Parkin DM, Srivatanakul P, Khlat M, et al. Liver cancer in Thailand. I. A case-control study of cholangiocarcinoma. Int J Cancer 1991;48(3):323–8. PubMed PMID: 1645697.
100. Shin HR, Oh JK, Masuyer E, et al. Epidemiology of cholangiocarcinoma: an update focusing on risk factors. Cancer Sci 2010;101(3):579–85. PubMed PMID: 20085587.
101. Wu W, Qian X, Huang Y, et al. A review of the control of clonorchiasis sinensis and *Taenia solium* taeniasis/cysticercosis in China. Parasitol Res 2012;111(5): 1879–84. PubMed PMID: 23052782.
102. Torbenson M, Yeh MM, Abraham SC. Bile duct dysplasia in the setting of chronic hepatitis C and alcohol cirrhosis. Am J Surg Pathol 2007;31(9):1410–3. PubMed PMID: 17721197.
103. Shaib YH, El-Serag HB, Nooka AK, et al. Risk factors for intrahepatic and extrahepatic cholangiocarcinoma: a hospital-based case-control study. Am J Gastroenterol 2007;102(5):1016–21. PubMed PMID: 17324130.
104. Wu ZF, Yang N, Li DY, et al. Characteristics of intrahepatic cholangiocarcinoma in patients with hepatitis B virus infection: clinicopathologic study of resected tumours. J Viral Hepat 2013;20(5):306–10. PubMed PMID: 23565611.

105. Zhang L, Cai JQ, Zhao JJ, et al. Impact of hepatitis B virus infection on outcome following resection for intrahepatic cholangiocarcinoma. J Surg Oncol 2010; 101(3):233–8. PubMed PMID: 20169539.
106. Zhou HB, Wang H, Li YQ, et al. Hepatitis B virus infection: a favorable prognostic factor for intrahepatic cholangiocarcinoma after resection. World J Gastroenterol 2011;17(10):1292–303. PubMed PMID: 21455328. PubMed Central PMCID: PMC3068264.
107. Chijiiwa K, Koga A. Surgical management and long-term follow-up of patients with choledochal cysts. Am J Surg 1993;165(2):238–42. PubMed PMID: 8427404.
108. Hewitt PM, Krige JE, Bornman PC, et al. Choledochal cysts in adults. Br J Surg 1995;82(3):382–5. PubMed PMID: 7796017.
109. Ishibashi T, Kasahara K, Yasuda Y, et al. Malignant change in the biliary tract after excision of choledochal cyst. Br J Surg 1997;84(12):1687–91. PubMed PMID: 9448616.
110. Lipsett PA, Pitt HA, Colombani PM, et al. Choledochal cyst disease. A changing pattern of presentation. Ann Surg 1994;220(5):644–52. PubMed PMID: 7979612. PubMed Central PMCID: 1234452.
111. Liu CL, Fan ST, Lo CM, et al. Choledochal cysts in adults. Arch Surg 2002; 137(4):465–8. PubMed PMID: 11926955.
112. Stain SC, Guthrie CR, Yellin AE, et al. Choledochal cyst in the adult. Ann Surg 1995;222(2):128–33. PubMed PMID: 7639580. PubMed Central PMCID: 1234770.
113. Tashiro S, Imaizumi T, Ohkawa H, et al. Pancreaticobiliary maljunction: retrospective and nationwide survey in Japan. J Hepatobiliary Pancreat Surg 2003;10(5):345–51. PubMed PMID: 14598134.
114. Voyles CR, Smadja C, Shands WC, et al. Carcinoma in choledochal cysts. Age-related incidence. Arch Surg 1983;118(8):986–8. PubMed PMID: 6870530.
115. Soreide K, Korner H, Havnen J, et al. Bile duct cysts in adults. Br J Surg 2004; 91(12):1538–48. PubMed PMID: 15549778.
116. Cheung KL, Lai EC. The management of intrahepatic stones. Adv Surg 1996;29: 111–29. PubMed PMID: 8719998.
117. Tsui WM, Chan YK, Wong CT, et al. Hepatolithiasis and the syndrome of recurrent pyogenic cholangitis: clinical, radiologic, and pathologic features. Semin Liver Dis 2011;31(1):33–48. PubMed PMID: 21344349.
118. Huang MH, Chen CH, Yen CM, et al. Relation of hepatolithiasis to helminthic infestation. J Gastroenterol Hepatol 2005;20(1):141–6. PubMed PMID: 15610459.
119. Deniz K, Torun E, Celikbilek M, et al. Combined hepatocellular and cholangiocarcinoma associated with hepatolithiasis: report of a case. Surg Today 2011; 41(4):591–5. PubMed PMID: 21431501.
120. Liu ZY, Zhou YM, Shi LH, et al. Risk factors of intrahepatic cholangiocarcinoma in patients with hepatolithiasis: a case-control study. Hepatobiliary Pancreat Dis Int 2011;10(6):626–31. PubMed PMID: 22146627.
121. Balamurali G, du Plessis DG, Wengoy M, et al. Thorotrast-induced primary cerebral angiosarcoma: case report. Neurosurgery 2009;65(1):E210–1 [discussion: E1]. PubMed PMID: 19574803.
122. Kato I, Kido C. Increased risk of death in thorotrast-exposed patients during the late follow-up period. Jpn J Cancer Res 1987;78(11):1187–92. PubMed PMID: 2826375.

Imaging of the Patient with a Biliary Tract or Primary Liver Tumor

Celia P. Corona-Villalobos, MD[a],
Timothy M. Pawlik, MD, MPH, PhD[b], Ihab R. Kamel, MD, PhD[a],*

KEYWORDS

- Biliary tract and primary liver tumors • Diffusion-weighted imaging
- Contrast-enhanced MRI • Volumetric functional MRI • Response to therapy

KEY POINTS

- Knowledge of the diverse manifestations and mimickers of biliary tract and primary liver tumors is essential for diagnosis and management.
- CT and MR imaging are essential in characterizing biliary tract and primary liver tumors, as well as defining potential involvement of surrounding structures.
- Volumetric functional MRI may be used to assess early response of biliary and primary liver tumors following intra-arterial therapy.

INTRODUCTION

Noninvasive imaging plays a critical role in the diagnosis, staging, and treatment of patients with biliary tract and primary liver tumors. In addition, imaging provides important information to assess tumor resectability as well as patient prognosis. Noninvasive imaging modalities, such as ultrasonography (US), computed tomography (CT), and magnetic resonance imaging (MRI), are the most common modalities used to image hepatobiliary diseases.

Imaging: Tumor Detection

Because biliary tract and primary liver tumors can vary significantly in location, growth pattern, and histologic subtype, these tumors can have a wide spectrum of radiologic

---

The authors have nothing to disclose.
[a] The Russell H. Morgan Department of Radiology and Radiological Sciences, The Johns Hopkins School of Medicine, 600 North Wolfe Street, MRI 143, Baltimore, MD 21287, USA;
[b] Division of Surgical Oncology, Department of Surgery, Johns Hopkins Hospital, 600 North Wolfe Street, Blalock 688, Baltimore, MD 21287, USA
* Corresponding author.
E-mail address: ikamel@jhmi.edu

Surg Oncol Clin N Am 23 (2014) 189–206
http://dx.doi.org/10.1016/j.soc.2013.10.002
1055-3207/14/$ – see front matter © 2014 Elsevier Inc. All rights reserved.

appearances. Noninvasive cross-sectional imaging is critical to characterize biliary tract and primary liver tumors, as well as define their location to critical adjacent structures. Knowledge of the radiologic manifestations of the various possible biliary and primary liver tumors, as well as potential mimickers, is important in the accurate diagnosis and management of these tumors.

Imaging: Tumor Staging

Although US is sometimes the primary modality used in the evaluation of biliary tract and primary liver tumors, the accuracy of US varies according to the equipment and experience of the operator. Although the sensitivity of color Doppler US for portal vein occlusion is 100% and for portal vein infiltration is 83% with 100% specificity,[1] US is less accurate in the estimation of tumor spread and the determination of tumor resectability compared with CT or MRI.[1] CT and MRI have the advantage of 2- and 3-dimensional visualization, which is particularly useful to define vascular involvement, tumor extent, and spread to adjacent structures. Given that this information is crucial for tumor staging and treatment planning, CT or MRI is the preferred imaging modality for patients with suspected biliary or primary liver tumors.

Imaging: Treatment Response Assessment

CT and MRI are commonly used to evaluate treatment response among patients with biliary tract and primary liver tumors. Treatment response after locoregional therapies remains challenging given the limitations of using current available criteria for tumor assessment and treatment response, such as Response Evaluation Criteria in Solid Tumors (RECIST) and Modified RECIST (mRECIST). Alternative methods such as functional CT and MRI have been proposed. Contrast-enhanced CT can provide an estimation of perfusion (blood flow) and tumoral angiogenesis.[2,3] In addition to perfusion, treatment response assessed by functional MRI with volumetric enhancement and apparent diffusion coefficient (ADC) are promising tools for early tumor assessment and patient prognosis.[4,5]

HEPATOCELLULAR CARCINOMA

Hepatocellular carcinoma (HCC) is the most common primary liver neoplasm. The incidence of HCC is increasing, and the disease most commonly afflicts patients with viral hepatitis, chronic liver disease, and cirrhosis.[6] The appearance of HCC on US can be variable; an HCC mass may appear hypoechoic, mixed, or echogenic. Most small HCCs are hypoechoic to isoechoic with a peripheral hypoechoic halo, which corresponds to a fibrous capsule (**Fig. 1**). Contrast-enhanced US with microbubbles often demonstrates tumor vascularization in the arterial phase and washout in the portal phase. Contrast-enhanced US may also have a role in assessing response after treatment.[7,8]

HCC typically presents as an arterial enhancing lesion of CT or MRI. The HCC most commonly shows increased perfusion in the arterial phase, with higher perfusion reported in well-differentiated tumors.[2,3] On CT and MRI most small HCC will enhance after contrast administration and display a "washout" of contrast material during the portal-venous phase (**Fig. 2**). Features of HCC on MRI can vary as lesions may appear hypointense, isointense, or hyperintense compared with the normal liver parenchyma (**Fig. 3**). Part of the reason for the varied appearance of the HCC lesion on MRI can be due to different signal intensity related to the underlying cirrhotic liver parenchyma.

Most HCC patients are not eligible for curative treatment because of advanced disease or poor liver function. These patients often receive intra-arterial therapy such as

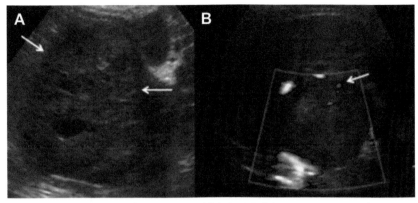

Fig. 1. Imaging appearance of HCC varies widely by US. (*A*) Heterogeneous echogenic mass (*arrows*) with hypoechoic areas involving both hepatic lobes. (*B*) Isoechoic mass with peripheral hypoechoic halo showing internal vascularity (*arrow*) on Doppler US.

transarterial chemoembolization (TACE) or Yyttrium-90 therapy to treat the HCC and delay tumor progression. Recent studies have shown decreased vascularization of the index HCC after TACE therapy,[9,10] yet higher flow values on any remaining viable tumor.[11] In the assessment of tumor response to therapy, the use of size or

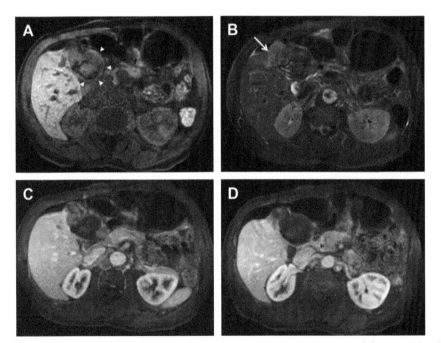

Fig. 2. Moderately differentiated HCC in a 77-year-old man. Precontrast (*A*) T1-weighted image shows a heterogeneous slightly hypointense mass surrounded by an isointense halo (*arrowheads*). (*B*) T2-weighted fat-suppressed image shows heterogeneity of the mass with a hyperintense area (*arrow*). After contrast administration on late arterial phase (*C*), there is enhancement of the mass, with washout on the portal venous phase (*D*).

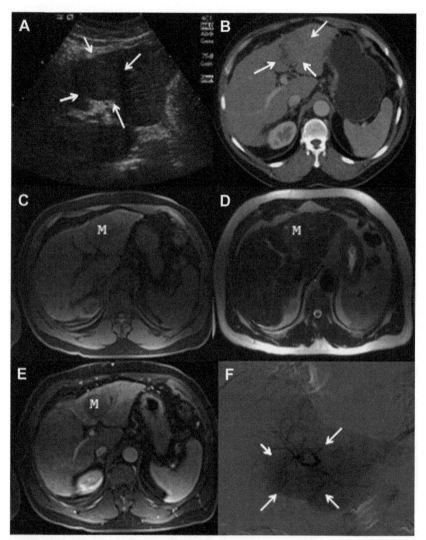

Fig. 3. HCC in a 57-year-old man. (*A*) US shows a 4 × 4 cm isoechoic mass with a peripheral hypoechoic halo (*arrows*) on background cirrhotic liver. (*B*) CT in the portal venous phase depicts a slightly hypointense heterogeneous mass (*arrows*). (*C*) T1-weighted hypointense (M) and (*D*) T2-weighted hyperintense mass (M) with heterogeneous enhancement (M) after contrast administration (*E*). (*F*) Angiogram shows abnormal vascularity (*arrows*) in the left hepatic lobe.

enhancement criteria in the axial plane using RECIST, mRECIST, and European Association for the Study of the Liver (EASL) may not accurately represent the true amount of viable tumor using a single slice (**Fig. 4**). Therefore, new techniques for diagnostic criteria combining anatomic and functional imaging techniques are needed.

CT is limited in the evaluation of lipiodol-containing TACE whereby high lipiodol density interferes with response assessment. On the other hand, the high concentration of lipiodol does not affect the signal intensity on fat-saturated T1-weighted MRI (**Fig. 5**).

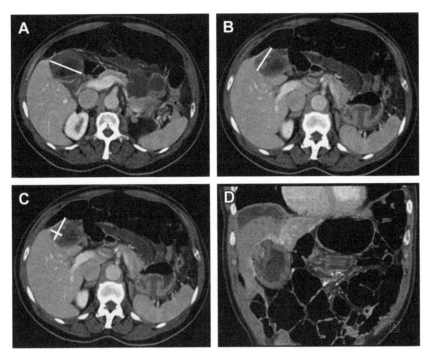

Fig. 4. HCC in a 76-year-old man. Treatment response as measured by (*A*) RECIST, (*B*) mRECIST, and (*C*) EASL. (*D*) Limitations of conventional metrics: RECIST, mRECIST, and EASL measure response in a single axial plane, whereas other planes are not taken into account. Therefore, these measurements may not represent tumor response in the entire tumor.

Specifically, diffusion-weighted imaging provides indirect assessment of tissue properties, such as cellularity, perfusion, and cellular necrosis, giving a qualitative and quantitative analysis by ADC maps of the HCC (**Fig. 6**). Studies have shown that diffusion-weighted imaging can improve the detection of HCC in cirrhotic livers.[12,13]

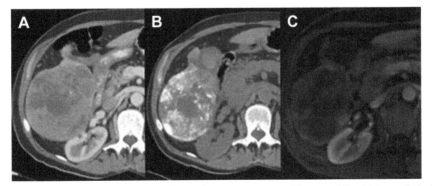

Fig. 5. (*A*) Pretreatment contrast-enhanced CT in a 65-year-old man with a history of cholangiocarcinoma. (*B*) Nonenhanced CT ensures that lipiodol was deposited in the tumor, but is of limited value in assessing enhancement and viability because of the high density of the deposited lipiodol. (*C*) Contrast-enhanced MRI shows areas of necrosis with minimal viable rim of enhancement after TACE. Lipiodol does not impair assessment of tissue enhancement on MRI.

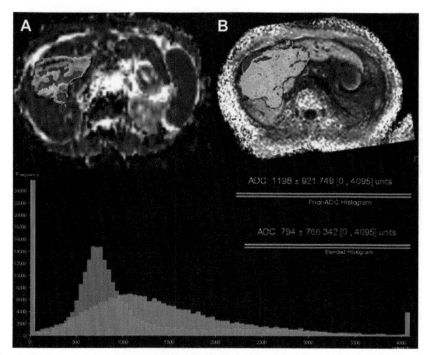

Fig. 6. Treatment response assessed by functional MRI with volumetric ADC. (A) Baseline study (*blue*, ADC map) demonstrates a tumor with ADC of 1.19×10^{-3} mm²/s. (B) Follow-up study posttreatment (*orange*, ADC map) demonstrates significant increase in ADC to 0.74×10^{-3} mm²/s, which indicates poor response to treatment.

In addition, there is significant correlation between histologic grade and ADC values.[14] Another study suggested that volumetric increase in ADC and decrease in venous enhancement after TACE[6] can provide early response to therapy.

FIBROLAMELLAR CARCINOMA

Fibrolamellar carcinoma (FLC) is an HCC variant that occurs in young adults most commonly without elevated α-fetoprotein level or underlying hepatic liver disease.[15] In fact, 85% of patients are less than 35 years of age.[16] Clinical manifestations may include gynecomastia, jaundice, venous compression, or thrombosis[16,17] that are frequently associated with abdominal pain or an abdominal mass.

FLC often appears as a large circumscribed nonencapsulated mass with a coalescent fibrous scar in up to 60% to 70% of cases.[17,18] Other FLC presentations include satellite lesions, a bilobulated mass, or multiple masses.[17]

US can demonstrate a solitary circumscribed mass with heterogeneous echotexture that is predominantly isoechoic to the liver parenchyma.[17] The central scar is hyperechoic and may contain calcifications depicted as shadowing echoes.

CT shows similar findings with FLC appearing as a hypoattenuating density compared with the surrounding liver. After contrast administration, the tumor is hyperdense compared with the adjacent liver in the arterial phase with variable density in the portal venous phase. The central scar is hypodense compared with the rest of the tumor. On MRI, FLC appears as a mass that is T1-weighted hypointense to isointense and T2-weighted hyperintense to isointense with a central fibrotic scar that is T1-hypointense and T2-hypointense. Unlike focal nodular hyperplasia the central fibrous scar in FLC does not enhance after contrast administration (**Fig. 7**).

LYMPHOMA OF THE LIVER

Primary lymphoma of the liver is extremely rare and usually manifests as a solitary focal mass; however, primary hepatic lymphoma can also present as multiple liver lesions or a diffuse process infiltrating the entire liver.[19] On imaging, the differential diagnosis of primary lymphoma versus metastatic disease can be challenging.

On US primary hepatic lymphoma is generally hypoechoic relative to the normal liver. CT shows low-attenuation foci compared with the normal liver parenchyma with variable enhancement after contrast administration.[20] MRI demonstrates T1-weighted hypointense foci that are hyperintense on T2-weighted images. However, the appearance of primary lymphoma on MRI varies and may be isointense on T1-weighted images. OnT2-weighted images the tumor can be hyperintense, hypointense, or isointense to normal liver.[21]

CHOLANGIOCARCINOMA

Cholangiocarcinomas originate from the biliary epithelium within either the liver or the extrahepatic biliary tree. Cholangiocarcinoma is often a firm hypovascular tumor due to its fibrous stroma, and most commonly histologically is an adenocarcinoma with desmoplasia. Risk factors associated with cholangiocarcinoma are infection with liver flukes and hepatolithiases, which are endemic in certain geographic areas. The most common risk factors for cholangiocarcinoma include primary sclerosing cholangitis, hepatic cirrhosis, chronic hepatitis C, hepatitis B, Epstein-Barr virus infection, alcoholic liver disease, chronic inflammatory bowel disease, and diabetes.[22,23] Nitrosamine compounds associated with parasitic infections act as cofactors owing to a carcinogenic effect on the proliferation of epithelial cells of the bile ducts.[24]

Imaging patterns and the radiologic manifestations of cholangiocarcinoma are diverse because tumors vary in location, growth pattern, and histologic type. US may be the initial imaging modality used in patients with an elevated bilirubin level. US imaging of cholangiocarcinoma is often limited and typically only is helpful in

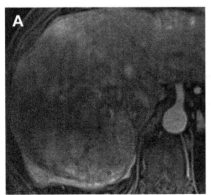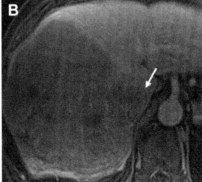

Fig. 7. MRI of a 78-year-old man with fibrolamellar infiltrative HCC. (*A*) Arterial phase depicts a large heterogeneous infiltrating enhancing mass on the right hepatic lobe. (*B*) The mass shows washout on portal venous phase and is invading the inferior vena cava (*arrow*).

detecting the level of obstruction. US is particularly limited in tumor staging. Doppler US may be helpful in differentiating vessels from dilated ducts. In contrast, CT has become the diagnostic test of choice for detailed evaluation and staging of cholangio-carcinoma in many centers. CT can provide information about local disease and metastatic spread to lymph nodes and distant organs. In other centers, MRI is the preferred imaging modality of choice for cholangiocarcinoma. On MRI, cholangiocarcinoma shows variable intensities depending on the amount of mucinous material, fibrous tissue, hemorrhage, and necrosis within the tumor. Diffusion-weighted imaging improves the diagnostic yield of MRI and may be useful in assessing early response to treatment.[4] Magnetic resonance cholangiopancreatography (MRCP) has an added value in the evaluation of cholangiocarcinoma. Specifically, MRCP can help delineate the biliary tree and gallbladder with comparable diagnostic accuracy to endoscopic retrograde cholangiopancreatography.[25] Accuracy of MRCP in localizing the site of obstruction has been reported to be 100%, with 95% accuracy in determining the cause of biliary obstruction.[26] In general, cholangiocarcinoma is classified as either intrahepatic or extrahepatic in location.

Intrahepatic Cholangiocarcinoma

Intrahepatic cholangiocarcinoma (ICC) is the second most common primary malignancy of the liver. Based on growth pattern and tumor morphology, ICC has been classified into 3 subgroups: mass forming, intraductal growth pattern, and periductal infiltrating type (PIT).[27]

US is often the initial imaging modality for evaluation of biliary dilatation and can reveal a mass when ICC is present.

On unenhanced CT, ICCs are noted to hypoattenuating or isoattenuating lesions. After contrast administration, most cholangiocarcinomas remain hypoattenuating during arterial and portal venous phase and show enhancement during delayed phases.

Contrast-enhanced MRI depicts early rim enhancement and persistent delayed enhancement of the tumor. These characteristic findings reflect the fibrous content within the tumor.[28] Gadoxetic acid–enhanced images in the hepatobiliary phase depict the tumor as a hypointense lesion without liver-specific contrast uptake.[29]

Mass forming type

Mass forming type (MFT) of ICC typically presents as a homogenous mass with irregular, well-defined margins often associated with dilatation of the biliary tree in the periphery. On US, MFT appears as hyperechoic (>3 cm), hypoechoic, isoechoic (<3 cm), or of mixed echogenicity.[30] By CT, MFT ICC appears homogeneous in attenuation, with irregular peripheral enhancement that gradually becomes centripetal in pattern. On MRI MFT demonstrates irregular margins with variable high signal intensity on T2-weighted images and low signal intensity on T1-weighted images. Postcontrast images show an irregular peripheral enhancement with concentric filling,[31] and significant central enhancement can be seen on delayed phase (20 minutes) MRI. Associated MFT findings are capsular retraction, satellite nodules, hepatolithiasis, and vascular encasement without gross tumor thrombus formation.

PIT

PIT ICC presents as a growth along a dilated or narrowed bile duct without mass formation. PIT can also present as an elongated or branchlike abnormality. On imaging, it is crucial to differentiate benign from malignant strictures, and the presence of an irregular margin, asymmetric narrowing, lymph node enlargement, enhancing ducts, or periductal soft tissue lesions should raise suspicion for a malignant stricture.[32]

By US PIT appears as a small solitary masslike lesion or may be seen as diffuse bile duct thickening with or without obliteration of the bile duct lumen. Occasionally PIT may cause a diffusely abnormal liver echotexture that sometimes mimics HCC or metastases.[33] On CT and MRI, PIT presents as diffuse periductal thickening and increased enhancement because of tumor infiltration with abnormal dilated or irregular narrow duct and peripheral ductal dilatation (**Fig. 8**).[34]

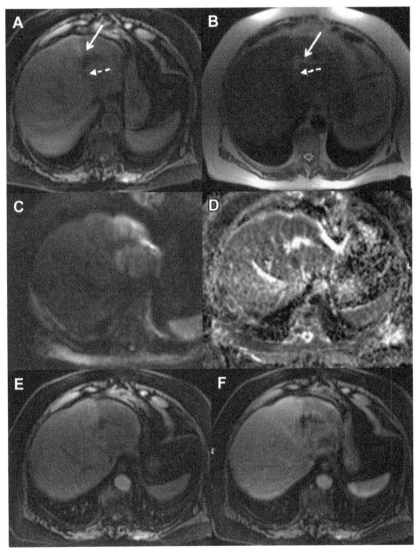

Fig. 8. A 73-year-old man with a diagnosis of cholangiocarcinoma. There is intrahepatic biliary dilatation (*arrow*) with atrophy of the left hepatic lobe. The biliary dilatation terminates at a (*A*) T1-weighted hypointense (*B*) T2-weighted hyperintense area within the left lobe (*dotted arrow*). (*C*) Diffusion-weighted images and (*D*) ADC map of the cholangiocarcinoma show restricted diffusion, and (*E*) arterial and (*F*) portal phase demonstrate heterogeneous enhancement.

Intraductal growing type

Intraductal growing type (IGT) has a significantly better prognosis compared with mass MFT or PIT. Several imaging features are suggestive of IGT. For example, features such as a papillary or irregular polypoid shape, lack of constriction of the tumor-bearing segment, hypo-enhancement of the tumor relative to the liver during the equilibrium phase, tumor multiplicity, upstream and downstream bile duct dilatation, and no bile duct wall thickening adjacent to the tumor all suggest IGT.[35] On US IGT tumors are often present as localized or diffuse duct ectasia with or without an echogenic intraductal polypoid lesion.[30] By CT, IGT can appear as diffuse and marked ductal dilatation with an intraductal mass that is hypoattenuating or isoattenuating relative to the surrounding liver parenchyma.[30] On MRI IGT most often shows washout, whereas MFT ICC more often shows gradual persistent or progressive enhancement, which can help in differentiating between the 2 subtypes of tumors. MRCP is superior to CT for the assessment of IGT (**Fig. 9**).[35] MRCP depicts intrahepatic and extrahepatic ducts helping to determine the origin of the tumor, as well as define the margins of the tumor facilitating treatment planning.

Extrahepatic Cholangiocarcinoma

Extrahepatic cholangiocarcinoma (ECC) arises from the ductal epithelium of the extrahepatic bile duct. Tumor location and extent of the ECC are the most important factors influencing outcome and patient survival.[24] MRI is one of the most important diagnostic imaging modalities used in assessing the longitudinal and lateral spread of a tumor, thereby helping determine resectability. The enhancement pattern of ECC is similar to that of ICC except ECC are often less heterogeneous because they typically present as smaller infiltrating tumors. ECC are hypovascular and enhance slowly with peak enhancement on delayed phase. ECC typically presents as an abnormal circumferential extrahepatic bile duct wall thickening and enhancement is best visualized at 1 to 5 minutes after gadolinium injection.[36] Diffusion-weighted imaging of ECC demonstrates different levels of high signal intensity and low signal intensity in ADC maps and has very good sensitivity in detection of ECC comparable to MRCP.[37]

Perihilar Cholangiocarcinoma

Hilar cholangiocarcinomas (PCC) are adenocarcinomas that arise at the confluence of the right and left hepatic bile ducts. PCC has been categorized into 4 types by the modified Bismuth-Corlette classification adapted from the original classification.[38]

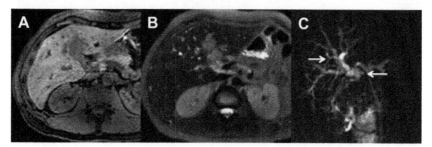

Fig. 9. A 44-year-old man with diagnosis of extrahepatic adenocarcinoma. There is a mass that is hypointense on T1-weighted image (*A*) and hyperintense on T2-weighted image (*B*). The mass extends to the right and left hepatic lobes and the gallbladder fossa. (*C*) MRCP depicts intrahepatic and extrahepatic biliary dilatation (*arrows*). The gallbladder is not visualized.

On most imaging modalities, PCC demonstrates circumferential growth and spreads along the bile duct with poor conspicuity on noncontrast images.[39]

US shows dilatation and disruption of the confluence of the right and left hepatic duct at the porta hepatis. Dilatation can be associated with hepatic lobar atrophy, contralateral lobar hypertrophy, and crowding of the bile ducts. MRI and MRCP are probably the best modalities for evaluating PCC and can provide accurate preoperative staging of the biliary tree, liver parenchyma, and vascular involvement for assessment of resectability. On MRI, PCC presents with the same signal intensity as PIT on T1-weighted and T2-weighted images; however, after contrast administration PCC shows different enhancement patterns. Most of the lesions are hypovascular compared with the adjacent liver parenchyma with heterogeneous enhancement that gradually peaks on delayed phase images because of the high fibrous content of the tumor.[40] Some lesions show periductal enhancement and very few PCC show delayed hypervascular enhancement.

GALLBLADDER CARCINOMA

Primary gallbladder carcinoma is the fifth most common gastrointestinal tumor.[41] Eighty percent of gallbladder carcinomas are associated with cholelithiasis and the risk seems to be also associated with stone size.[11] Gallbladder carcinoma has a predilection for women, which is thought to be associated with the higher incidence of gallstones in women. Chronic inflammation of the gallbladder by bile fluid components may also play a pathogenic role in malignant transformation.[42] Other risk factors include polypoid lesions (>10 mm) with a prevalence of 3% to 6%, anomalous junction of the pancreatobiliary ducts in approximately 10% of patients, and perhaps porcelain gallbladder in up to 20% of gallbladder carcinomas. Less significant factors associated with gallbladder cancer are bacterial infections (*Escherichia coli*, *Oposthorchis viverrini*), typhoid carriers (*Salmonella typhi* or *Salmonella paratyphi*), and hormonal changes. Gallbladder carcinoma is typically classified according to its appearance as (1) intramural polypoid mass, (2) focal or diffuse asymmetrical gallbladder wall thickening, and (3) occupying the gallbladder fossa (**Fig. 10**).[43]

US aids in differentiating sludge from an intraluminal mass. Enhanced CT aids in distinguishing complicated cholecystitis from gallbladder carcinoma. MRI is useful in cases of focal or diffuse mural thickening to distinguish gallbladder carcinoma from adenomyomatosis[44] and chronic cholecystitis.[45]

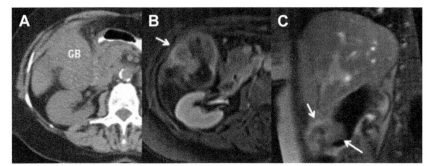

Fig. 10. Gallbladder carcinoma in a 70-year-old woman. (*A*) Noncontrast CT shows localized thickening and modularity in the gallbladder fossa (GB). (*B*) Contrast-enhanced T1-weighted (*arrow*) and (*C*) coronal plane MR images show a mass like thickening (*arrows*) involving the gallbladder funds with the presence of enhancement after contrast administration.

Intramural Polypoid Mass

An intramural polypoid mass is the least common form of gallbladder carcinoma, representing only 15% to 25% of cases.[46] This form of gallbladder cancer is usually confined to the muscular layer and tends to expand into the gallbladder lumen before invading the wall. On cross-sectional imaging, the intramural polypoid mass appears as a well-defined, round or oval-shaped polypoid lesion. US typically demonstrates that the intraluminal mass is immobile with changes in patient position. By CT the mass has the appearance of a hypoattenuating or isoattenuating lesion. On T1-weighted images a polypoid mass arising from a thickened gallbladder wall is often seen and typically has intermediate signal intensity. On T2-weighted images the polypoid mass is hyperintense. After contrast administration, the intramural polypoid lesions shows moderately early enhancement that persists through the portal venous phase.[47]

Focal or Diffuse Asymmetric Gallbladder Wall Thickening

This form of gallbladder carcinoma represents up to 20% to 30% of cases. Focal or diffuse thickening of the gallbladder wall that is equal or more than 10 mm is highly suspicious. On CT and MRI the tumor is seen as a diffuse asymmetric thickened wall. The tumor often is characterized by heterogeneous hyperintensity compared with the liver parenchyma on T2-weighted images and hypointense or isointense on T1-weighted images. After contrast administration the tumor shows irregular conspicuous arterial enhancement[48] that persists or becomes isointense to the liver during the portal venous phase.[49]

Subhepatic Mass Occupying the Gallbladder

A subhepatic mass occupying the gallbladder is the most common form of gallbladder carcinoma representing 40% to 65% of cases.[43] This form of gallbladder carcinoma tends to occupy the entire lumen of the gallbladder invading the surrounding liver parenchyma.

By US the gallbladder has irregular margins and heterogeneous echotexture reflecting varying degrees of tumor necrosis. Echogenic foci and acoustic shadowing associated with the tumor may be related to coexisting gallstones or calcifications.[50] Contrast-enhanced CT demonstrates a hypoattenuating or isoattenuating mass within the gallbladder fossa and soft tissue invasion of the liver. The low-attenuation areas within the tumor mass or thickened gallbladder wall may appear nodular.[51] Associated frequent findings include biliary obstruction at the level of the porta hepatis and enlarged metastatic lymph nodes. On MRI, the T1-weighted images of the tumor reveal hypointense to isointense signal intensity and the tumor mass is frequently heterogeneously hyperintense in signal on T2-weighted images.[43] During arterial enhancement, the tumor shows avid irregular enhancement on the periphery and tends to maintain the enhancement throughout the portal and delayed phase.

LYMPHOMA OF THE GALLBLADDER

Gallbladder lymphoma is extremely rare, with most reported cases being diffuse large B cell or mucosa-associated lymphoid tissue types. Reported cases are in elderly patients and most present with clinical symptoms of cholecystitis or cholelithiasis. Radiological findings in previous reports have noted wall thickening associated with intramural mass formation.[52] On MRI T1-weighted images show loss of signal intensity on fat-suppression images and high signal intensity on T2-weighted fat-suppression images. T2-weighted images show a hypointense homogenous signal commonly in the presence of enlarged lymph nodes.

PERIAMPULLARY TUMORS

Periampullary tumors include pancreatic head carcinoma, intrapancreatic bile duct carcinoma, and periampullary duodenal carcinoma. Most common imaging findings are pancreaticobiliary duct dilatation, double duct sign, 3-segment sign (a dilated proximal bile duct, a nondilated distal bile duct, and a dilated or nondilated pancreatic duct), 4-segment sign (when 2 proximal and 2 distal pancreatic and biliary ducts appear as 4 separate ducts) and shape, and increased wall thickness of the distal margin of the common bile duct and main pancreatic duct (**Fig. 11**).[53] CT scans are commonly used to diagnosis these images. Similar to ampullary carcinomas, periampullary tumors involve the papilla, resulting in papillary bulging. MRI can also be used to assess periampullary tumors. On T1-weighted images periampullary tumors appear as low signal intensity masses, and most lesions are hypovascular. However, a thin peripheral rim of enhancement can be depicted on fat-suppressed images.

AMPULLARY CARCINOMA

Ampullary tumors arise from the ampulla of Vater, often causing biliary obstruction. According to gross morphologic features, ampullary carcinomas are divided into 3 types: protruded, ulcerative, and mixed. Usually ampullary carcinomas manifest as small tumors at the time of diagnosis because of the early onset of symptoms and often they are not apparent at CT. When ampullary carcinomas are seen on CT, it is because the tumor protrudes into the duodenum. Classic imaging findings include an ampullary mass, papillary bulging, irregular and asymmetric common bile duct narrowing, and biliary dilatation.[53]

MRCP can detect ampullary carcinomas with a high sensitivity (100%) but limited specificity (up to 63%).[54] A recent study showed that diffusion-weighted imaging can improve the detection of ampullary carcinoma.[55]

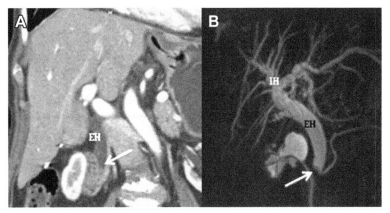

Fig. 11. (*A*) Coronal contrast-enhanced CT in the portal venous phase shows dilatation of the common bile duct with abrupt truncation because of enhancing soft tissue (*arrow*). (*B*) MRCP shows intrahepatic (IH) and extrahepatic (EH) ductal dilatation of the common bile duct to the level of the pancreatic head. The common bile duct is dilated with abrupt truncation (*arrow*) at the level of the pancreatic head, associated with a filling defect.

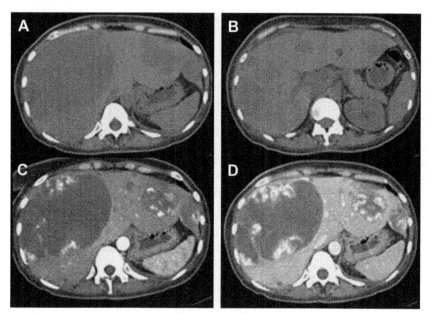

Fig. 12. A 45-year-old woman. CT shows multiple (*A, B*) hypodense masses within the right and left hepatic lobe. After contrast-enhanced (*C*) in arterial phase centripetal enhancement is depicted. (*D*) During portal venous phase there are areas of central necrosis without central filling compatible with patient's history of angiosarcoma.

VASCULAR TUMORS
Angiosarcoma

Angiosarcoma is a rare tumor of vascular origin, frequently affecting elderly men between 60 and 70 years of age, although it can occur in younger patients.[56] This tumor is usually related to toxic exposures such as thorium dioxide (Thorotrast) or vinyl chloride. At the time of diagnosis metastatic disease is present in up to 60% of patients.[56,57] Tumor patterns include (1) multiple nodules, (2) large dominant mass, (3) mixture of dominant mass with multiple nodules, and less commonly, (4) micronodular infiltration of the liver (**Fig. 12**).[56]

The echogenicity of angiosarcoma varies by US according to the amount of hemorrhagic or necrotic change. On CT, nodules are often hypodense to normal liver but may contain hyperdense areas corresponding to acute hemorrhage.[56,57] After contrast administration angiosarcomas are hypointense during arterial and venous phase and occasionally show early heterogeneous central enhancement or ring enhancement. On delayed images enhancement persists but complete centripetal fill is not seen. T1-weighted MRIs demonstrate a hypointense lesion with hyperintense foci representing intramural hemorrhage. On T2-weighted images angiosarcoma is heterogeneously hyperintense and may contain dark septa or fluid levels consistent with hemorrhage.[56]

After contrast administration there is heterogeneous enhancement that progresses centrally on delayed images with lack of central filling.

SUMMARY

Biliary tumors are diverse in growth patterns, histologic types, and tumor location. In turn, imaging manifestations of biliary tumors and primary liver tumors are varied.

Accurate detection, characterization, and assessment of tumor extent are the primary goals of radiological imaging. Knowledge about various manifestations and mimickers of biliary and primary liver tumors is essential for tumor diagnosis and suitable management.

REFERENCES

1. Neumaier CE, Bertolotto M, Perrone R, et al. Staging of hilar cholangiocarcinoma with ultrasound. J Clin Ultrasound 1995;23(3):173–8.
2. Sahani DV, Holalkere NS, Mueller PR, et al. Advanced hepatocellular carcinoma: CT perfusion of liver and tumor tissue–initial experience. Radiology 2007;243(3): 736–43.
3. Ippolito D, Sironi S, Pozzi M, et al. Perfusion CT in cirrhotic patients with early stage hepatocellular carcinoma: assessment of tumor-related vascularization. Eur J Radiol 2010;73(1):148–52.
4. Halappa VG, Bonekamp S, Corona-Villalobos CP, et al. Intrahepatic cholangiocarcinoma treated with local-regional therapy: quantitative volumetric apparent diffusion coefficient maps for assessment of tumor response. Radiology 2012; 264(1):285–94.
5. Bonekamp S, Halappa VG, Geschwind JF, et al. Unresectable hepatocellular carcinoma: MR imaging after intraarterial therapy. Part II. Response stratification using volumetric functional criteria after intraarterial therapy. Radiology 2013; 268(2):431–9.
6. Bonekamp S, Jolepalem P, Lazo M, et al. Hepatocellular carcinoma: response to TACE assessed with semiautomated volumetric and functional analysis of diffusion-weighted and contrast-enhanced MR imaging data. Radiology 2011; 260(3):752–61.
7. Xia Y, Kudo M, Minami Y, et al. Response evaluation of transcatheter arterial chemoembolization in hepatocellular carcinomas: the usefulness of sonazoid-enhanced harmonic sonography. Oncology 2008;75(Suppl 1):99–105.
8. Meloni MF, Livraghi T, Filice C, et al. Radiofrequency ablation of liver tumors: the role of microbubble ultrasound contrast agents. Ultrasound Q 2006;22(1): 41–7.
9. Ippolito D, Sironi S, Pozzi M, et al. Perfusion computed tomographic assessment of early hepatocellular carcinoma in cirrhotic liver disease: initial observations. J Comput Assist Tomogr 2008;32(6):855–8.
10. Koh TS, Thng CH, Hartono S, et al. Dynamic contrast-enhanced CT imaging of hepatocellular carcinoma in cirrhosis: feasibility of a prolonged dual-phase imaging protocol with tracer kinetics modeling. Eur Radiol 2009;19(5): 1184–96.
11. Sheth S, Bedford A, Chopra S. Primary gallbladder cancer: recognition of risk factors and the role of prophylactic cholecystectomy. Am J Gastroenterol 2000;95(6):1402–10.
12. Lee MH, Kim SH, Park MJ, et al. Gadoxetic acid-enhanced hepatobiliary phase MRI and high-b-value diffusion-weighted imaging to distinguish well-differentiated hepatocellular carcinomas from benign nodules in patients with chronic liver disease. AJR Am J Roentgenol 2011;197(5):W868–75.
13. Nasu K, Kuroki Y, Tsukamoto T, et al. Diffusion-weighted imaging of surgically resected hepatocellular carcinoma: imaging characteristics and relationship among signal intensity, apparent diffusion coefficient, and histopathologic grade. AJR Am J Roentgenol 2009;193(2):438–44.

14. Nakanishi M, Chuma M, Hige S, et al. Relationship between diffusion-weighted magnetic resonance imaging and histological tumor grading of hepatocellular carcinoma. Ann Surg Oncol 2012;19(4):1302–9.
15. Levy AD. Malignant liver tumors. Clin Liver Dis 2002;6(1):147–64.
16. Torbenson M. Review of the clinicopathologic features of fibrolamellar carcinoma. Adv Anat Pathol 2007;14(3):217–23.
17. McLarney JK, Rucker PT, Bender GN, et al. Fibrolamellar carcinoma of the liver: radiologic-pathologic correlation. Radiographics 1999;19(2):453–71.
18. Liu S, Chan KW, Wang B, et al. Fibrolamellar hepatocellular carcinoma. Am J Gastroenterol 2009;104(10):2617–24 [quiz: 2625].
19. Ryan J, Straus DJ, Lange C, et al. Primary lymphoma of the liver. Cancer 1988; 61(2):370–5.
20. Zornoza J, Ginaldi S. Computed tomography in hepatic lymphoma. Radiology 1981;138(2):405–10.
21. Weinreb JC, Brateman L, Maravilla KR. Magnetic resonance imaging of hepatic lymphoma. AJR Am J Roentgenol 1984;143(6):1211–4.
22. Shaib YH, El-Serag HB, Davila JA, et al. Risk factors of intrahepatic cholangiocarcinoma in the United States: a case-control study. Gastroenterology 2005; 128(3):620–6.
23. Welzel TM, Graubard BI, El-Serag HB, et al. Risk factors for intrahepatic and extrahepatic cholangiocarcinoma in the United States: a population-based case-control study. Clin Gastroenterol Hepatol 2007;5(10):1221–8.
24. Khan SA, Thomas HC, Davidson BR, et al. Cholangiocarcinoma. Lancet 2005; 366(9493):1303–14.
25. Fernandez-Esparrach G, Gines A, Sanchez M, et al. Comparison of endoscopic ultrasonography and magnetic resonance cholangiopancreatography in the diagnosis of pancreatobiliary diseases: a prospective study. Am J Gastroenterol 2007;102(8):1632–9.
26. Romagnuolo J, Bardou M, Rahme E, et al. Magnetic resonance cholangiopancreatography: a meta-analysis of test performance in suspected biliary disease. Ann Intern Med 2003;139(7):547–57.
27. Yamasaki S. Intrahepatic cholangiocarcinoma: macroscopic type and stage classification. J Hepatobiliary Pancreat Surg 2003;10(4):288–91.
28. Menias CO, Surabhi VR, Prasad SR, et al. Mimics of cholangiocarcinoma: spectrum of disease. Radiographics 2008;28(4):1115–29.
29. Peporte AR, Sommer WH, Nikolaou K, et al. Imaging features of intrahepatic cholangiocarcinoma in Gd-EOB-DTPA-enhanced MRI. Eur J Radiol 2013; 82(3):e101–6.
30. Chung YE, Kim MJ, Park YN, et al. Varying appearances of cholangiocarcinoma: radiologic-pathologic correlation. Radiographics 2009;29(3):683–700.
31. Maetani Y, Itoh K, Watanabe C, et al. MR imaging of intrahepatic cholangiocarcinoma with pathologic correlation. AJR Am J Roentgenol 2001;176(6): 1499–507.
32. Park HJ, Kim YK, Park MJ, et al. Small intrahepatic mass-forming cholangiocarcinoma: target sign on diffusion-weighted imaging for differentiation from hepatocellular carcinoma. Abdom Imaging 2012;38(4):793–801.
33. Colli A, Cocciolo M, Mumoli N, et al. Peripheral intrahepatic cholangiocarcinoma: ultrasound findings and differential diagnosis from hepatocellular carcinoma. Eur J Ultrasound 1998;7(2):93–9.
34. Han JK, Lee JM. Intrahepatic intraductal cholangiocarcinoma. Abdom Imaging 2004;29(5):558–64.

35. Kim JE, Lee JM, Kim SH, et al. Differentiation of intraductal growing-type chol-angiocarcinomas from nodular-type cholangiocarcinomas at biliary MR imaging with MR cholangiography. Radiology 2010;257(2):364–72.

36. Vanderveen KA, Hussain HK. Magnetic resonance imaging of cholangiocarci-noma. Cancer Imaging 2004;4(2):104–15.

37. Cui XY, Chen HW. Role of diffusion-weighted magnetic resonance imaging in the diagnosis of extrahepatic cholangiocarcinoma. World J Gastroenterol 2010; 16(25):3196–201.

38. Bismuth H, Nakache R, Diamond T. Management strategies in resection for hilar cholangiocarcinoma. Ann Surg 1992;215(1):31–8.

39. Manfredi R, Masselli G, Maresca G, et al. MR imaging and MRCP of hilar chol-angiocarcinoma. Abdom Imaging 2003;28(3):319–25.

40. Kassahun WT, Hauss J. Management of combined hepatocellular and cholan-giocarcinoma. Int J Clin Pract 2008;62(8):1271–8.

41. Roberts JW, Daugherty SF. Primary carcinoma of the gallbladder. Surg Clin North Am 1986;66(4):743–9.

42. Weiss KM, Ferrell RE, Hanis CL, et al. Genetics and epidemiology of gallbladder disease in New World native peoples. Am J Hum Genet 1984;36(6):1259–78.

43. Levy AD, Murakata LA, Rohrmann CA Jr. Gallbladder carcinoma: radiologic-pathologic correlation. Radiographics 2001;21(2):295–314 [questionnaire: 549–55].

44. Yoshimitsu K, Honda H, Jimi M, et al. MR diagnosis of adenomyomatosis of the gallbladder and differentiation from gallbladder carcinoma: importance of showing Rokitansky-Aschoff sinuses. AJR Am J Roentgenol 1999;172(6): 1535–40.

45. Demachi H, Matsui O, Hoshiba K, et al. Dynamic MRI using a surface coil in chronic cholecystitis and gallbladder carcinoma: radiologic and histopathologic correlation. J Comput Assist Tomogr 1997;21(4):643–51.

46. Reid KM, Ramos-De la Medina A, Donohue JH. Diagnosis and surgical manage-ment of gallbladder cancer: a review. J Gastrointest Surg 2007;11(5):671–81.

47. Gore RM, Yaghmai V, Newmark GM, et al. Imaging benign and malignant dis-ease of the gallbladder. Radiol Clin North Am 2002;40(6):1307–23, vi.

48. Catalano OA, Sahani DV, Kalva SP, et al. MR imaging of the gallbladder: a picto-rial essay. Radiographics 2008;28(1):135–55 [quiz: 324].

49. Yoshimitsu K, Honda H, Kaneko K, et al. Dynamic MRI of the gallbladder lesions: differentiation of benign from malignant. J Magn Reson Imaging 1997;7(4): 696–701.

50. Weiner SN, Koenigsberg M, Morehouse H, et al. Sonography and computed to-mography in the diagnosis of carcinoma of the gallbladder. AJR Am J Roent-genol 1984;142(4):735–9.

51. Chun KA, Ha HK, Yu ES, et al. Xanthogranulomatous cholecystitis: CT features with emphasis on differentiation from gallbladder carcinoma. Radiology 1997; 203(1):93–7.

52. Ono A, Tanoue S, Yamada Y, et al. Primary malignant lymphoma of the gall-bladder: a case report and literature review. Br J Radiol 2009;82(973):e15–9.

53. Kim JH, Kim MJ, Chung JJ, et al. Differential diagnosis of periampullary carci-nomas at MR imaging. Radiographics 2002;22(6):1335–52.

54. Chung YE, Kim MJ, Kim HM, et al. Differentiation of benign and malignant ampullary obstructions on MR imaging. Eur J Radiol 2011;80(2):198–203.

55. Jang KM, Kim SH, Lee SJ, et al. Added value of diffusion-weighted MR imaging in the diagnosis of ampullary carcinoma. Radiology 2013;266(2):491–501.

56. Koyama T, Fletcher JG, Johnson CD, et al. Primary hepatic angiosarcoma: findings at CT and MR imaging. Radiology 2002;222(3):667–73.
57. Buetow PC, Buck JL, Ros PR, et al. Malignant vascular tumors of the liver: radiologic-pathologic correlation. Radiographics 1994;14(1):153–66 [quiz: 167–8].

Endoscopic and Percutaneous Approaches to the Treatment of Biliary Tract and Primary Liver Tumors: Controversies and Advances

Kevin N. Shah, MD, Bryan M. Clary, MD*

KEYWORDS

- Cholangiocarcinoma • Hepatocellular carcinoma • Biliary stenting • Ampullectomy
- Radiofrequency ablation

KEY POINTS

- Primary tumors of the bile ducts and liver often carry unfavorable prognoses and present several clinical and therapeutic challenges.
- Advances in percutaneous and endoscopic techniques have improved preoperative selection and optimization, as well as offering alternatives to traditionally morbid surgical therapies.
- However, these advances are controversial and include questions about the role of routine preoperative biliary drainage, endoscopic versus surgical resection of ampullary tumors, and the use of ablative techniques to treat primary liver tumors.

INTRODUCTION

Primary tumors of the bile ducts and liver often carry unfavorable prognoses and present several clinical and therapeutic challenges. Selecting the correct intervention to perform is only part of this challenge, because many of these patients have underlying comorbidities that exacerbate the already high morbidity of potentially curative operations. Careful selection of patients and preoperative optimization are therefore important considerations. Further complicating management is that individual diseases like cholangiocarcinoma and hepatocellular carcinoma (HCC) do not represent a uniform disease. Variations in location, size, and multicentricity mandate tailored approaches. Although these are serious and difficult diseases to cure, new technologies have added to the armamentarium, offering some less invasive alternatives to traditionally

Division of Surgical Oncology, Duke University Medical Center, 10 Searle Drive, 485 Seeley Mudd Building, DUMC 3247, Durham, NC 27710, USA
* Corresponding author.
E-mail address: bryan.clary@dm.duke.edu

Surg Oncol Clin N Am 23 (2014) 207–230
http://dx.doi.org/10.1016/j.soc.2013.10.003
1055-3207/14/$ – see front matter © 2014 Elsevier Inc. All rights reserved.
surgonc.theclinics.com

morbid therapeutic options. This article highlights controversies and recent advances in the use of endoscopic and percutaneous approaches to the treatment of bile duct and liver tumors. The following issues are discussed:

1. The role of preoperative biliary drainage: the arguments for and against its routine use, as well as the best modality for performing it (percutaneous or endoscopic approaches, plastic or metal stents).
2. Local resections of ampullary tumors: the role endoscopic ampullectomy (EA) plays in the treatment of ampullary neoplasms, technical issues and strategies to minimize post-EA complications, and the role of surgical ampullectomy in the era of advanced endoscopic techniques.
3. Endoluminal treatments like photodynamic therapy as a palliative option for patients with unresectable cholangiocarcinoma.
4. The use of ablative therapies in the treatment of primary liver tumors: evaluation of popular thermal ablative types, percutaneous versus laparoscopic approaches, and the efficacy of ablation relative to surgical resection.

BILIARY DRAINAGE
Indications for Preoperative Biliary Drainage

Among patients with obstructive jaundice who have unresectable patterns of disease or are otherwise not candidates for surgery, biliary drainage, either endoscopic or percutaneous, has become a mainstay of palliation. In treating resectable disease, there are also several situations in which there is little controversy regarding the importance of preoperative biliary drainage (PBD). For example, PBD plays an essential role in the treatment of cholangitis and severe hepatic/renal dysfunction related to obstructive jaundice. Preoperative drainage is also required in any situation that results in a delay to surgery, whether it is planned neoadjuvant therapy, a delay while awaiting patient transfer to a high-volume center, or issues related to scheduling. Although PBD is indicated in several situations, the role of universal PBD in patients who are candidates for resection is the subject of some controversy. Several small studies published in the 1980s indicated that PBD resulted in lower postoperative morbidity.[1–5] These data, along with the increasing availability of both endoscopic and percutaneous methods of biliary drainage, have led to the adoption of routine preresection biliary drainage at some centers. However, the data regarding universal PBD are heterogeneous, and most modern reports do not support indiscriminant PBD. A meta-analysis by Sewnath and colleagues[6] analyzed 5 randomized controlled trials (RCTs) and 18 nonrandomized reviews of PBD versus early surgery and did not find convincing evidence that PBD was beneficial. There was no clear difference in postoperative morbidity between the PBD group and the early surgery group. Furthermore, when drainage-related complications were added, the rate of morbidity was in favor of the non-PBD group. There are several criticisms of this study that should be noted when interpreting its results. Some clinicians have criticized the randomized trials included in this meta-analysis (all from the 1980s) because they were all small studies without the methodological rigor marked by more modern randomized trials.[7] In addition, these conclusions are difficult to interpret, because most of the included studies did not distinguish between proximal and distal biliary strictures. Because the issues surrounding the management of proximal and distal bile duct strictures are distinct, the use of PBD is best understood by discussing the management of distal obstructing lesions and more proximal lesions separately.

Distal Bile Duct Strictures

Several more recent studies (summarized in **Table 1**) have attempted to address some of the deficiencies seen in older reports of PBD in patients undergoing pancreaticoduodenectomy (PD) for mid to distal bile duct strictures.[6,8–17] In 2010, van der Gaag and colleagues[8] published the results of the Drainage versus Operation trial with the aim of reporting a larger and more rigorous trial than previous randomized studies. The trial recruited patients with distal bile duct strictures and hyperbilirubinemia ranging between 2.3 and 14.7 mg/dL. A total of 202 patients were enrolled (6 excluded from analysis) with 94 being randomized to the early PD group (without drainage) and 102 patients assigned to the PBD group (surgery 4–6 weeks after drainage). Endoscopic drainage with plastic stents was successfully performed on the first attempt in 75% of patients and in 94% of patients after multiple endoscopic or percutaneous attempts. Drainage-related complications were observed in 47 patients (46%), with 27 (26%) developing cholangitis. There was 1 drainage-related mortality. The overall rate of severe complications was 39% in the early surgery group and 74% in the PBD group (relative risk [RR] for early surgery, 0.54). The rate of postoperative complications was again in favor of the early surgery group: 37% versus 47% in the PBD group (RR for early surgery, 0.79), and the PBD group had significantly more hospital readmissions (39% vs 19%). There was no significant difference in mortality. Based on these findings, the investigators recommended against routine PBD in patients undergoing PD.

Table 1 Summary of recent studies comparing PBD with no PBD for distal strictures undergoing pancreaticoduodenectomy					
Author, Year	N (Total)	Mortality (%)	Morbidity (%)	Intra-abdominal Infection (%)	Wound Infection (%)
Cavell et al,[10] 2013	SEMS 71	0	63.4	NR	31.0[a,b]
	PS 149	0	55.0		12.8[a,b]
	No PBD 289	1.4	51.2		6.2[a]
van der Gaag et al,[8] 2010	PBD 102	15	47[a]	2	13
	Non-PBD 96	13	37[a]	3	7
Garcea et al,[12] (review) 2010	PBD 2856	3.5	40	4.6	7.7[a]
	No PBD 2332	4.4	31.3	3.1	3.3[a]
Mezhir et al,[13] 2009	PBD 94	0	51	12[a]	20[a]
	No PBD 94	5	41	3[a]	7[a]
Coates et al,[14] 2009	PBD 90	4	38	7	5
	No PBD 34	15	47	12	9
Sewnath et al,[6] 2002	PBD 232	1.3	50	15.5	7.3
	No PBD 58	0	55	15.5	8.6
Srivastava et al,[15] 2001	PBD 54	15	48	28[a]	43[a]
	No PBD 67	12	46	15[a]	24[a]
Martignoni et al,[16] 2001	PBD 99	1.9	50	0	5.1
	No PBD 158	3.0	45	2.5	6.1
Pisters et al,[17] 2001	PBD 172	1	88	6	13[a]
	No PBD 93	1	86	11	4[a]

Abbreviations: NR, not reported; PS, plastic stent; SEMS, self-expanding metal stent.
[a] Statistically significant difference between PBD and no PBD groups.
[b] Statistically significant difference between SEMS and PS.

There are several criticisms of this study. Baron and Kozarek[18] wrote in response to van der Gaag and colleagues'[8] findings that the rate of postdrainage complications was higher than that observed in other studies. They noted in particular the substantial number of patients who experienced cholangitis after PBD and stated that this rate likely could have been reduced with the use of self-expanding metal stents (SEMSs). Others have also stated that routine use of antibiotics before endoscopic retrograde cholangiopancreatography (ERCP) may also have reduced the incidence of PBD-related cholangitis.[19] Another issue with this trial is the exclusion of patients with severe hyperbilirubinemia (>14.7 mg/dL), because these patients are at higher risk for cholangitis and would theoretically benefit the most from PBD.[20]

Despite these criticisms, most modern studies favor selective rather than routine PBD. Several studies summarized in **Table 1** show a higher incidence of postoperative infectious complications as a result of PBD. Even among those studies that do not show evidence of increased postoperative infections, few show any decisive advantage in favor of PBD. The importance of selective PBD highlights the need for multidisciplinary coordination. Invasive procedures should be delayed, if possible, until discussion between the surgeon, gastroenterologist, medical oncologist, and radiation oncologist takes place. The primary indications for PBD in distal bile duct strictures are:

1. Severe hyperbilirubinemia with present or impending renal failure and coagulopathy
2. Cholangitis
3. Planned neoadjuvant therapy or scheduling difficulty that results in delay of surgery

Proximal Bile Duct Strictures

Despite the many advances in intraoperative and perioperative management, the mortality of en-bloc partial hepatectomy and bile duct excision when performed for perihilar cholangiocarcinoma remains between 7% and 10%. The principal driver of this excess mortality (compared with other indications for hepatectomy) is postoperative liver failure, which is largely explained by the frequent need for extended hepatectomies and the damage associated with prolonged biliary obstruction.[21,22] These facts highlight the need for optimization of resectable patients (and future liver remnant [FLR]) before surgery. Optimization of the FLR plays a critical role in minimizing postoperative hepatic failure and has more recently included maximizing FLR volume with portal vein embolization and PBD of the FLR. Several studies from Memorial Sloan Kettering have found that the absence of PBD in patients with small FLR (<30%) is associated with increased mortality and postoperative liver failure.[23,24] Sixty patients who underwent liver resection for hilar cholangiocarcinoma (HCCA) were included, with an overall mortality of 10% and a hepatic failure rate of 8%. When stratified by FLR volume, patients with FLR less than 30% had mortality and liver failure rates of 19% and 24% compared with 5% and 0% respectively for the group with FLR greater than 30%. In the group with less than 30% FLR, PBD was associated with significantly lower rates of hepatic failure (0% vs 42%) and mortality (0% vs 33%). This advantage of PBD was not seen in the larger FLR group: there were no cases of postoperative hepatic failure or mortality in the undrained group, but a 9% mortality in the PBD group was noted (with no cases of hepatic failure), indicating that, although PBD is important in augmenting marginal FLRs, routine use may not be of benefit in larger FLRs.

There is generally a consensus among surgeons and gastroenterologists that PBD is indicated for small FLR and cholangitic patients. However, the literature supporting routine PBD in all patients with proximal obstructing biliary lesions has been more heterogeneous and lacking in RCTs. To help answer this question, Liu and colleagues[25] performed a systematic review of studies comparing PBD with no PBD in patients undergoing resection of HCCA. In analyzing postoperative morbidity, 1 prospective and 9 retrospective studies were identified. A total of 442 patients underwent PBD and 233 had no PBD. The rate of postoperative morbidity was significantly higher in the PBD group (36.4%–100% for the PBD group vs 28.6%–72.2% for the non-PBD group; odds ratio [OR], 1.67). When infectious complications were analyzed, the rate in the PBD group (18.2%–52.4%) was again significantly higher than in the nondrainage group (0%–27.6%; OR, 2.17). With regard to mortality, there was no significant difference between the PBD (13.2%) and non-PBD (13.9%) groups. Based on these data, the investigators concluded that PBD should be reserved for specific indications and that it may increase infectious complications. They did note that the heterogeneity of the studies (differing methods of drainage, varying duration of PBD) placed limitations on the conclusions, and that larger RCTs were needed.

Although there are several studies indicating that infectious complications may be increased by routine PBD in resectable proximal strictures,[26,27] many investigators (particularly in Japan and Korea), remain staunch advocates of PBD. They state that adopting strategies like bile replacement and preoperative probiotics may help decrease infectious complications.[28,29] They have also noted that normalization of hepatic function does not occur immediately and longer duration of PBD may be required to reap its benefits. Koyama and colleagues[30] showed that greater than 6 weeks of PBD can be required before normal hepatic mitochondrial function is restored, despite return of bilirubin levels to normal. Extending the PBD window raises several potential issues, including tube-related complications (in percutaneous drainage), cholangitis, and delay of potentially curative operations.

Sugawara and colleagues[31] recently published a retrospective review of 587 patients who underwent liver resection with hepaticojejunostomy for treatment of HCCA between 2001 and 2011. Most of these patients (N = 475) underwent PBD, and 112 did not. Only patients without jaundice (bilirubin <2.0 mg/dL) or without evidence of biliary dilatation in the FLR were left undrained. The method of PBD was predominantly percutaneous before 2005, after which time the preferred approach became nasobiliary drainage and percutaneous drainage was reserved for nasobiliary drainage failures. All patients had weekly bile cultures drawn and perioperative antibiotics were tailored according to culture results. Antibiotics were continued for 3 days after surgery. Patients were also treated with preoperative synbiotics for at least 2 weeks. All externally drained bile, regardless of culture positivity, was replaced either via oral or nasojejunal routes.

In comparing the PBD and non-PBD groups, the patients who underwent PBD had an increased likelihood to have more complex operations including hepatectomy combined with PD and venous or arterial resection. This finding may indicate more advanced tumors in the PBD group, and these patients had higher blood loss and need for transfusion, and longer operative times. With regard to overall morbidity and mortality, there was no significant difference between the two groups. When considering infectious complications, there was again no difference. The investigators concluded that, with rigorous perioperative routines, postoperative infectious complications need not be increased after PBD. This study did not present evidence of a distinct advantage in favor of PBD, and the rates of cholangitis were significantly higher in the PBD group (16% vs 0%; P<.001). There was no difference in rates of hepatic failure, which may be caused by the difference in patient characteristics between the PBD (mean presenting bilirubin of 7.7 mg/dL) and the undrained (presenting bilirubin of 0.9 mg/dL) groups.

The evidence in the debate over PBD in proximal bile duct strictures is less clear than for distal lesions. Patients with compromised FLR seem to benefit the most from PBD. There are infectious concerns with PBD that may be able to be mitigated through careful surveillance of bile cultures and use of adjunctive therapies. Percutaneous drainage does have a small, but real, risk of tumor seeding, therefore judicious use of PBD of the FLR in patients undergoing hepatobiliary resections is warranted.

Endoscopic Versus Percutaneous Drainage

In Europe and the Americas, PBD is achieved predominantly through either endoscopic or percutaneous means. Many Asian investigators have advocated nasobiliary drainage because it has a lower incidence of cholangitis, but the discomfort of having a nasal tube for several weeks has made this a less attractive option in Western countries.[1] Both ERCP and percutaneous transhepatic biliary drainage (PTBD) have strengths and weaknesses, as summarized in **Table 2**. In general, stenting of mid to distal bile duct strictures should be performed via ERCP unless this is technically not feasible because such lesions are readily accessible from an endoscopic approach. Restoration of bilioenteric continuity is more physiologic and avoids the inconvenience of an external drain. In contrast, proximal strictures are, in the author's opinion (BC), more easily accessed percutaneously and the risk for cholangitis seems to be lower than with ERCP stenting. High-quality rotational cholangiography is more readily performed, adding anatomic information that is valuable to operative planning even in some patients with prior magnetic resonance cholangiopancreatography. In addition, percutaneous drains are more easily appreciated during surgery when palpating the hilum and/or during the transection phase of the operation. Many surgeons use postoperative drainage across the biliary-enteric anastomoses by using the preoperatively placed percutaneous drain, and for this reason advocate preoperative drainage.

Plastic Versus Metal Stents

Both plastic and SEMSs have advantages and disadvantages.[35,36] Plastic stents are inexpensive, easy to place, and can be manipulated after placement. However, they are less durable and typically need to be replaced every 3 months to avoid stent obstruction and cholangitis. The need for repeat stent changes offsets much of the initial cost savings with plastic stent use. In contrast, metal stents are more durable and maintain patency for 12 months or longer. Once placed, they are difficult to

Table 2 Advantages and disadvantages of PTBD and ERCP in achieving PBD	
Advantages	**Disadvantages**
PTBD	
High success rate on first attempt[32] Quality of cholangiography Ability to selectively drain liver segments or multiple segments with multiple drains Easily palpated at surgery and can be easily used to stent across the new anastomoses	Higher complication rate, particularly severe complications like vascular injury[33] Risk for tumor seeding (4%)[33] Discomfort of external drain
ERCP	
Internal biliary drainage is more physiologic Lack of external tubes	Higher risk of cholangitis[34] More difficult to drain more proximal lesions or drain bilateral hilar strictures

manipulate endoscopically. Surgeons have traditionally been wary of using SEMS before resection because of concerns that SEMS placement may make the operation more technically challenging and may compromise the ability to achieve an R0 resection. Cavell and colleagues[10] compared their experience with plastic and SEMS in patients undergoing PD and found that, although there was an increased incidence of infectious complications in the SEMS group, there was no difference in margin negativity, local unresectability, mortality, or severe morbidity. SEMS should therefore not be contraindicated in candidates for PD, and should be the stent of choice in patients undergoing neoadjuvant therapy because its improved patency results in fewer stent-related disruptions to therapy. The long patency times also make SEMS preferable as a palliative option in unresectable patients. Plastic stents are better used when the diagnosis of malignancy is not clear and only short-term biliary drainage is required.

EA
The Case for Local Resection of Ampullary Neoplasms

Accounting for less than 5% of all new gastrointestinal neoplasms per year, lesions of the ampulla of Vater are rare but their management raises several challenges.[37] Although there is little debate that pancreaticoduodenectomy (PD) remains the preferred approach for periampullary adenocarcinomas, benign adenomas can undergo malignant transformation and therefore also require adequate treatment. Pancreaticoduodenectomy has previously been considered the gold standard for ampullary adenomas as well, but the morbidity of the procedure has led to increasing interest in more limited resections for treatment of benign lesions. From this interest, the local treatment strategies of surgical ampullectomy (SA) and EA have emerged as alternatives to PD.

Although SA has been established for more than a century as a potential alternative to PD, its adequacy in treating ampullary adenomas relative to PD has been controversial. Proponents of PD contrast the low rate of local recurrence of ampullary neoplasms after PD with the rate of local recurrence (up to 25%) seen in contemporary SA series (**Table 3**). Use of local resection strategies for the treatment of ampullary adenocarcinoma has been described in select situations, but these recurrence data combined with the possibility of lymph node metastasis even in T1 ampullary

| Table 3 | | | |
| **Results of studies for SA** | | | |
Author, Year	**N**	**Mortality/Morbidity (%)**	**Recurrence (%)**
Ceppa et al,[39] 2013	41	0/42	9
Winter et al,[54] 2010	15	0/33	20
Tien et al,[55] 2009	20	0/10	NR
Grobmyer et al,[56] 2008	29	3/45	8
Ouaissi et al,[57] 2006	26	0/8	15
Roggin et al,[58] 2005	29	0/31	NR
Demetriades et al,[59] 2006	20	0/10	0
Dixon et al,[60] 2005	19	0/37	25
Miossec et al,[61] 2004	8	0/75	0
Heidecke et al,[62] 2002	20	0/40	11
Posner et al,[63] 2000	21	0/62	11
Clary et al,[64] 2000	18	0/29	0

adenocarcinomas have led most investigators to promote SA primarily in the treatment of benign ampullary lesions.[38,39] Pancreaticoduodenectomy should, with rare exceptions (as in elderly patients with severe comorbidities), be the centerpiece in treating malignant ampullary lesions. In carefully selected benign ampullary lesions, local resection with either SA or EA may still be appropriate.

Critics of local approaches have stated that such selection cannot be made reliably from endoscopic forceps biopsy, because most series note that the accuracy of preoperative endoscopic biopsy is in the range of 62% to 90% and false-negative rates of 17% to 40%.[40–42] This discordance between preoperative and final surgical disorders can lead to inappropriate selection of patients for local excision even when targeting patients with presumed benign disorders. However, preoperative biopsy should not be the sole determinant of amenability to local resection. Although size has not been shown to correlate reliably with malignancy, other gross features like a soft, non-friable, and nonulcerated appearance are more likely to represent a benign disorder.[43] In cases in which the suspicion for malignancy is higher, endoscopic ultrasound (EUS) can provide more detailed anatomic detail and T and N staging that is superior to those of computed tomography (CT). Accuracy of EUS T and N staging is 78% to 84% and 50% to 100% respectively, compared with 5% to 24% and 33% to 59% for CT.[44] The addition of ERCP provides critical information regarding biliary and pancreatic duct involvement. In using gross appearance and EUS/ERCP findings to mitigate the high false-negative rate seen on endoscopic forceps biopsy, Irani and colleagues[45] applied the following exclusion criteria to local resection (EA): ulceration, friability, greater than 50% lateral extension, duodenal infiltration, and greater than 1-cm intraductal extension. By using these characteristics in conjunction with biopsy results, only 5% of lesions deemed to be resectable by EA ultimately had an invasive component on pathology.

The principal purported advantage of SA compared with the more complex PD is that its rates of mortality and morbidity should be favorable. The rates of mortality for SA (see **Table 3**) are superior to the generally accepted 2% to 3% mortality for PD. In comparing lengths of stay, Ceppa and colleagues[39] noted a 10-day length of stay for SA versus 19 days for comparable patients who had PD. Some studies have noted lower postoperative morbidity rates for SA compared with PD, but others (see **Table 3**) are roughly comparable between SA and PD. Regardless of overall rate, the complication profiles of these two procedures are different. Pancreatic leak and hemorrhage are major components of post-PD morbidity, whereas dehydration and pancreatitis are commonly noted complications after SA. The shorter length of stay for SA also suggests decreased severity of post-SA complications relative to those of PD.[39]

Given the potential advantages shown by SA, interest in endoscopic resections began to grow as advances in endoscopic technology made performance of EA technically possible.

Basic EA Technique

EA typically begins with inspection of the major and minor papillae using a side-viewing endoscope, because this allows more thorough visualization of the ampulla than front-viewing instruments. Once an ampullary disorder has been visually identified, EUS can be useful in more accurately assessing the lesion's size and relationship to adjacent structures.[46,47] Some investigators think that, for small (<1–2 cm), asymptomatic, and grossly benign-appearing ampullary lesions, EUS is not required before proceeding with EA.[45,48] Cholangiography and pancreatography provide important data regarding involvement of the pancreatic and common bile ducts and should routinely be performed. If involvement of the pancreatic or bile duct is observed, EUS should be performed to further evaluate the lesion.[48,49] After performing a modest sphincterotomy, most investigators suggest routine placement of pancreatic duct stents to minimize the risk of postprocedure pancreatitis.[42,48,50,51] Harewood and colleagues[51] performed a prospective randomized controlled trial to evaluate the effect of prophylactic pancreatic stent placement on post-EA pancreatitis. Of the 19 patients enrolled, 10 underwent pre-EA pancreatic stenting and 9 were assigned to the nonstented group. No patients in the stented group developed postprocedural pancreatitis and 3 of 9 nonstented patients (33%) developed pancreatitis ($P = .02$) with a median hospital stay of 2 days. Stent selection should focus on using small (3–5 Fr), short stents, largely because such stents are more likely to migrate out of the duct and pass spontaneously, eliminating the need for repeat endoscopy and stent retrieval.[48,51]

Once the anatomic features of the lesion have been assessed and it has been determined to be amenable to EA, resection is performed with a polypectomy snare. Some investigators advocate injecting a dilute epinephrine solution to create a submucosal fluid cushion that elevates the lesion and may aid in hemostasis.[52,53] Ampullary lesions should ideally be resected in an en bloc fashion using a polypectomy snare and applying blended current. Large lesions that cannot be resected en bloc (typically >2 cm) should be excised in a piecemeal fashion because this minimizes the risk of inadvertently involving deeper layers in the resection.[42,45,48] Any remaining adenomatous tissue can be ablated using an argon plasma coagulator or another thermal device.

EA Versus SA

Given that endoscopic interventions are even less invasive, the advantage of SA compared with PD in mortality, morbidity profile, and length of stay is extended even further with EA. The results of recent EA series are summarized in **Table 4**. Ceppa and colleagues[39] recently published the first retrospective comparison of outcomes between SA and EA. Over a 20-year period, 68 patients who underwent EA and 41 who were treated with SA were identified. With the exception of higher rates of morbid obesity and hyperlipidemia in the EA group, there was no significant difference in comorbid conditions between the EA and SA groups. Patients who underwent SA had a higher incidence of pancreatitis, jaundice, and cholangitis as presenting symptoms. Patients were considered for EA if preampullectomy biopsy was benign and there were no features concerning for malignancy on endoscopic, EUS, or ERCP examination. By combining histologic studies with various endoscopic modalities, there were no unexpected cases of malignancy observed on final pathology in the EA group. The rates of margin positivity (20% EA vs 10% SA) and reoperation/reintervention (26% EA vs 15% SA) trended toward being higher in the EA group, but this did not reach significance. The principal reason for repeat intervention in the EA group was margin positivity, followed by postprocedure bleeding. No EA required more than a second endoscopy to achieve margin negativity. Reoperations in the SA group were the result of wound dehiscence, incisional hernia, and need for feeding tube placement.

There were no mortalities in either group, but there was a clear difference in length of stay and postoperative morbidity. By avoiding a laparotomy, EA can be safely performed as an outpatient procedure giving the EA group (average length of stay 0.6 days) a significant advantage over SA (10 days) and PD (19 days). Morbidity was also significantly lower in the EA group (18% vs 42%; $P = .0006$). Post-EA pancreatitis and hemorrhage were each observed in 9% of patients. The most common

Table 4
Results of recent studies of EA

Author, Year	N	Mortality/ Morbidity (%)	Recurrence (%)	Common Complications
Ceppa et al,[39] 2013	68	0/18	20	Pancreatitis 9%, hemorrhage 9%
Laleman et al,[49] 2013	71	0/25	18	Pancreatitis 15%, hemorrhage 12%, cholangitis 5%
Salmi et al,[65] 2012	43	0/18	NR	Pancreatitis 10%, hemorrhage 5%, perforation 3%
Patel et al,[66] 2011	38	0/16	16	Pancreatitis 8%, hemorrhage 5%
Jeanniard-Malet et al,[67] 2011	42	0/21	18	Pancreatitis 15%, hemorrhage 7%, cholangitis 2%
Irani et al,[45] 2009	102	0/21	8	Pancreatitis 10%, hemorrhage 5%, stenosis 3%, perforation 2%
Jung et al,[68] 2009	22	0/22	45	Pancreatitis 18%, hemorrhage 5%
Boix et al,[69] 2009	21	0/24	74	Pancreatitis 19%, hemorrhage 5%
Katsinelos et al,[70] 2006	14	0/14	18	Pancreatitis 7%, hemorrhage 7%
Bohnacker et al,[71] 2005	106	0/NR	15	Pancreatitis 12%, hemorrhage 13%
Catalano et al,[72] 2004	103	0/10	20	Pancreatitis 5%, stenosis 3%, bleeding 2%
Cheng et al,[73] 2004	27	0/15	33	Pancreatitis 9%, hemorrhage 7%, perforation 2%
Norton et al,[74] 2002	26	0/27	10	Pancreatitis 15%, stenosis 8%, perforation 4%
Desilets et al,[52] 2001	13	0/8	10	Pancreatitis 8%
Zadorova et al,[75] 2001	16	0/13	19	Pancreatitis 13%, hemorrhage 13%

complications after SA were dehydration requiring readmission (12%), wound infection (12%), and symptomatic pancreatitis (10%).

In using a combination of histologic, gross, EUS, and ERCP features, the investigators concluded that benign ampullary lesions could be appropriately selected for local resection. The morbidity, length of stay, and readmission advantages in favor of EA make it the treatment of choice for benign lesions amenable to endoscopic treatment. The investigators noted that there was a higher rate of margin positivity and reintervention in the EA group, but that the advantages of EA likely outweigh this. A second endoscopy to achieve clear margins is generally preferable to a repeat laparotomy or extended length of stay, especially considering the benign disorders typically encountered with EA. Furthermore, should the final pathologic specimen reveal an invasive component after EA, this does not preclude definitive treatment with PD.

Because of the advantages of EA, the investigators reviewed why the patients in the SA group were treated surgically rather than endoscopically. Ten lesions (24%) treated by SA were not considered for EA because they were done before 2000, when EA was not being performed routinely at our hospital. Twenty-two of the remaining 31 lesions had anatomic features that were unfavorable for EA: 17 had proximal extension, 3 were too large for snare resection, and 2 appeared to involve the sphincter. The remaining 9 patients were treated by SA because the lesion could not be identified at the time of attempted EA, because of malignancy on biopsy (and patient refusing PD), or because they required an operation for an additional indication.

INTRALUMINAL THERAPIES FOR CHOLANGIOCARCINOMA

Although surgical resection remains the only potentially curative treatment of primary hepatobiliary tumors, these tumors are often unresectable at the time of presentation, particularly in the case of hilar cholangiocarcinomas. Systemic therapies typically provide limited survival and palliative benefits, and several adjunctive therapies have been tried in attempts to improve outcomes for unresectable cholangiocarcinomas. Both external beam radiation and intraluminal brachytherapy techniques have yielded mixed results. Some early studies did not show a survival advantage for brachytherapy alone, but several more recent reports suggest that brachytherapy in combination with external beam radiation offers improved stent patency as well as improved survival.[76–78] Shinohara and colleagues[79] used the Surveillance, Epidemiology, and End Results (SEER) database to examine a total of 193 patients with cholangiocarcinoma who were treated with brachytherapy. Median survival was 11 months in patients treated with brachytherapy, compared with 4 months without brachytherapy. Brachytherapy was associated with better survival on multivariate analysis, and, on subset analysis, the investigators thought that this was driven predominantly by the combined brachytherapy/external beam group rather than the brachytherapy-only group.

Photodynamic therapy (PDT) offers another intraluminal palliative option in the treatment of locally unresectable cholangiocarcinoma. PDT relies on the preferential accumulation of photosensitizing drugs in malignant cells rather than normal bile duct cells. After administration of the photosensitizing agent (typically a hematoporphyrin derivative), ERCP or percutaneous biliary access is obtained so that a specific wavelength of light energy can be delivered via an endoluminal fiber that is positioned across the lesion.[80,81] Activation of the photosensitizing agent by light energy results in cell death via several incompletely understood mechanisms, including induction of apoptosis secondary to free radical formation, tissue hypoxia, and immunomodulatory effects including increase in interleukin 6 production.

These tumoricidal effects are most pronounced within a 4-mm to 5-mm depth, and, once a tumor depth of 7 to 9 mm is reached, only incomplete tumor eradication is achieved. For this reason, patients with bulky tumors, as well as those with distant metastases, are typically not ideal to be treated with PDT. Given these factors, several appropriate indications of PDT have been suggested[82]:

1. Neoadjuvant or palliative treatment of sclerosing variant or superficial spreading type with the papillary variant
2. After resection for treatment of positive margins

Leggett and colleagues[83] recently published a meta-analysis of studies comparing PDT plus biliary stenting with stenting alone. Length of survival was significantly increased in the patients treated with PDT, and, although the sizes of the studies included were modest, the investigators thought that the current body of evidence suggests greater than a 10-month survival advantage in favor of palliative PDT. This meta-analysis included the only 2 RCTs performed to date. The first was by Ortner and colleagues,[84] comparing 20 patients who underwent combined PDT and stenting with 19 who underwent stenting alone for unresectable cholangiocarcinoma. Median survival in the PDT group was 493 days versus 98 days for the stent-only group (P<.0001). The investigators also noted that the PDT group had an improvement in Karnofsky performance status compared with the stent-only patients. The study was terminated early because the investigators thought that the decisive advantage of PDT compared with stenting alone made continued randomization unethical. A second RCT, performed by Zoepf and colleagues,[85] randomized 32 patients with unresectable cholangiocarcinoma to PDT plus stenting or stenting alone. Median survival in the PDT group was 21 months compared with 7 months for drainage alone (P = .0109). The advantage in quality of life that was observed by Ortner and colleagues[84] was not duplicated by this RCT, but the baseline performance status of patients in both groups was higher in the study by Zoepf and colleagues[85] than in the study by Ortner and colleagues.[84]

Beyond survival advantage, there is also some evidence that stent patency is improved with PDT. In a retrospective study of 33 patients with unresectable cholangiocarcinoma, Lee and colleagues[86] found that stent patency was significantly longer when PDT was combined with stenting versus stenting alone (median 244 ± 66 days vs 177 ± 45 days; P = .002). The investigators suggested that the ability of PDT to destroy cancer cells and lessen cholestasis may have contributed to stent patency. Cheon and colleagues similarly found that median stent patency time was longer in patients treated with PDT plus stenting (215 days vs 181 days; P = .018). With the improvement in survival and stent patency, intraluminal ablative therapies are useful palliative options in patients with unresectable cholangiocarcinoma.

PERCUTANEOUS ABLATIVE THERAPIES FOR PRIMARY LIVER TUMORS

HCCs account for about 90% of all primary liver tumors and are the fifth most common cancer worldwide. Surgical resection can result in improved survival for patients with HCC, but less than 20% of patients meet appropriate criteria for resection, limited often by tumor burden and underlying liver disease. Sorafenib has been shown to improve survival in patients with advanced HCC, but outcomes are still dismal with systemic therapy alone.[87] Although in many ways transplantation offers the ideal approach to HCC, the number of transplant candidates is limited by organ availability as well as age and other comorbidities. These concerns have spurred interest in local-regional transarterial and ablative therapies. Early ablative strategies relied on injection of ethanol or acetic acid to chemically ablate primary and metastatic liver tumors. Thermal ablative methods have largely replaced chemical approaches after several reports and RCTs showed the superiority of thermal ablation to percutaneous ethanol injection in local control and overall survival.[88,89] Radiofrequency (RFA) and microwave ablation (MWA) have largely supplanted cryoablation as the preferred thermal ablative modalities, largely because of their improved local control and morbidity profiles.[90]

RFA creates protein denaturation and cell death by creating extreme heat. The heat is generated as a result of an alternating current that results in molecular and ionic friction. As the temperature increases, tissue charring and desiccation occur. The size of the ablation zone depends on several factors including current, duration of ablation, and the amount of heat transmitted through the tissue. Heat loss through convection can be amplified by local blood flow (the heat sink effect), and as a result ablating near large vessels can result in incomplete ablations or thrombosis of the vessel.[91] There is some evidence, both in experimental animal models and in clinical studies, that vascular occlusion may help achieve more complete ablation, particularly when used for large tumors.[92] Animal studies have shown that the increased intra-abdominal pressure associated with laparoscopy can reduce hepatic flow and that higher pressures are associated with larger ablation defects.[93] In surgical approaches to RFA, the Pringle maneuver provides excellent vascular occlusion. Although there is no access to the hilum in the percutaneous approach, vascular occlusion is achievable via angiography and balloon catheter occlusion with similar increases in ablation defects.[94]

MWA

The heat generation and tissue destruction achieved by MWA occurs through an active heating process that depends on water and other dielectric molecules that respond to the electromagnetic field created by the microwave antenna.[95] Vibratory energy and heat are produced as water molecules rapidly change their orientation to match the electromagnetic field. Because the coagulative necrosis is generated by an electromagnetic field rather than the flow of current, rapid and homogeneous heating of tissue occurs. Advocates of MWA think that these characteristics contribute to faster, larger, and more predictable ablation zones compared with monopolar RFA, and that they decrease the impact of heat sinking.[95]

Several clinical trials have evaluated the efficacy of MWA in treating HCC. A phase II trial performed by Iannitti and colleagues[96] enrolled 87 patients whose liver tumors (both metastatic and primary tumors were included in the study) were treated with MWA. A total of 224 lesions with a mean diameter of 3.6 cm were treated. The overall mortality was 2.3% with no procedure-related deaths and the local recurrence rate was 2.7% at 19 months of follow-up. Shibata and colleagues[97] performed a randomized trial in 72 patients with small HCCs and reported that there was no significant difference in achieving complete ablation between MWA (89%) and RFA (96%, $P = .26$), although it required significantly more treatment sessions to achieve this with MWA than with RFA (2.4 vs 1.1; $P<.001$). There was no significant difference in morbidity or recurrence between the two groups (RFA 8% vs MWA 17%; $P = .2$). Most series to date have been smaller, single-institution studies, and, although there is some variability in the rates of local recurrence and morbidity, these rates seem to be roughly comparable with outcomes observed with historical RFA data.[95,98–100]

Although there are no data at present that clearly establish one method as superior to the other, MWA does offer some physical advantages compared with RFA. The amount of heat generated and the speed of ablation are greater in MWA, allowing a larger ablation zone and potentially the ability to more effectively treat larger tumors. Furthermore, MWA seems to be less effected by issues of heat sink, and thus may be better suited to treat lesions near vessels. Although MWA is an effective and safe ablative strategy that seems to be comparable with RFA, this article is confined to RFA because it is the current standard and it has the largest collection of safety and efficacy data.

Selection Criteria/Assessing Response

Candidates for RFA are typically in one of the following categories: (1) high-risk surgical candidates secondary to underlying liver disease or medical comorbidities,

(2) technically unresectable disease because of anatomic distribution or inadequate FLR volume, (3) candidates for liver transplantation who need local control as a bridge to transplantation.[101] For patients in the first 2 categories, RFA often represents definitive treatment. Local recurrence and survival are determined by several factors, the most critical of which is size. RFA can provide excellent local control for small lesions. Livraghi and colleagues[102] used RFA to treated 218 patients with small (<2 cm), technically resectable HCCs. At a median follow-up of 31 months, sustained complete response was seen in 97.2% of patients and the 5-year survival was 68.5%. As lesions become larger and begin to exceed the size of the ablation zone, it becomes increasingly difficult to achieve complete tumor necrosis. Lesions more than 5 cm in diameter have higher recurrence rates, largely because the overlapping ablation zones required to achieve complete tumor necrosis is technically more difficult to achieve.

Tumor location also plays an important role in determining appropriateness of RFA. Caution must be exercised when treating tumors situated close to major bile ducts because damage to these structures can lead to biliary stricture or fistula. Treating tumors located near large blood vessels is problematic for issues related to heat sinking, as noted earlier. In addition to the risk of incomplete treatment, complications related to venous thrombosis can occur.

As is discussed later in greater detail, RFA can provide local control for patients with HCC with tumor burden that is within transplantation criteria. The use of RFA can provide local control while the patient is awaiting organ availability and has thus been used as a bridge to transplantation. A prospective study by Porrett and colleagues[103] comparing the use of locoregional therapies as bridge to transplantation versus no pretransplant therapy failed to show a benefit for pretransplant treatment. However, the wait times for transplant were short (2–6 months) and this may in part contribute to the result. DuBay and colleagues[104] examined patients within Milan Criteria undergoing transplants for HCC between 1999 and 2007. Seventy-seven patients were treated with pretransplant RFA, whereas 93 received no treatment. There was no difference in 5-year survival or tumor-free survival between the two groups despite a longer median wait time in the RFA group (9.5 months vs 5 months), suggesting that RFA can provide adequate local control while awaiting organ availability. Regions with longer pretransplant wait times are therefore most likely to benefit from bridging pretransplant locoregional therapy.

Laparoscopic Versus Percutaneous Ablation

The optimal technique for delivering ablative therapy depends on both on institutional factors and tumor characteristics. Like most medical procedures, the appropriate technique is tied closely to the training and expertise of the practicing physicians. In the ideal setting, a single institution would have both surgeons and interventional radiologists experienced with ablative techniques, allowing appropriate selection on a case-by-case basis after discussion at a multidisciplinary tumor board. However, this is not feasible at all hospitals.

Each technique (percutaneous, laparoscopic, and open) has its individual strengths and weaknesses, as summarized in **Table 5**. In general, the least invasive technique is the best choice and open ablation should be reserved for cases in which laparotomy is required for another indication. Although the limited invasiveness of percutaneous ablation makes it most attractive, there are some disadvantages to this approach. Percutaneous ablation has been associated with thermal injury to adjacent structures when treating subcapsular and peripheral lesions, and is thus limited by tumor location. Proponents of the percutaneous approach think that this risk can be mitigated through the use of specialized techniques. Diaphragmatic injury when treating hepatic

Table 5
Advantages and weaknesses of different ablative approaches

Technique	Advantages	Weaknesses
Percutaneous	Least invasive Can perform without general anesthesia Outpatient/overnight hospitalization Potentially lower cost[106]	Potential injury to adjacent structures when treating superficial/peripheral/dome lesions May have increased local recurrence rates
Laparoscopic	Shorter hospital stay and less invasive than open Increased sensitivity of laparoscopic ultrasound rather than percutaneous ultrasound and CT[107,108] Direct visual inspection of peritoneal cavity Lower local recurrence compared with percutaneous Ability to treat larger tumors (>5 cm) Ability to decrease heat sink effect via Pringle-induced and pneumoperitoneum-induced decreased hepatic perfusion	Requires general anesthesia Increased cost
Open	Greatest access to abdomen/ease of Pringle Ease of placing probe Decreases potential track-seeding risk	Most invasive Longest hospital stay

dome lesions and injury to adjacent intra-abdominal organs and skin when treating superficial/peripheral lesions can be decreased by the instillation of pneumoperitoneum or artificial ascites before ablation.[105]

Local recurrence rates are a concern for all modes of ablation. The data from individual studies comparing percutaneous and surgical approaches have been mixed, with some showing an advantage for laparoscopic ablations and others showing no difference. Mulier and colleagues[92] performed a meta-analysis of local recurrence rates after undergoing RFA. Ninety-five series with a total of 5224 treated tumors were included in the analysis. Ablation was performed percutaneously in 67.9%, laparoscopically in 11.6%, and as an open procedure in 20.5%. Local recurrence occurred significantly more frequently after percutaneous ablation compared with laparoscopic cases, regardless of tumor size (16.4% vs 5.8%; $P<.001$). The investigators offered several explanations for this difference, the first being that laparoscopic ultrasound offered superior resolution to CT and transcutaneous ultrasound.[62,63] The improved visualization allows more precise electrode placement, as well as greater appreciation of margins and satellite lesions. There is also greater flexibility in placing the electrodes via a surgical approach and this further increases precision of probe placement as well as allowing parallel reinsertions and overlapping ablation zones when required.

Local anesthesia (with or without sedation) was also associated with higher local failure rates (14.3% vs 6.2% for general anesthesia; $P<.001$). When this analysis was repeated only with tumors treated percutaneously, there was no significant difference. Despite this, the investigators hypothesized that the increased pain and incomplete respiratory hold in local anesthesia may result in suboptimal ablation. The increased recurrence rate in percutaneous ablations may in part be caused by the mode of anesthesia used, and there may therefore be a benefit to using general anesthesia even in the percutaneous approach for difficult lesions that may need multiple RFA treatments and subcapsular lesions that are often more painful to ablate.

Long-term Outcomes Versus Resection

RFA and other ablative therapies initially began as palliative therapies for patients who were not candidates for extirpation. Surgical resection has been considered the gold standard in HCC treatment and the guidelines discussed earlier all consider ablation as an adjunction therapy rather than a competitive alternative to resection. The growing experience with RFA has resulted in a body of literature examining the survival and local recurrence implications of RFA as they relate to resection. The results of RCTs comparing RFA with resection are summarized in **Table 6**. An additional RCT was performed by Lu and colleagues[109] but is not discussed here because it was not published in English. The data from these RCTs are conflicting. Chen and colleagues[110] studied 161 patients with solitary tumors less than 5 cm in size. Seventy-one patients were treated by percutaneous RFA and 90 were treated by resection. There were no significant differences in overall survival (OS) or disease-free survival

Table 6
Summary of RCTs comparing RFA with resection

Author	Inclusion Criteria	N	Results
Feng et al,[111] 2012	<4 cm max <2 tumors Childs A/B	RFA 84 SR 84	1- and 3-y OS: SR- 96.0%, 74.8% RFA- 93.1%, 67.2% ($P = .342$)
			RFS, 1- and 3-y: SR- 90.6%, 61.1% RFA- 86.2, 49.6 ($P = .122$)
Huang et al,[112] 2010	Within Milan Criteria Childs A/B	Single tumor <3 cm RFA 57 SR 45	Single tumor <3 cm OS 3-, 5-y RFA 77.2%, 61.4% SR 95.6%, 82.2% ($P = .03$)
		Single tumor >3 cm and <5 cm RFA 27 SR 44	Single tumor >3 cm and <5 cm OS 3-, 5-y RFA- 66.7%, 51.5% SR- 95.5%, 72.3% ($P = .046$)
		Multifocal <3 cm RFA 31 SR 26	Multifocal <3 cm OS 3-, 5-y RFA- 58.1%, 45.2% SR- 80.8%, 69.2% ($P = .042$)
Chen et al,[110] 2006	<5 cm Single tumor	RFA 71 SR 90	OS 1-, 3- and 4 y RFA 95.8%, 71.4%, 67.9% SR 93.3%, 73.4%, 64.0%
			RFS 1-, 3- and 4 y RFA 85.9%, 64.1%, 46.4% SR 86.6%, 69%, 51.6%

Abbreviations: DFS, disease-free survival; OS, overall survival; RES, resection; RFS, recurrence free survival; SR, surgical resection.

(DFS) between the two groups. When stratifying by tumor size, there was no difference either for small tumors (<3 cm) or for those between 3 cm and 5 cm. There was an increased incidence of major morbidity in the resection group (55% vs 4%; $P<.05$), as well as increased length of stay and postoperative pain. Feng and colleagues[111] similarly found no significant differences in OS or DFS between 84 patients treated with RFA and 84 undergoing resection. Both of these studies concluded that percutaneous RFA may achieve oncologic equivalency to surgical resection in selected patients.

However, the RCT performed by Huang and colleagues[112] found that, in patients with Child A or B cirrhosis and tumor burden within Milan Criteria, surgical resection offered an advantage. This advantage was preserved regardless of tumor size or multifocality. These conflicting reports make it difficult to state confidently that resection is superior oncologically to RFA for small HCC lesions. Cucchetti and colleagues[113] explored this matter further in a systematic review that included the previously mentioned RCTs as well as 16 retrospective studies. For small tumors (<2 cm), local control rates were similar to those of surgical resection. For larger tumors (>3 cm) there was a higher local failure rate.

Given that most patients diagnosed with HCC are not surgical candidates, either because of distribution of disease or underlying liver dysfunction, ablative therapies are critical tools in the armamentarium of HCC treatments. Ablation can provide excellent local control for small tumors and, in patients who have underlying cirrhosis, serve as a bridge to transplantation. Given the presently available data, surgical resection should still be considered the oncologic benchmark and preferred option in patients with resectable HCC, particularly for large lesions (>3 cm), for which achieving complete ablation is more technically demanding. Even peripheral/superficial lesions that require only a modest volume resection are probably best treated with resection through a laparoscopic or minimally invasive approach. However, there are certain circumstances in which RFA or MWA can be considered as a first-line therapy for technically resectable disease. Small, central tumors that would otherwise require formal or large-volume resections may be treated by ablation rather than resection, particularly in patients with multiple medical comorbidities. It is in these patients in whom the limited morbidity and invasiveness, as well as the preservation of hepatic function, is most advantageous.

SUMMARY

Primary tumors of the liver and bile duct are best understood as a group of heterogeneous diseases that require a tailored approach to their management. Surgical extirpation is the gold standard of treatment and usually represents the best chance for cure, but resection of these tumors typically requires challenging operations that carry substantial risk for postoperative complications. Advances in percutaneous and endoscopic techniques have allowed better preoperative selection and optimization, as well as alternatives to traditionally morbid surgical therapies. However, these advances are controversial.

With regard to PBD, most studies do not support routine PBD in patients with distal bile duct strictures who are candidates for pancreaticoduodenectomy. When required, PBD should be performed by ERCP and should be reserved for patients with cholangitis, severe hyperbilirubinemia, and those undergoing neoadjuvant therapy. In patients with more proximal tumors who require combined hepatic and bile duct resection for cure, the risk for postoperative hepatic failure requires adequate optimization of the FLR. For small FLRs, PBD is mandatory, but in those with larger remnant volume the benefit is not as clear and may carry a higher rate of infectious complications.

EA allows local resection of ampullary lesions and avoids the morbidity of PD. With rare exceptions, it should be reserved for benign tumors given that it has higher recurrence rates than PD. SA should typically be reserved for patients who have a benign ampullary mass that is not technically resectable endoscopically, or for patients with small cancers that are not candidates for PD.

Ablative techniques can be used as palliative therapy; as a bridge to transplantation; or, in select situations, as definitive therapy. Local control and survival depend largely on tumor size, and for very small tumors RFA rivals the local recurrence rates achieved by surgery. Although resection is still the gold standard and should be the preferred approach when possible (even for small tumors), RFA can be used as definitive therapy or as a bridge to transplantation in patients who have severe underlying liver dysfunction or medical comorbidities that contraindicate a major hepatectomy.

REFERENCES

1. Iacono C, Ruzzenente A, Campagnaro T, et al. Role of preoperative biliary drainage in jaundiced patients who are candidates for pancreatoduodenectomy or hepatic resection: highlights and drawbacks. Ann Surg 2013; 257(2):191–204.
2. Smith RC, Pooley M, George CR, et al. Preoperative percutaneous transhepatic internal drainage in obstructive jaundice: a randomized, controlled trial examining renal function. Surgery 1985;97(6):641–8.
3. Denning DA, Ellison EC, Carey LC. Preoperative percutaneous transhepatic biliary decompression lowers operative morbidity in patients with obstructive jaundice. Am J Surg 1981;141(1):61–5.
4. Lygidakis NJ, van der Heyde MN, Lubbers MJ. Evaluation of preoperative biliary drainage in the surgical management of pancreatic head carcinoma. Acta Chir Scand 1987;153(11–12):665–8.
5. Gundry SR, Strodel WE, Knol JA, et al. Efficacy of preoperative biliary tract decompression in patients with obstructive jaundice. Arch Surg 1984;119(6): 703–8.
6. Sewnath ME, Karsten TM, Prins MH, et al. A meta-analysis on the efficacy of preoperative biliary drainage for tumors causing obstructive jaundice. Ann Surg 2002;236(1):17–27.
7. Kim JH, Won HJ, Shin YM, et al. Radiofrequency ablation for the treatment of primary intrahepatic cholangiocarcinoma. AJR Am J Roentgenol 2011;196(2): W205–9.
8. van der Gaag NA, Rauws EA, van Eijck CH, et al. Preoperative biliary drainage for cancer of the head of the pancreas. N Engl J Med 2010;362(2):129–37.
9. Watanabe F, Noda H, Kamiyama H, et al. Risk factors for intra-abdominal infection after pancreaticoduodenectomy - a retrospective analysis to evaluate the significance of preoperative biliary drainage and postoperative pancreatic fistula. Hepatogastroenterology 2012;59(116):1270 3.
10. Cavell LK, Allen PJ, Vinoya C, et al. Biliary self-expandable metal stents do not adversely affect pancreaticoduodenectomy. Am J Gastroenterol 2013;108(7): 1168–73.
11. Ngu W, Jones M, Neal CP, et al. Preoperative biliary drainage for distal biliary obstruction and post-operative infectious complications. ANZ J Surg 2013; 83(4):280–6.
12. Garcea G, Chee W, Ong SL, et al. Preoperative biliary drainage for distal obstruction: the case against revisited. Pancreas 2010;39(2):119–26.

13. Mezhir JJ, Brennan MF, Baser RE, et al. A matched case-control study of preoperative biliary drainage in patients with pancreatic adenocarcinoma: routine drainage is not justified. J Gastrointest Surg 2009;13(12):2163–9.
14. Coates JM, Beal SH, Russo JE, et al. Negligible effect of selective preoperative biliary drainage on perioperative resuscitation, morbidity, and mortality in patients undergoing pancreaticoduodenectomy. Arch Surg 2009;144(9):841–7.
15. Srivastava S, Sikora SS, Kumar A, et al. Outcome following pancreaticoduodenectomy in patients undergoing preoperative biliary drainage. Dig Surg 2001; 18(5):381–7.
16. Martignoni ME, Wagner M, Krahenbuhl L, et al. Effect of preoperative biliary drainage on surgical outcome after pancreatoduodenectomy. Am J Surg 2001;181(1):52–9 [discussion: 87].
17. Pisters PW, Hudec WA, Hess KR, et al. Effect of preoperative biliary decompression on pancreaticoduodenectomy-associated morbidity in 300 consecutive patients. Ann Surg 2001;234(1):47–55.
18. Baron TH, Kozarek RA. Preoperative biliary stents in pancreatic cancer–proceed with caution. N Engl J Med 2010;362(2):170–2.
19. Jaganmohan S, Lynch PM, Raju RP, et al. Endoscopic management of duodenal adenomas in familial adenomatous polyposis–a single-center experience. Dig Dis Sci 2012;57(3):732–7.
20. Gruttadauria S, Li Petri S, Echeverri GJ, et al. Liver abscess and septic shock as an unusual complication after endoscopic ampullectomy. Endoscopy 2011; 43(Suppl 2 UCTN):E158–9.
21. Regimbeau JM, Fuks D, Le Treut YP, et al. Surgery for hilar cholangiocarcinoma: a multi-institutional update on practice and outcome by the AFC-HC study group. J Gastrointest Surg 2011;15(3):480–8.
22. Hemming AW, Reed AI, Fujita S, et al. Surgical management of hilar cholangiocarcinoma. Ann Surg 2005;241(5):693–9 [discussion: 699–702].
23. Rocha FG, Matsuo K, Blumgart LH, et al. Hilar cholangiocarcinoma: the Memorial Sloan-Kettering Cancer Center experience. J Hepatobiliary Pancreat Sci 2010;17(4):490–6.
24. Kennedy TJ, Yopp A, Qin Y, et al. Role of preoperative biliary drainage of liver remnant prior to extended liver resection for hilar cholangiocarcinoma. HPB (Oxford) 2009;11(5):445–51.
25. Liu F, Li Y, Wei Y, et al. Preoperative biliary drainage before resection for hilar cholangiocarcinoma: whether or not? A systematic review. Dig Dis Sci 2011; 56(3):663–72.
26. Hochwald SN, Burke EC, Jarnagin WR, et al. Association of preoperative biliary stenting with increased postoperative infectious complications in proximal cholangiocarcinoma. Arch Surg 1999;134(3):261–6.
27. Ferrero A, Lo Tesoriere R, Vigano L, et al. Preoperative biliary drainage increases infectious complications after hepatectomy for proximal bile duct tumor obstruction. World J Surg 2009;33(2):318–25.
28. Kamiya S, Nagino M, Kanazawa H, et al. The value of bile replacement during external biliary drainage: an analysis of intestinal permeability, integrity, and microflora. Ann Surg 2004;239(4):510–7.
29. Sugawara G, Nagino M, Nishio H, et al. Perioperative synbiotic treatment to prevent postoperative infectious complications in biliary cancer surgery: a randomized controlled trial. Ann Surg 2006;244(5):706–14.
30. Koyama K, Takagi Y, Ito K, et al. Experimental and clinical studies on the effect of biliary drainage in obstructive jaundice. Am J Surg 1981;142(2):293–9.

31. Sugawara G, Ebata T, Yokoyama Y, et al. The effect of preoperative biliary drainage on infectious complications after hepatobiliary resection with cholangiojejunostomy. Surgery 2013;153(2):200–10.

32. Kanai M, Nimura Y, Kamiya J, et al. Preoperative intrahepatic segmental cholangitis in patients with advanced carcinoma involving the hepatic hilus. Surgery 1996;119(5):498–504.

33. Kawakami H, Kuwatani M, Eto K, et al. Endoscopic nasobiliary drainage should be initially selected for preoperative biliary drainage in patients with perihilar bile duct cancer. World J Surg 2012;36(9):2265–6 [author reply: 2267–8].

34. Rerknimitr R, Angsuwatcharakon P, Ratanachu-ek T, et al. Asia-Pacific consensus recommendations for endoscopic and interventional management of hilar cholangiocarcinoma. J Gastroenterol Hepatol 2013;28(4): 593–607.

35. Kaassis M, Boyer J, Dumas R, et al. Plastic or metal stents for malignant stricture of the common bile duct? Results of a randomized prospective study. Gastrointest Endosc 2003;57(2):178–82.

36. Soderlund C, Linder S. Covered metal versus plastic stents for malignant common bile duct stenosis: a prospective, randomized, controlled trial. Gastrointest Endosc 2006;63(7):986–95.

37. Branum GD, Pappas TN, Meyers WC. The management of tumors of the ampulla of Vater by local resection. Ann Surg 1996;224(5):621–7.

38. Askew J, Connor S. Review of the investigation and surgical management of resectable ampullary adenocarcinoma. HPB 2013. [Epub ahead of print].

39. Ceppa EP, Burbridge RA, Rialon KL, et al. Endoscopic versus surgical ampullectomy: an algorithm to treat disease of the ampulla of Vater. Ann Surg 2013; 257(2):315–22.

40. Arendt LM, McCready J, Keller PJ, et al. Obesity promotes breast cancer by CCL2-mediated macrophage recruitment and angiogenesis. Cancer Res 2013;73(19):6080–93.

41. Seewald L, Hurley L, Crane LA, et al. Things are not as bad as they seem: physicians' ability to predict their clinical practice when a new vaccine becomes available. Health Policy 2013;8(4):71–85.

42. Patel R, Varadarajulu S, Wilcox CM. Endoscopic ampullectomy: techniques and outcomes. J Clin Gastroenterol 2012;46(1):8–15.

43. Seewald S, Omar S, Soehendra N. Endoscopic resection of tumors of the ampulla of Vater: how far up and how deep down can we go? Gastrointest Endosc 2006;63(6):789–91.

44. Menzel J, Hoepffner N, Sulkowski U, et al. Polypoid tumors of the major duodenal papilla: preoperative staging with intraductal US, EUS, and CT–a prospective, histopathologically controlled study. Gastrointest Endosc 1999; 49(3 Pt 1):349–57.

45. Irani S, Arai A, Ayub K, et al. Papillectomy for ampullary neoplasm: results of a single referral center over a 10-year period. Gastrointest Endosc 2009;70(5): 923–32.

46. Skordilis P, Mouzas IA, Dimoulios PD, et al. Is endosonography an effective method for detection and local staging of the ampullary carcinoma? A prospective study. BMC Surg 2002;2:1.

47. Roberts KJ, McCulloch N, Sutcliffe R, et al. Endoscopic ultrasound assessment of lesions of the ampulla of Vater is of particular value in low-grade dysplasia. HPB (Oxford) 2013;15(1):18–23.

48. Baillie J. Endoscopic ampullectomy. Am J Gastroenterol 2005;100(11):2379–81.

49. Laleman W, Verreth A, Topal B, et al. Endoscopic resection of ampullary lesions: a single-center 8-year retrospective cohort study of 91 patients with long-term follow-up. Surg Endosc 2013;27(10):3865–76.
50. Baillie J. Endoscopic ampullectomy: does pancreatic stent placement make it safer? Gastrointest Endosc 2005;62(3):371–3.
51. Harewood GC, Pochron NL, Gostout CJ. Prospective, randomized, controlled trial of prophylactic pancreatic stent placement for endoscopic snare excision of the duodenal ampulla. Gastrointest Endosc 2005;62(3):367–70.
52. Desilets DJ, Dy RM, Ku PM, et al. Endoscopic management of tumors of the major duodenal papilla: refined techniques to improve outcome and avoid complications. Gastrointest Endosc 2001;54(2):202–8.
53. Pandolfi M, Martino M, Gabbrielli A. Endoscopic treatment of ampullary adenomas. JOP 2008;9(1):1–8.
54. Winter JM, Cameron JL, Olino K, et al. Clinicopathologic analysis of ampullary neoplasms in 450 patients: implications for surgical strategy and long-term prognosis. J Gastrointest Surg 2010;14(2):379–87.
55. Tien YW, Yeh CC, Wang SP, et al. Is blind pancreaticoduodenectomy justified for patients with ampullary neoplasms? J Gastrointest Surg 2009;13(9): 1666–73.
56. Grobmyer SR, Stasik CN, Draganov P, et al. Contemporary results with ampullectomy for 29 "benign" neoplasms of the ampulla. J Am Coll Surg 2008; 206(3):466–71.
57. Ouaissi M, Panis Y, Sielezneff I, et al. Long-term outcome after ampullectomy for ampullary lesions associated with familial adenomatous polyposis. Dis Colon Rectum 2005;48(12):2192–6.
58. Roggin KK, Yeh JJ, Ferrone CR, et al. Limitations of ampullectomy in the treatment of nonfamilial ampullary neoplasms. Ann Surg Oncol 2005;12(12):971–80.
59. Demetriades H, Zacharakis E, Kirou I, et al. Local excision as a treatment for tumors of ampulla of Vater. World J Surg Oncol 2006;4:14.
60. Dixon E, Vollmer CM Jr, Sahajpal A, et al. Transduodenal resection of periampullary lesions. World J Surg 2005;29(5):649–52.
61. Miossec S, Parc R, Paye F. Ampullectomy in benign lesion: indications and results. Ann Chir 2004;129(2):73–8 [in French].
62. Heidecke CD, Rosenberg R, Bauer M, et al. Impact of grade of dysplasia in villous adenomas of Vater's papilla. World J Surg 2002;26(6):709–14.
63. Posner S, Colletti L, Knol J, et al. Safety and long-term efficacy of transduodenal excision for tumors of the ampulla of Vater. Surgery 2000;128(4):694–701.
64. Clary BM, Tyler DS, Dematos P, et al. Local ampullary resection with careful intraoperative frozen section evaluation for presumed benign ampullary neoplasms. Surgery 2000;127(6):628–33.
65. Salmi S, Ezzedine S, Vitton V, et al. Can papillary carcinomas be treated by endoscopic ampullectomy? Surg Endosc 2012;26(4):920–5.
66. Patel R, Davitte J, Varadarajulu S, et al. Endoscopic resection of ampullary adenomas: complications and outcomes. Dig Dis Sci 2011;56(11):3235–40.
67. Jeanniard-Malet O, Caillol F, Pesenti C, et al. Short-term results of 42 endoscopic ampullectomies: a single-center experience. Scand J Gastroenterol 2011;46(7–8):1014–9.
68. Jung MK, Cho CM, Park SY, et al. Endoscopic resection of ampullary neoplasms: a single-center experience. Surg Endosc 2009;23(11):2568–74.
69. Boix J, Lorenzo-Zuniga V, Moreno de Vega V, et al. Endoscopic resection of ampullary tumors: 12-year review of 21 cases. Surg Endosc 2009;23(1):45–9.

70. Katsinelos P, Paroutoglou G, Kountouras J, et al. Safety and long-term follow-up of endoscopic snare excision of ampullary adenomas. Surg Endosc 2006;20(4): 608–13.

71. Bohnacker S, Seitz U, Nguyen D, et al. Endoscopic resection of benign tumors of the duodenal papilla without and with intraductal growth. Gastrointest Endosc 2005;62(4):551–60.

72. Catalano MF, Linder JD, Chak A, et al. Endoscopic management of adenoma of the major duodenal papilla. Gastrointest Endosc 2004;59(2):225–32.

73. Cheng CL, Sherman S, Fogel EL, et al. Endoscopic snare papillectomy for tumors of the duodenal papillae. Gastrointest Endosc 2004;60(5):757–64.

74. Norton ID, Gostout CJ, Baron TH, et al. Safety and outcome of endoscopic snare excision of the major duodenal papilla. Gastrointest Endosc 2002; 56(2):239–43.

75. Zadorova Z, Dvofak M, Hajer J. Endoscopic therapy of benign tumors of the papilla of Vater. Endoscopy 2001;33(4):345–7.

76. Takamura A, Saito H, Kamada T, et al. Intraluminal low-dose-rate 192Ir brachytherapy combined with external beam radiotherapy and biliary stenting for unresectable extrahepatic bile duct carcinoma. Int J Radiat Oncol Biol Phys 2003;57(5):1357–65.

77. Alden ME, Mohiuddin M. The impact of radiation dose in combined external beam and intraluminal Ir-192 brachytherapy for bile duct cancer. Int J Radiat Oncol Biol Phys 1994;28(4):945–51.

78. Turaga KK, Tsai S, Wiebe LA, et al. Novel multimodality treatment sequencing for extrahepatic (mid and distal) cholangiocarcinoma. Ann Surg Oncol 2013; 20(4):1230–9.

79. Shinohara ET, Guo M, Mitra N, et al. Brachytherapy in the treatment of cholangiocarcinoma. Int J Radiat Oncol Biol Phys 2010;78(3):722–8.

80. Allison RR, Zervos E, Sibata CH. Cholangiocarcinoma: an emerging indication for photodynamic therapy. Photodiagnosis Photodyn Ther 2009;6(2):84–92.

81. Tomizawa Y, Tian J. Photodynamic therapy for unresectable cholangiocarcinoma. Dig Dis Sci 2012;57(2):274–83.

82. Lee TY, Cheon YK, Shim CS. Current status of photodynamic therapy for bile duct cancer. Clin Endosc 2013;46(1):38–44.

83. Leggett CL, Gorospe EC, Murad MH, et al. Photodynamic therapy for unresectable cholangiocarcinoma: a comparative effectiveness systematic review and meta-analyses. Photodiagnosis Photodyn Ther 2012;9(3):189–95.

84. Ortner ME, Caca K, Berr F, et al. Successful photodynamic therapy for nonresectable cholangiocarcinoma: a randomized prospective study. Gastroenterology 2003;125(5):1355–63.

85. Zoepf T, Jakobs R, Arnold JC, et al. Palliation of nonresectable bile duct cancer: improved survival after photodynamic therapy. Am J Gastroenterol 2005; 100(11):2426–30.

86. Lee TY, Cheon YK, Shim CS, et al. Photodynamic therapy prolongs metal stent patency in patients with unresectable hilar cholangiocarcinoma. World J Gastroenterol 2012;18(39):5589–94.

87. Peck-Radosavljevic M, Greten TF, Lammer J, et al. Consensus on the current use of sorafenib for the treatment of hepatocellular carcinoma. Eur J Gastroenterol Hepatol 2010;22(4):391–8.

88. Bouza C, Lopez-Cuadrado T, Alcazar R, et al. Meta-analysis of percutaneous radiofrequency ablation versus ethanol injection in hepatocellular carcinoma. BMC Gastroenterol 2009;9:31.

89. Orlando A, Leandro G, Olivo M, et al. Radiofrequency thermal ablation vs. percutaneous ethanol injection for small hepatocellular carcinoma in cirrhosis: meta-analysis of randomized controlled trials. Am J Gastroenterol 2009; 104(2):514–24.

90. Pearson AS, Izzo F, Fleming RY, et al. Intraoperative radiofrequency ablation or cryoablation for hepatic malignancies. Am J Surg 1999;178(6):592–9.

91. Strasberg SM, Linehan D. Radiofrequency ablation of liver tumors. Curr Probl Surg 2003;40(8):459–98.

92. Mulier S, Ni Y, Jamart J, et al. Local recurrence after hepatic radiofrequency coagulation: multivariate meta-analysis and review of contributing factors. Ann Surg 2005;242(2):158–71.

93. Smith MK, Mutter D, Forbes LE, et al. The physiologic effect of the pneumoperitoneum on radiofrequency ablation. Surg Endosc 2004;18(1):35–8.

94. Chinn SB, Lee FT Jr, Kennedy GD, et al. Effect of vascular occlusion on radiofrequency ablation of the liver: results in a porcine model. AJR Am J Roentgenol 2001;176(3):789–95.

95. Lloyd DM, Lau KN, Welsh F, et al. International multicentre prospective study on microwave ablation of liver tumours: preliminary results. HPB (Oxford) 2011; 13(8):579–85.

96. Iannitti DA, Martin RC, Simon CJ, et al. Hepatic tumor ablation with clustered microwave antennae: the US Phase II trial. HPB (Oxford) 2007;9(2):120–4.

97. Shibata T, Iimuro Y, Yamamoto Y, et al. Small hepatocellular carcinoma: comparison of radio-frequency ablation and percutaneous microwave coagulation therapy. Radiology 2002;223(2):331–7.

98. Kawamoto C, Ido K, Isoda N, et al. Long-term outcomes for patients with solitary hepatocellular carcinoma treated by laparoscopic microwave coagulation. Cancer 2005;103(5):985–93.

99. Martin RC, Scoggins CR, McMasters KM. Safety and efficacy of microwave ablation of hepatic tumors: a prospective review of a 5-year experience. Ann Surg Oncol 2010;17(1):171–8.

100. Dong B, Liang P, Yu X, et al. Percutaneous sonographically guided microwave coagulation therapy for hepatocellular carcinoma: results in 234 patients. AJR Am J Roentgenol 2003;180(6):1547–55.

101. Gervais DA, Goldberg SN, Brown DB, et al. Society of Interventional Radiology position statement on percutaneous radiofrequency ablation for the treatment of liver tumors. J Vasc Interv Radiol 2009;20(Suppl 7):S342–7.

102. Livraghi T, Meloni F, Di Stasi M, et al. Sustained complete response and complications rates after radiofrequency ablation of very early hepatocellular carcinoma in cirrhosis: is resection still the treatment of choice? Hepatology 2008;47(1):82–9.

103. Porrett PM, Peterman H, Rosen M, et al. Lack of benefit of pre-transplant locoregional hepatic therapy for hepatocellular cancer in the current MELD era. Liver Transpl 2006;12(4):665–73.

104. DuBay DA, Sandroussi C, Kachura JR, et al. Radiofrequency ablation of hepatocellular carcinoma as a bridge to liver transplantation. HPB (Oxford) 2011; 13(1):24–32.

105. Raman SS, Aziz D, Chang X, et al. Minimizing diaphragmatic injury during radiofrequency ablation: efficacy of intraabdominal carbon dioxide insufflation. AJR Am J Roentgenol 2004;183(1):197–200.

106. Cassera MA, Potter KW, Ujiki MB, et al. Computed tomography (CT)-guided versus laparoscopic radiofrequency ablation: a single-institution comparison of morbidity rates and hospital costs. Surg Endosc 2011;25(4):1088–95.

107. Foroutani A, Garland AM, Berber E, et al. Laparoscopic ultrasound vs triphasic computed tomography for detecting liver tumors. Arch Surg 2000; 135(8):933–8.
108. Siperstein A, Garland A, Engle K, et al. Local recurrence after laparoscopic radiofrequency thermal ablation of hepatic tumors. Ann Surg Oncol 2000;7(2): 106–13.
109. Lu MD, Kuang M, Liang LJ, et al. Surgical resection versus percutaneous thermal ablation for early-stage hepatocellular carcinoma: a randomized clinical trial. Zhonghua Yi Xue Za Zhi 2006;86(12):801–5 [in Chinese].
110. Chen MS, Li JQ, Zheng Y, et al. A prospective randomized trial comparing percutaneous local ablative therapy and partial hepatectomy for small hepatocellular carcinoma. Ann Surg 2006;243(3):321–8.
111. Feng K, Yan J, Li X, et al. A randomized controlled trial of radiofrequency ablation and surgical resection in the treatment of small hepatocellular carcinoma. J Hepatol 2012;57(4):794–802.
112. Huang J, Yan L, Cheng Z, et al. A randomized trial comparing radiofrequency ablation and surgical resection for HCC conforming to the Milan criteria. Ann Surg 2010;252(6):903–12.
113. Cucchetti A, Piscaglia F, Cescon M, et al. Systematic review of surgical resection vs radiofrequency ablation for hepatocellular carcinoma. World J Gastroenterol 2013;19(26):4106–18.

Intrahepatic Cholangiocarcinoma

Kimberly M. Brown, MD[a],*, Abhishek D. Parmar, MD[a,b],
David A. Geller, MD[c],*

KEYWORDS

- Intrahepatic cholangiocarcinoma • Peripheral cholangiocarcinoma
- Cholangiocarcinoma • Bile duct neoplasms • Intrahepatic bile duct cancer

KEY POINTS

- Intrahepatic cholangiocarcinomas (ICCs) are aggressive, locally invasive tumors with limited 5-year survival. Multifocality, vascular invasion, lymphatic spread, and tumor histology are all determinants of staging and prognosis.
- Both the incidence and the mortality of ICCs have risen over the past several decades.
- Surgical resection is the only viable treatment option for patients who present with ICCs. Minimally invasive hepatectomy is increasingly becoming a valid option in select cases.

INTRODUCTION: NATURE OF THE PROBLEM
Epidemiology

Intrahepatic cholangiocarcinoma (ICC) is a subtype of a family of aggressive cholangiocarcinomas, tumors that arise from cholangiocytes of the biliary tree. There are several key epidemiologic considerations of ICC:

- ICCs are rare, accounting for 20% to 25% of all cholangiocarcinomas; perihilar (50%–60%) or distal common bile duct (20%–25%) tumors are more common (**Fig. 1**).[1] They are still the second most common primary liver malignancy, following hepatocellular carcinoma.[2]
- The incidence rate of ICCs for Americans has increased from 3.2 per 1,000,000 in 1975 to 1979 to 8.5 per 1,000,000 in 1995 to 1999,[3,4] but this trend has stabilized over the last decade.[5]
- The reasons underlying this increasing incidence are unclear, but potential reasons include changes in the classification system[6] or a recent increase in the

Funding: Supported by grants from the UTMB Clinical and Translational Science Award no. UL1TR000071 and NIH T-32 Grant no. 5T32DK007639.
Disclosures: None.
[a] Department of Surgery, University of Texas Medical Branch, 301 University Boulevard, Galveston, TX 77555-0541, USA; [b] Department of Surgery, University of California San Francisco-East Bay, 1411 East 31st Street, Oakland, CA 94602, USA; [c] Liver Cancer Center, University of Pittsburgh School of Medicine, 3459 Fifth Avenue, Pittsburgh, PA 15213-2582, USA
* Corresponding authors.
E-mail addresses: km3brown@utmb.edu; gellerda@upmc.edu

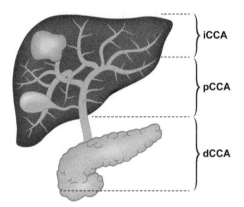

Fig. 1. Anatomic distribution of cholangiocarcinomas. Intrahepatic lesions such as the lesion in the right lobe of the liver shown in this image are many times asymptomatic and as a result present at a later stage. dCCA, distal cholangiocarcinoma; iCCA, intrahepatic cholangiocarcinoma; pCCA, perihilar cholangiocarcinoma.

incidence of Hepatitis C.[7] This increased incidence does not seem to be related to increased tumor detection, as there has been no change in the proportion of early stage or smaller tumors detected over time.[3]

- Population-based data demonstrate that men are 1.5 times as likely to develop ICCs as women in the United States.
- The average age of diagnosis worldwide is 50 years old, and patients are rarely diagnosed younger than age 40.[3,8]
- ICCs are lethal malignancies with more aggressive tumor biology than the more common liver malignancy, hepatocellular carcinoma.[9] Overall 3-year and 5-year survival rates are a dismal 30% and 18%, respectively.[10]
- Mortality from ICCs has risen over the last several decades. Data from the World Health Organization database indicate that although mortality has improved for extrahepatic biliary tumors, mortality has actually increased worldwide for ICCs since the 1970s.[11] For the United States, age-adjusted mortality has risen from 0.7 per 1,000,000 in 1973 to 6.9 per 1,000,000 in 1997, paralleling the rising incidence of ICCs (**Fig. 2**).[4]

Risk Factors

Risk factors for ICC can range from established precursors such as choledochal cysts, cholangitis, and toxin exposure to potential associations such as smoking and diabetes.[12] Patients with chronic inflammatory processes such as primary sclerosing cholangitis and patients infected with the parasites *Opisthorchis viverrini* or *Clonorchis sinensis* are at particularly increased risk for ICC.[13] Other risk factors are listed in **Box 1**. Although these factors are key considerations in the diagnosis of ICC, most of these cancers occur de novo in the absence of any underlying liver disease.[7,14]

Subtypes

The Liver Cancer Study Group of Japan has distinguished 3 different histologic subtypes of ICCs: mass-forming, periductal infiltrating, and intraductal growth (**Fig. 3**).[15]

- Mass-forming ICCs are the most common and are characteristically solid nodules that are discrete from the surrounding liver parenchyma. Intrahepatic metastases are more commonly observed with this subtype.[16]

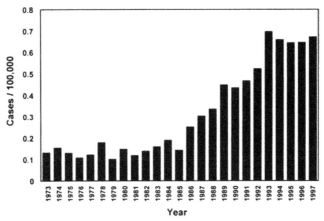

Fig. 2. Age-adjusted mortality for ICC, 1973–1997. (*From* Patel T. Increasing incidence and mortality of primary intrahepatic cholangiocarcinoma in the United States. Hepatology 2001;33(6):1354; with permission.)

- Periductal infiltrating ICCs invade the liver parenchyma along portal structures and metastasize to hilar lymph nodes; this subtype rarely forms a discrete liver mass. A combined mass-forming–periductal-infiltrating tumor type is an aggressive subtype correlating with decreased survival in the Japanese series,[17,18] but this finding has not been observed in Western populations.[19]

Box 1
Risk factors for cholangiocarcinoma
Established risk factors
Primary sclerosing cholangitis
Choledochal cyst
Parasitic infection (Opisthorchis viverrini or Clonorchis sinensis)
Inflammatory bowel disease
Drug or toxin exposure (thorotrast)
Biliary cirrhosis
Cholelithiasis
Bile duct adenoma and biliary papillomatosis
Alcoholic liver disease
Associated risk factors
Diabetes
Thyrotoxicosis
Chronic pancreatitis
Obesity
Nonalcoholic liver disease
Hepatitis B/C infection
Typhoid
Smoking

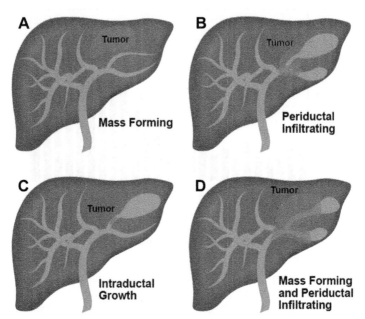

Fig. 3. Histologic subtypes of ICC. Mass-forming types (*A*) are the most common type, typically presenting as a mass lesion. Periductal infiltrating (*B*) are the next most common and infiltrate the hepatic parenchyma along portal structures. Intraductal growth types (*C*) carry the best prognosis but are the least common. Mass-forming periductal infiltrating mixed type (*D*) have been suggested to be the most aggressive of these subtypes.

- Intraductal growth ICCs are the least common subtype and can be characterized by growth into the biliary tract lumen. These ICCS may represent less aggressive variants with a more favorable prognosis.[20]

CLINICAL PRESENTATION AND DIAGNOSIS
Clinical Presentation

The clinical presentation of ICCs is usually nonspecific, and symptoms can include generalized abdominal pain, or less commonly, weight loss and jaundice.

- In a retrospective review of a 31-year experience at Johns Hopkins University, patients with ICC most commonly presented with abdominal pain and were less likely to experience jaundice or weight loss than patients with extrahepatic cholangiocarcinoma.[21] This finding was confirmed in other studies.[22,23]
- Because these tumors are discrete from the main bile ducts and rarely cause obstructive jaundice, clinical diagnoses are rare, and many patients initially present with advanced disease.[13,24] In addition, incidental diagnoses of ICCs in asymptomatic patients are also relatively common, accounting for 12% to 30% of diagnoses in some series.[14,25]
- A single-institution retrospective review at the Memorial Sloan Kettering Cancer Center demonstrated that 54% of these tumors are unresectable at presentation.[23]

Diagnosis and Initial Evaluation

The nonspecific, aggressive presentation of ICC, coupled with its relatively rare incidence, makes the initial diagnosis challenging. ICCs are most commonly identified on cross-sectional imaging, which is also used for staging and determining tumor resectability. Determining the diagnosis before intervention has significant treatment implications given the unique tumor biology of these cancers relative to others (hepatocellular carcinoma, metastatic adenocarcinoma). Laboratory tests are rarely helpful, with occasional exceptions:

- CA 19-9 is the most widely used laboratory test, but it is nonspecific and may be elevated in any number of benign or malignant diseases.[26,27] It may serve a role as an ancillary test in patients with PSC who present with a suspicious intrahepatic lesion. In these patients a value greater than 100 U/mL carries a sensitivity and specificity of 89% and 86%, respectively, for the diagnosis of cholangiocarcinoma.[28]
- α-Fetoprotein is similarly controversial and has been suggested to play a role in differentiating ICCs from hepatocellular carcinoma.[29] In one study by Koh and colleagues[9] these values were typically lower or normal in patients with ICCs compared with patients with hepatocellular carcinoma, but this finding was not statistically significant.
- On ultrasound there are no characteristic findings to differentiate these lesions from secondary metastases or hepatocellular carcinoma.[30,31]
- Cross-sectional imaging with computed tomography (CT) or magnetic resonance imaging (MRI) rarely identifies any pathognomonic features of ICC compared with other liver lesions. As a result, neither is superior to the other in the initial diagnosis of these tumors.[32] However, there are findings on these studies that can aid in the diagnosis, particularly when the 2 modalities are used in conjunction.
- Characteristic findings of ICC on CT include the following:
  - Thin rimlike contrast enhancement on both arterial and portal venous phases;
  - Areas of low attenuation within the tumor with areas of high attenuation scattered throughout, also on both phases[33];
  - Delayed contrast enhancement, which may also correlate with poor prognosis. In a retrospective comparison of patients with tumors with delayed contrast enhancement versus those without enhancement, patients in the former group experienced worse overall survival.[34]
- Characteristic findings of ICC on MRI include the following:
  - Hypointensity on T1-weighted imaging and hyperintensity on T2-weighted imaging;
  - Peripheral enhancement, progressive concentric filling, and contrast pooling on delayed images in contrast-enhanced MRI.[29]
- The utility of PET-CT in the initial diagnosis and staging of suspected ICC is unclear. Studies have been mixed, with some finding a sensitivity and specificity greater than 85%,[35,36] whereas others observed limited specificity in the presence of infectious or inflammatory processes.[37,38]
- Patients who present with a hepatic lesion, biopsy-proven to be adenocarcinoma with an unknown primary lesion, represent special diagnostic cases. In these patients the aim is to discern primary ICC from secondary metastases, and patients should undergo a thorough evaluation to identify a potential primary lesion. These evaluations should include cross-sectional imaging of the chest, abdomen, and pelvis, upper and lower endoscopy, mammography, and gynecologic evaluation as indicated.

STAGING AND PROGNOSIS
7th Edition AJCC Staging

Previous iterations of the American Joint Committee on Cancer (AJCC) staging for ICCs had been based on data from patients with hepatocellular carcinoma. Findings from population-based studies[5] and basic science literature[39,40] have demonstrated that ICCs are pathologic entities with a more aggressive tumor biology and distinct phenotype than hepatocellular carcinoma. Recognizing this, Nathan and colleagues[10] used Surveillance, Epidemiology, and End Results-Medicare data from 1988 to 2004 to (1) assess the validity of the 6th edition staging system and (2) identify prognostic findings from pathologically confirmed ICCs. The authors observed that tumor size as defined by the previous staging classification had no prognostic value, whereas vascular invasion, number of tumors, and extent of lymph node invasion had significant prognostic significance. Based on these findings, the AJCC revised the previous classification system to construct the 7th edition staging classification, the first novel staging system for patients with ICCs (**Table 1**).[41]

- In a multi-institutional study of 12 tertiary academic centers, the AFC-IHCC-2009 study group validated the AJCC 7th edition staging classification as a discriminatory system in which each TNM stage was associated with significantly varying survival outcomes (**Fig. 4**).[42]
- Another single-institutional Japanese study recognized in a multivariate analysis that this system has some limitations and ignores or underestimates the influence of tumor histology and multiplicity while overemphasizing the influence of periductal invasion.[43]
- Wang and colleagues[44] conducted a multivariate analysis to construct a prognostic nomogram for overall 3-year and 5-year survival. This study confirmed the prognostic implications of tumor multiplicity, vascular invasion, and

Table 1
Staging classification for intrahepatic cholangiocarcinoma

Classification	Description
T1	Solitary tumor without vascular invasion[a]
T2a	Solitary tumor with vascular invasion[a]
T2b	Multiple tumors, with or without vascular invasion[a]
T3	Tumor perforating visceral peritoneum or involving local extrahepatic structures by direct invasion
T4	Tumor with periductal invasion[b]
N0	No regional lymph node metastasis
N1	Regional lymph node metastasis[c]
M0	No distant metastasis
M1	Distant metastasis
Stage groupings	
Stage I	T1 N0 M0
Stage II	T2 N0 M0
Stage III	T3 N0 M0
Stage IVA	T4 N0 M0, any T N1 M0
Stage IVB	Any T, any N M1

[a] Includes major vascular invasion (portal vein or hepatic vein) and microvascular invasion.
[b] Includes tumors with periductal-infiltrating or mixed mass-forming and periductal-infiltrating growth pattern.
[c] Nodal involvement of the celiac, periaortic, or caval lymph nodes is considered to be distant metastasis (M1).
Adapted from Edge SB, Byrd DR, Compton CC, et al, editors. AJCC cancer staging manual. 7th edition. New York: Springer; 2010; with permission.

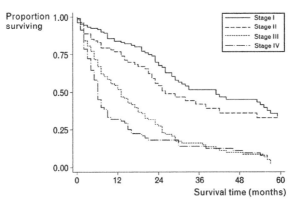

Fig. 4. Kaplan-Meier survival curve of patients with cholangiocarcinoma. (*From* Nathan H, Pawlik TM. Staging of intrahepatic cholangiocarcinoma. Curr Opin Gastroenterol 2010;26(3):271; with permission.)

lymphatic spread, all of which are included in the current AJCC staging system. However, in this retrospective review the addition of carcinoembryonic antigen (CEA) and CA 19-9 levels resulted in improved staging accuracy.

MANAGEMENT AND TREATMENT

Although there have been some developments in adjuvant therapies, surgical resection remains the only potentially curative treatment modality for patients with ICCs.[21,45,46] This section deals with the considerations of operative resection, including the extent of resection, minimally invasive surgical techniques, and orthotopic liver transplantation (OLT). Finally, the role of other nonsurgical therapies is discussed.

Preoperative Preparation

The preoperative evaluation of a patient with suspected ICC should include high-quality cross-sectional imaging of the liver to determine tumor resectability but should also include a detailed evaluation to exclude metastatic or occult primary disease in the chest, abdomen, and pelvis. A discussion of all of the considerations involved in hepatic parenchymal resection is outside the scope of this article, but a few salient points are mentioned:

- Resectability in ICC is defined as the ability to resect tumor to negative margins while preserving adequate functioning liver with intact arterial, portal venous, and hepatic venous flow, and biliary-enteric drainage.
- Preservation of an adequate functioning liver is a central tenet in liver surgery but predicting the amount and function of viable future liver remnant is sometimes difficult. Most authors have suggested 20% to 25% of future liver remnant[47–49] or 40% future liver remnant in patients with compromised liver function[50] as standard cutoff values.
- Preoperative portal venous embolization has been developed as a technique to stimulate hypertrophy in the future liver remnant by interrupting flow to tumor-bearing segments, thereby mitigating the risks of postoperative liver failure. The data on this technique in patients with ICCs are limited but studies in other populations have demonstrated that it is safe and can reduce the incidence of postoperative liver failure.[50,51]

Staging Laparoscopy

Staging laparoscopy has been demonstrated to reduce unnecessary laparotomy for patients with hepatopancreaticobiliary malignancies. However, in the largest series of staging laparoscopy for ICC (53 patients), the sensitivity of staging laparoscopy was only 55%.[52] A smaller study of 11 patients also demonstrated a high false-negative rate with laparoscopy for ICCs, but this finding is inconclusive given the small sample size.[53] Unresectability is often determined by local involvement of vascular supply or biliary drainage of the future liver remnant, which may not be evident on laparoscopic exploration, contributing to the low yield for laparoscopy. As a result, routine staging laparoscopy is not currently recommended in these patients.

Hepatic Resection

- Morbidity and mortality after hepatectomy have declined over the past several decades, owing to improved surgical technique, perioperative care, and advances in hemostasis.[54] For ICCs, perioperative morbidity and mortality range from 1% to 14%[21,23,25,52,55–59] and 6% to 43%,[21,23,25,52,55–59] respectively. Studies of survival after resection and factors associated with survival are illustrated in **Table 2**.
- R0 resection (resection of both gross and microscopic disease) is the aim of curative intent surgery[60] and is associated with favorable outcomes,[19,21,22,25,52,58,60,61] but is achieved in only 45% to 96% of attempted resections.[19,21–23,25,52,55–57,60,61]
- R0 resection only improves survival in cases where regional lymphatic spread has not already occurred and has been confirmed in 2 multi-institutional studies.[19,60]
- Five-year overall survivals after resection range from 17% to 44%, with median survivals of 12 to 43 months.[19,21,23,25,55,57,59,62]

Lymphadenectomy

The lymphatic drainage of the liver is generally predictable, and the left lobe of the liver generally drains toward the lesser curve and cardia of the stomach, whereas the right lobe drains to the hepatoduodenal ligament.[63] However, for ICC there are some important considerations with regards to lymph node disease:

- In a study mapping the lymphatic drainage of patients with left-sided ICC, 46% of tumor deposits were identified in the hepatoduodenal ligament, where right-sided tumor metastases normally occur.[64]
- Although lymphatic involvement is a clear prognostic factor, there is no evidence that routine lymphadenectomy confers any survival benefit.[65] Although this finding has been observed in only small single-institution studies, most large series demonstrate that routine lymphadenectomy is rarely performed in practice.[19,23,52,57]
- Lymphadenectomy with surgical resection is recommended in patients with grossly positive lymphatic disease, but spread beyond the regional lymph node basins is a contraindication to resection.[66]

Vascular Resection

- Because ICCs are locally invasive tumors, vascular invasion is a relatively common occurrence, and vascular resections are required in 9% to 14% of hepatectomies.[23,25,52,55,57,58,61]

Table 2
Factors associated with disease-free survival and overall survival after resection for ICC

First Author/Year	N	R0 Resection	LN Positivity	Tumor Size	Multifocality	Vascular Invasion	Median Survival (mo)	1-y OS (%)	5-y OS (%)
Madariaga et al,[58] 1998	34	Yes-OS	No	No	Yes	No	19	67	35
Weber et al,[52] 2001	33	Yes	No	Yes-DFS	No	Yes-OS	37	—	31
Nakagawa et al,[61] 2005	44	Yes-OS	Yes-OS	No	Yes-OS	No	22	66	26
DeOliveira et al,[21] 2007	44	Yes	Yes	No	No	No	28	—	40
Paik et al,[22] 2008	97	Yes-DFS	Yes-DFS	Yes-DFS	Yes-DFS	No	53	75	31
Endo et al,[23] 2008	77	No	Yes-RFS	Yes	Yes-RFS	No	36 (DSS)	—	—
Guglielmi et al,[56] 2009	62	Yes	Yes	No	N/A	Yes	41	—	26
Lang et al,[59] 2009	83	Yes	No	No	No	No	26	71	21
Nathan et al,[10] 2009	598	N/A	Yes	No	Yes	Yes	21	—	18
Shen et al,[25] 2009	429	Yes-OS	Yes-OS	Yes-OS	No	No	12	51	17
de Jong et al,[19] 2011	449	Yes-OS	Yes-OS	No	Yes	Yes	27	78	31
Farges et al,[42,60] 2011	212	Yes-OS in N0	No	No	Yes-OS	No	28	77	28

Abbreviations: DSS, disease-specific survival; OS, overall survival.

- Vascular resection is feasible in experienced centers. In a single-institution review by the Mayo Clinic, 12% of patients underwent major vascular resection.[55] There was no difference in achievable R0 resections in patients who required vascular resection compared with patients who did not require vascular resection. In addition, there were no differences in perioperative morbidity and mortality. As a result, overall 5-year survival did not differ between groups (44% in the vascular resection group vs 23% in the nonresected group, $P = .268$).

Minimally Invasive Surgery

Since the advent of minimally invasive surgical techniques for hepatic resection in the early 1990s, many of the initial questions of the feasibility of minimally invasive hepatic resection have been answered. Although there have been no randomized controlled trials comparing minimally invasive liver resection to open techniques, there are several observational studies that support the use of the minimally invasive approach.[67]

- Minimally invasive hepatic resection is associated with decreased narcotic pain medication requirement, decreased hospital length of stay, and comparable morbidity and mortality when compared with open resection.[68–71]
- In small case-control series of patients with hepatic malignancy, minimally invasive hepatectomy was not associated with margin positivity or decreased disease-free survival.[70,72] However, the conclusions of these observational studies should be approached with caution as they are subject to selection bias. Prospective studies are needed to determine the true impact of minimally invasive techniques on the adequacy of hepatic resection for patients with cancer.
- Robotic resections of hepatic malignancies are currently being investigated with promising results,[73–75] but long-term data are lacking and these resections should only be undertaken at high-volume centers with specialized expertise in robotic surgery.

Transplant

Given the locally aggressive nature of ICCs, OLT has been attempted as a treatment option. Potential indications for OLT in this population include locally advanced unresectable disease or the presence of advanced cirrhosis that would preclude partial hepatectomy.

- In one of the earliest experiences with OLT for ICC at the University of Pittsburgh, investigators observed similar tumor-free survival and recurrence rates in a small retrospective series (N = 54) of patients who underwent hepatectomy versus OLT.[76]
- However, similar patterns in disease-free survival have not been consistently reproduced. Other experiences with OLT have found dismally low disease-free survival rates of 40% at 1 year,[77] or high recurrence rates of 51% to 80%.[78,79] The University of California, Los Angeles OLT experience for ICCs actually observed a trend toward improved recurrence-free survival with OLT compared with hepatectomy.[80]
- In a retrospective review of United Network for Organ Sharing database from 1987 to 2005, 1-year and 5-year survival for 280 patients who underwent OLT for ICCs were 74% and 38%, respectively.[81]
- Nearly all of these studies included some form of adjuvant or neoadjuvant therapy in conjunction with OLT. Based on these mixed data and the potential likelihood for high tumor recurrence in patients with ICCs, OLT for ICC should only be considered in the context of clinical trials.

- Noteworthy, the Mayo Clinic team has reported excellent results with OLT for early-stage Klaskin cholangiocarcinoma tumors, typically in the setting of PSC, with 5-year OS rate of ~70%.[82]

Medical Therapy

Nonsurgical therapies for ICCs have not been demonstrated to improve survival or decrease recurrence independently. Because of the relative rarity of ICCs, data on chemotherapy in the adjuvant setting are lacking, but chemotherapy may serve a role in select populations:

- For patients with unresectable ICCs, combination chemotherapy with cisplatin and gemcitabine may provide a survival benefit. In a prospective randomized controlled trial of unresectable biliary tract cancers, Valle and colleagues[83] observed a modest survival benefit (~3 months) with combined cisplatin-gemcitabine therapy compared with gemcitabine alone. In a subgroup analysis of patients with ICC, patients treated with combination therapy experienced a survival benefit (hazard ratio [HR] for mortality 0.57, 95% CI 0.34–0.94).
- Studies of other adjuvant therapies have been limited by small sample size or retrospective design.
- Radiation therapy in conjunction with surgery was suggested to improve survival when compared with resection alone in a retrospective population-based study,[84] but this observation is subject to unmeasured confounding and should be interpreted with caution.
- Transarterial chemoembolization (TACE) is a promising therapy with limited side effects[85] that may improve survival in patients with unresectable ICC.[86] In one nonrandomized study, treatment with gemcitabine-cisplatin combination TACE resulted in significantly longer survival (13.8 months) compared with TACE with gemcitabine alone (6.3 months).[87] TACE has had limited impact in the adjuvant setting.[88]

SUMMARY

ICCs are aggressive malignancies that have been increasing in incidence and mortality over time. Few patients present with resectable disease at the time of presentation, and diagnosis is often difficult because of the occult nature and anatomic position of ICCs. Prognostic features, such as multifocality, vascular invasion, lymphatic spread, and histopathology, should be considered in the management and treatment of these patients. However, because of the relative rarity of ICCs, little is known of the optimal treatment strategy beyond surgical resection. Prospective data are needed to better characterize the efficacy of minimally invasive techniques, transplantation, chemotherapeutic regimens, and other adjuvant therapies on patients who present with this lethal disease.

REFERENCES

1. Khan SA, Davidson BR, Goldin R, et al. Guidelines for the diagnosis and treatment of cholangiocarcinoma: consensus document. Gut 2002;51(Suppl 6): VI1–9.
2. Khan SA, Toledano MB, Taylor-Robinson SD. Epidemiology, risk factors, and pathogenesis of cholangiocarcinoma. HPB (Oxford) 2008;10(2):77–82.
3. Shaib Y, El-Serag HB. The epidemiology of cholangiocarcinoma. Semin Liver Dis 2004;24(2):115–25.

4. Patel T. Increasing incidence and mortality of primary intrahepatic cholangiocarcinoma in the United States. Hepatology 2001;33(6):1353–7.
5. Everhart JE, Ruhl CE. Burden of digestive diseases in the United States Part III: liver, biliary tract, and pancreas. Gastroenterology 2009;136(4):1134–44.
6. Khan SA, Emadossadaty S, Ladep NG, et al. Rising trends in cholangiocarcinoma: is the ICD classification system misleading us? J Hepatol 2012;56(4): 848–54.
7. Sempoux C, Jibara G, Ward SC, et al. Intrahepatic cholangiocarcinoma: new insights in pathology. Semin Liver Dis 2011;31(1):49–60.
8. Altaee MY, Johnson PJ, Farrant JM, et al. Etiologic and clinical characteristics of peripheral and hilar cholangiocarcinoma. Cancer 1991;68(9):2051–5.
9. Koh KC, Lee H, Choi MS, et al. Clinicopathologic features and prognosis of combined hepatocellular cholangiocarcinoma. Am J Surg 2005;189(1): 120–5.
10. Nathan H, Aloia TA, Vauthey JN, et al. A proposed staging system for intrahepatic cholangiocarcinoma. Ann Surg Oncol 2009;16(1):14–22.
11. Patel T. Worldwide trends in mortality from biliary tract malignancies. BMC Cancer 2002;2:10.
12. Yang J, Yan LN. Current status of intrahepatic cholangiocarcinoma. World J Gastroenterol 2008;14(41):6289–97.
13. de Groen PC, Gores GJ, LaRusso NF, et al. Biliary tract cancers. N Engl J Med 1999;341(18):1368–78.
14. Dhanasekaran R, Hemming AW, Zendejas I, et al. Treatment outcomes and prognostic factors of intrahepatic cholangiocarcinoma. Oncol Rep 2013;29(4): 1259–67.
15. Yamasaki S. Intrahepatic cholangiocarcinoma: macroscopic type and stage classification. J Hepatobiliary Pancreat Surg 2003;10(4):288–91.
16. Sasaki A, Aramaki M, Kawano K, et al. Intrahepatic peripheral cholangiocarcinoma: mode of spread and choice of surgical treatment. Br J Surg 1998; 85(9):1206–9.
17. Shimada K, Sano T, Sakamoto Y, et al. Surgical outcomes of the mass-forming plus periductal infiltrating types of intrahepatic cholangiocarcinoma: a comparative study with the typical mass-forming type of intrahepatic cholangiocarcinoma. World J Surg 2007;31(10):2016–22.
18. Yamamoto J, Kosuge T, Takayama T, et al. Surgical treatment of intrahepatic cholangiocarcinoma: four patients surviving more than five years. Surgery 1992;111(6):617–22.
19. de Jong MC, Nathan H, Sotiropoulos GC, et al. Intrahepatic cholangiocarcinoma: an international multi-institutional analysis of prognostic factors and lymph node assessment. J Clin Oncol 2011;29(23):3140–5.
20. Suh KS, Roh HR, Koh YT, et al. Clinicopathologic features of the intraductal growth type of peripheral cholangiocarcinoma. Hepatology 2000;31(1):12–7.
21. DeOliveira ML, Cunningham SC, Cameron JL, et al. Cholangiocarcinoma: thirty-one-year experience with 564 patients at a single institution. Ann Surg 2007; 245(5):755–62.
22. Paik KY, Jung JC, Heo JS, et al. What prognostic factors are important for resected intrahepatic cholangiocarcinoma? J Gastroenterol Hepatol 2008;23(5): 766–70.
23. Endo I, Gonen M, Yopp AC, et al. Intrahepatic cholangiocarcinoma: rising frequency, improved survival, and determinants of outcome after resection. Ann Surg 2008;248(1):84–96.

24. Blechacz B, Komuta M, Roskams T, et al. Clinical diagnosis and staging of chol-angiocarcinoma. Nat Rev Gastroenterol Hepatol 2011;8(9):512–22.
25. Shen WF, Zhong W, Xu F, et al. Clinicopathological and prognostic analysis of 429 patients with intrahepatic cholangiocarcinoma. World J Gastroenterol 2009;15(47):5976–82.
26. Chen CY, Shiesh SC, Tsao HC, et al. The assessment of biliary CA 125, CA 19-9 and CEA in diagnosing cholangiocarcinoma–the influence of sampling time and hepatolithiasis. Hepatogastroenterology 2002;49(45):616–20.
27. Mann DV, Edwards R, Ho S, et al. Elevated tumour marker CA19-9: clinical inter-pretation and influence of obstructive jaundice. Eur J Surg Oncol 2000;26(5): 474–9.
28. Nichols JC, Gores GJ, LaRusso NF, et al. Diagnostic role of serum CA 19-9 for cholangiocarcinoma in patients with primary sclerosing cholangitis. Mayo Clin Proc 1993;68(9):874–9.
29. Miller G, Schwartz LH, D'Angelica M. The use of imaging in the diagnosis and staging of hepatobiliary malignancies. Surg Oncol Clin N Am 2007;16(2):343–68.
30. Wibulpolprasert B, Dhiensiri T. Peripheral cholangiocarcinoma: sonographic evaluation. J Clin Ultrasound 1992;20(5):303–14.
31. Colli A, Cocciolo M, Mumoli N, et al. Peripheral intrahepatic cholangiocarci-noma: ultrasound findings and differential diagnosis from hepatocellular carci-noma. Eur J Ultrasound 1998;7(2):93–9.
32. Zhang Y, Uchida M, Abe T, et al. Intrahepatic peripheral cholangiocarcinoma: comparison of dynamic CT and dynamic MRI. J Comput Assist Tomogr 1999; 23(5):670–7.
33. Kim TK, Choi BI, Han JK, et al. Peripheral cholangiocarcinoma of the liver: two-phase spiral CT findings. Radiology 1997;204(2):539–43.
34. Asayama Y, Yoshimitsu K, Irie H, et al. Delayed-phase dynamic CT enhance-ment as a prognostic factor for mass-forming intrahepatic cholangiocarcinoma. Radiology 2006;238(1):150–5.
35. Anderson CD, Rice MH, Pinson CW, et al. Fluorodeoxyglucose PET imaging in the evaluation of gallbladder carcinoma and cholangiocarcinoma. J Gastrointest Surg 2004;8(1):90–7.
36. Kim YJ, Yun M, Lee WJ, et al. Usefulness of 18F-FDG PET in intrahepatic chol-angiocarcinoma. Eur J Nucl Med Mol Imaging 2003;30(11):1467–72.
37. Fevery J, Buchel O, Nevens F, et al. Positron emission tomography is not a reli-able method for the early diagnosis of cholangiocarcinoma in patients with pri-mary sclerosing cholangitis. J Hepatol 2005;43(2):358–60.
38. Fritscher-Ravens A, Bohuslavizki KH, Broering DC, et al. FDG PET in the diag-nosis of hilar cholangiocarcinoma. Nucl Med Commun 2001;22(12):1277–85.
39. Andersen JB, Spee B, Blechacz BR, et al. Genomic and genetic characteriza-tion of cholangiocarcinoma identifies therapeutic targets for tyrosine kinase in-hibitors. Gastroenterology 2012;142(4):1021–31.e15.
40. Sia D, Hoshida Y, Villanueva A, et al. Integrative molecular analysis of intrahe-patic cholangiocarcinoma reveals 2 classes that have different outcomes. Gastroenterology 2013;144(4):829–40.
41. Edge SB, Compton CC. The American Joint Committee on Cancer: the 7th edi-tion of the AJCC cancer staging manual and the future of TNM. Ann Surg Oncol 2010;17(6):1471–4.
42. Farges O, Fuks D, Le Treut YP, et al. AJCC 7th edition of TNM staging accurately discriminates outcomes of patients with resectable intrahepatic cholangiocarci-noma: by the AFC-IHCC-2009 study group. Cancer 2011;117(10):2170–7.

43. Igami T, Ebata T, Yokoyama Y, et al. Staging of peripheral-type intrahepatic chol-angiocarcinoma: appraisal of the new TNM classification and its modifications. World J Surg 2011;35(11):2501–9.

44. Wang Y, Li J, Xia Y, et al. Prognostic nomogram for intrahepatic cholangiocarci-noma after partial hepatectomy. J Clin Oncol 2013;31(9):1188–95.

45. Nakeeb A, Pitt HA, Sohn TA, et al. Cholangiocarcinoma. A spectrum of intrahepatic, perihilar, and distal tumors. Ann Surg 1996;224(4):463–73 [discussion: 473–5].

46. Morise Z, Sugioka A, Tokoro T, et al. Surgery and chemotherapy for intrahepatic cholangiocarcinoma. World J Hepatol 2010;2(2):58–64.

47. Vauthey JN, Chaoui A, Do KA, et al. Standardized measurement of the future liver remnant prior to extended liver resection: methodology and clinical associ-ations. Surgery 2000;127(5):512–9.

48. Abdalla EK, Barnett CC, Doherty D, et al. Extended hepatectomy in patients with hepatobiliary malignancies with and without preoperative portal vein emboliza-tion. Arch Surg 2002;137(6):675–80 [discussion: 680–1].

49. Kishi Y, Abdalla EK, Chun YS, et al. Three hundred and one consecutive extended right hepatectomies: evaluation of outcome based on systematic liver volumetry. Ann Surg 2009;250(4):540–8.

50. Ebata T, Yokoyama Y, Igami T, et al. Portal vein embolization before extended hepatectomy for biliary cancer: current technique and review of 494 consecu-tive embolizations. Dig Surg 2012;29(1):23–9.

51. Hemming AW, Reed AI, Howard RJ, et al. Preoperative portal vein emboliza-tion for extended hepatectomy. Ann Surg 2003;237(5):686–91 [discussion: 691–3].

52. Weber SM, Jarnagin WR, Klimstra D, et al. Intrahepatic cholangiocarcinoma: resectability, recurrence pattern, and outcomes. J Am Coll Surg 2001;193(4): 384–91.

53. Goere D, Wagholikar GD, Pessaux P, et al. Utility of staging laparoscopy in sub-sets of biliary cancers: laparoscopy is a powerful diagnostic tool in patients with intrahepatic and gallbladder carcinoma. Surg Endosc 2006;20(5):721–5.

54. Aloia TA, Fahy BN, Fischer CP, et al. Predicting poor outcome following hepatec-tomy: analysis of 2313 hepatectomies in the NSQIP database. HPB (Oxford) 2009;11(6):510–5.

55. Ali SM, Clark CJ, Zaydfudim VM, et al. Role of major vascular resection in pa-tients with intrahepatic cholangiocarcinoma. Ann Surg Oncol 2012;20(6): 2023–8.

56. Guglielmi A, Ruzzenente A, Campagnaro T, et al. Intrahepatic cholangiocarci-noma: prognostic factors after surgical resection. World J Surg 2009;33(6): 1247–54.

57. Konstadoulakis MM, Roayaie S, Gomatos IP, et al. Fifteen-year, single-center experience with the surgical management of intrahepatic cholangiocarcinoma: operative results and long-term outcome. Surgery 2008;143(3):366–74.

58. Madariaga JR, Iwatsuki S, Todo S, et al. Liver resection for hilar and peripheral cholangiocarcinomas: a study of 62 cases. Ann Surg 1998;227(1):70–9.

59. Lang H, Sotiropoulos GC, Sgourakis G, et al. Operations for intrahepatic cholan-giocarcinoma: single-institution experience of 158 patients. J Am Coll Surg 2009;208(2):218–28.

60. Farges O, Fuks D, Boleslawski E, et al. Influence of surgical margins on outcome in patients with intrahepatic cholangiocarcinoma: a multicenter study by the AFC-IHCC-2009 study group. Ann Surg 2011;254(5):824–9 [discussion: 830].

61. Nakagawa T, Kamiyama T, Kurauchi N, et al. Number of lymph node metastases is a significant prognostic factor in intrahepatic cholangiocarcinoma. World J Surg 2005;29(6):728–33.

62. Nathan H, Pawlik TM, Wolfgang CL, et al. Trends in survival after surgery for cholangiocarcinoma: a 30-year population-based SEER database analysis. J Gastrointest Surg 2007;11(11):1488–96 [discussion: 1496–7].

63. Shirabe K, Shimada M, Harimoto N, et al. Intrahepatic cholangiocarcinoma: its mode of spreading and therapeutic modalities. Surgery 2002;131(Suppl 1): S159–64.

64. Okami J, Dono K, Sakon M, et al. Patterns of regional lymph node involvement in intrahepatic cholangiocarcinoma of the left lobe. J Gastrointest Surg 2003;7(7): 850–6.

65. Morine Y, Shimada M, Utsunomiya T, et al. Clinical impact of lymph node dissection in surgery for peripheral-type intrahepatic cholangiocarcinoma. Surg Today 2012;42(2):147–51.

66. Nguyen KT, Steel J, Vanounou T, et al. Initial presentation and management of hilar and peripheral cholangiocarcinoma: is a node-positive status or potential margin-positive result a contraindication to resection? Ann Surg Oncol 2009; 16(12):3308–15.

67. Reddy SK, Tsung A, Geller DA. Laparoscopic liver resection. World J Surg 2011; 35(7):1478–86.

68. Koffron AJ, Auffenberg G, Kung R, et al. Evaluation of 300 minimally invasive liver resections at a single institution: less is more. Ann Surg 2007;246(3): 385–92 [discussion: 392–4].

69. Buell JF, Thomas MJ, Doty TC, et al. An initial experience and evolution of laparoscopic hepatic resectional surgery. Surgery 2004;136(4):804–11.

70. Ito K, Ito H, Are C, et al. Laparoscopic versus open liver resection: a matched-pair case control study. J Gastrointest Surg 2009;13(12):2276–83.

71. Tsinberg M, Tellioglu G, Simpfendorfer CH, et al. Comparison of laparoscopic versus open liver tumor resection: a case-controlled study. Surg Endosc 2009;23(4):847–53.

72. Sarpel U, Hefti MM, Wisnievsky JP, et al. Outcome for patients treated with laparoscopic versus open resection of hepatocellular carcinoma: case-matched analysis. Ann Surg Oncol 2009;16(6):1572–7.

73. Packiam V, Bartlett DL, Tohme S, et al. Minimally invasive liver resection: robotic versus laparoscopic left lateral sectionectomy. J Gastrointest Surg 2012;16(12): 2233–8.

74. Choi GH, Choi SH, Kim SH, et al. Robotic liver resection: technique and results of 30 consecutive procedures. Surg Endosc 2012;26(8):2247–58.

75. Kitisin K, Packiam V, Bartlett DL, et al. A current update on the evolution of robotic liver surgery. Minerva Chir 2011;66(4):281–93.

76. Casavilla FA, Marsh JW, Iwatsuki S, et al. Hepatic resection and transplantation for peripheral cholangiocarcinoma. J Am Coll Surg 1997;185(5):429–36.

77. Goldstein RM, Stone M, Tillery GW, et al. Is liver transplantation indicated for cholangiocarcinoma? Am J Surg 1993;166(6):768–71 [discussion: 771–2].

78. Ghali P, Marotta PJ, Yoshida EM, et al. Liver transplantation for incidental cholangiocarcinoma: analysis of the Canadian experience. Liver Transpl 2005; 11(11):1412–6.

79. Meyer CG, Penn I, James L. Liver transplantation for cholangiocarcinoma: results in 207 patients. Transplantation 2000;69(8):1633–7.

80. Hong JC, Jones CM, Duffy JP, et al. Comparative analysis of resection and liver transplantation for intrahepatic and hilar cholangiocarcinoma: a 24-year experience in a single center. Arch Surg 2011;146(6):683–9.
81. Becker NS, Rodriguez JA, Barshes NR, et al. Outcomes analysis for 280 patients with cholangiocarcinoma treated with liver transplantation over an 18-year period. J Gastrointest Surg 2008;12(1):117–22.
82. Gores GJ, Darwish Murad S, Heimbach JK, et al. Liver transplantation for perihilar cholangiocarcinoma. Dig Dis 2013;31(1):126–9.
83. Valle J, Wasan H, Palmer DH, et al. Cisplatin plus gemcitabine versus gemcitabine for biliary tract cancer. N Engl J Med 2010;362(14):1273–81.
84. Shinohara ET, Mitra N, Guo M, et al. Radiation therapy is associated with improved survival in the adjuvant and definitive treatment of intrahepatic cholangiocarcinoma. Int J Radiat Oncol Biol Phys 2008;72(5):1495–501.
85. Vogl TJ, Naguib NN, Nour-Eldin NE, et al. Transarterial chemoembolization in the treatment of patients with unresectable cholangiocarcinoma: results and prognostic factors governing treatment success. Int J Cancer 2012;131(3):733–40.
86. Park SY, Kim JH, Yoon HJ, et al. Transarterial chemoembolization versus supportive therapy in the palliative treatment of unresectable intrahepatic cholangiocarcinoma. Clin Radiol 2011;66(4):322–8.
87. Gusani NJ, Balaa FK, Steel JL, et al. Treatment of unresectable cholangiocarcinoma with gemcitabine-based transcatheter arterial chemoembolization (TACE): a single-institution experience. J Gastrointest Surg 2008;12(1):129–37.
88. Shen WF, Zhong W, Liu Q, et al. Adjuvant transcatheter arterial chemoembolization for intrahepatic cholangiocarcinoma after curative surgery: retrospective control study. World J Surg 2011;35(9):2083–91.

Hilar Cholangiocarcinoma

Victor M. Zaydfudim, MD, MPH[a], Charles B. Rosen, MD[b],
David M. Nagorney, MD[c],*

KEYWORDS

- Hilar cholangiocarcinoma • Hepatic resection • Liver transplantation
- Vascular resection

KEY POINTS

- Margin-negative cancer extirpation is the only curative strategy for hilar cholangiocarcinoma.
- Bismuth-Corlette type I and II cholangiocarcinomas are rare and are occasionally resectable without a concomitant liver resection; Bismuth-Corlette type III cholangiocarcinoma requires a concomitant hepatectomy for a margin-negative resection.
- Resection and reconstruction of ipsilateral portal vein for a margin-negative resection is feasible and safe. Portal vein resections without direct tumor involvement and arterial resections as a routine resectional component for hilar cholangiocarcinoma have been promoted in a few specialized centers, but survival benefit remains unclear.
- Bismuth-Corlette type IV cholangiocarcinoma and cancers with major vascular involvement should be considered for neoadjuvant chemoradiation and liver transplantation. Liver resection and liver transplantation are mutually exclusive treatment pathways without possibility of crossover.
- Operative treatment of hilar cholangiocarcinoma is associated with greater perioperative mortality than any other elective hepatobiliary operation.

INTRODUCTION

Hilar cholangiocarcinoma remains a major focus for hepatobiliary surgeons worldwide.[1,2] Despite its relatively low incidence, aggressive tumor biology, lack of effective systemic therapy, and ongoing risks of hepatic failure and biliary sepsis have challenged the development of successful treatment strategies.[3] Margin-negative resection of hilar cholangiocarcinoma remains the only potentially curative therapy.

The past few decades have witnessed the evolution of 2 dominant resection strategies: (1) concomitant biliary and hepatic resection and regional lymphadenectomy for patients in whom a negative margin is expected based on modern imaging and (2) liver

[a] Department of Surgery, University of Virginia, 1300 Jefferson Park Avenue, Charlottesville, VA 22908, USA; [b] Division of Transplantation Surgery, Mayo Clinic, 200 1st Street Southwest, Rochester, MN 55905, USA; [c] Department of Surgery, Mayo Clinic, 200 1st Street Southwest, Rochester, MN 55905, USA
* Corresponding author.
E-mail address: nagorney.david@mayo.edu

Surg Oncol Clin N Am 23 (2014) 247–263
http://dx.doi.org/10.1016/j.soc.2013.10.005
1055-3207/14/$ – see front matter © 2014 Elsevier Inc. All rights reserved.

transplantation after neoadjuvant chemoradiation for patients with unresectable hilar cholangiocarcinoma in the absence of identifiable metastases.[4,5] In this article, we first discuss tumor pathology and staging, preoperative patient selection, and diagnostic techniques, and then focus on operative management and pertinent outcomes among patients with hilar cholangiocarcinoma.

TUMOR PATHOLOGY AND STAGING

There are 3 pathologic subtypes of extrahepatic bile duct adenocarcinoma: sclerosing, nodular, and papillary.[3] Sclerosing cholangiocarcinoma (>70%) is the most frequent subtype and is characterized by marked desmoplasia and neoplastic infiltration into surrounding tissues. Perineural and vascular invasion is frequent.[6] Nodular cholangiocarcinoma (~20%) shows local irregular infiltration into the bile duct. A combination of sclerosing and nodular features are observed with frequency and described as nodular-sclerosing. The sclerosing and nodular subtypes of cholangiocarcinoma have a predilection for radial and longitudinal extension along the mucosa and submucosa of the bile duct at times without extrabiliary evidence of tumor spread.[7] Microscopic extension of sclerosing and nodular cholangiocarcinomas must be anticipated during resection. Papillary cholangiocarcinomas are rare (~5%–10%) and are characterized by intraluminal mass with late transmural extension.[8]

Preoperative evaluation and definition of the anatomic location and extent of hilar cholangiocarcinoma is critical for operative planning. To this extent, the Bismuth-Corlette classification (**Fig. 1**) has been the most widely adopted system used to describe tumor location and biliary involvement.[9] The strength and utility of Bismuth-Corlette classification is its ability to conceptualize hilar cholangiocarcinoma into an operatively approachable scheme. In practice, neoplasia is a dynamic process with a spectrum of extension that defies exact categorization.

Patients with hilar cholangiocarcinoma at the level of the cystic duct, but below the bifurcation of the hepatic ducts (Bismuth-Corlette type I) or just at the bifurcation (Bismuth-Corlette type II) are best treated with resection of the extrahepatic bile duct, gallbladder, and regional lymph nodes and biliary reconstruction alone or with concomitant pancreaticoduodenectomy, depending on the distal extension of the cholangiocarcinoma. Occasionally, limited hepatic resection is required for type II

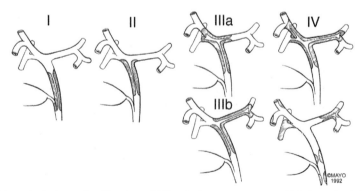

Fig. 1. Bismuth-Corlette classification of hilar cholangiocarcinoma: (I) below the bifurcation of right and left hepatic ducts; (II), at the bifurcation of right and left hepatic ducts; (IIIA) at the duct bifurcation with extension into the right hepatic duct; (IIIB) at the duct bifurcation with extension into the right hepatic duct; and (IV) extension into both right and left hepatic ducts or multicentric disease. (*Reprinted from* the Mayo Foundation; with permission.)

cholangiocarcinoma. However, clinically, Bismuth-Corlette types I and II tumors are rare, and most patients with hilar cholangiocarcinoma have extension into the biliary bifurcation or the right or the left hepatic ducts, or both. Classification of hilar cholangiocarcinoma involving one or both hepatic ducts is Bismuth-Corlette IIIa for right segmental extension, IIIb for left segmental extension, and IV for bilateral segmental extension or diffuse multifocal disease. Resection is possible for IIIa and IIIb cholangiocarcinomas by right or left hepatectomy, respectively, if the vasculature to the expected hepatic remnant is either uninvolved or resectable and reconstructable.

Patients who have unresectable hilar cholangiocarcinoma are best treated by neoadjuvant radiotherapy with chemosensitization and liver transplantation.[10–12] Although criteria for resectability vary widely, generally accepted criteria for unresectability are[2,12]:

1. Main portal or arterial involvement not amenable to reconstruction regardless of Bismuth-Corlette type
2. Unilateral segmental biliary extension with contralateral vascular involvement not amenable to reconstruction (Bismuth-Corlette types IIIa and IIIb)
3. Bilateral biliary involvement of secondary ducts (Bismuth-Corlette type IV)
4. An inadequate future liver remnant whether caused by atrophy or insufficient response to growth stimulation (portal vein [PV] ligation or embolization)

In addition, underlying chronic liver disease (especially primary sclerosing cholangitis [PSC]) may preclude hepatic resection. PSC is an idiopathic cholestatic chronic liver disease associated with progressive inflammatory destruction and fibrosis of the entire biliary system and cirrhosis.[13] PSC predisposes to cholangiocarcinoma throughout the biliary tract as a field defect with the potential for multiple cancers. Patients with PSC are best treated by neoadjuvant chemoradiation and liver transplantation rather than resection, even if they have otherwise potentially resectable tumors.[14,15] Although the diagnoses of cholangiocarcinoma and PSC may be established at the same time, 7% to 15% of patients with PSC develop cholangiocarcinoma during their lifetime.[16]

Adequate tumor staging has been historically challenging among patients with hilar cholangiocarcinoma. Unlike the previous editions, the seventh edition of the American Joint Committee on Cancer (AJCC) staging classification has separate staging schemes for intrahepatic, perihilar, and distal cholangiocarcinomas.[17] The AJCC seventh edition T stage has significantly improved granularity compared with previous AJCC editions. However, clinical usefulness of AJCC to predict survival has lacked consistency. Incorporation of a clinically adequate and relevant metric of radial tumor extent has been particularly difficult. One recently reported strategy has involved measurement of radial tumor extent during pathologic evaluation of the resected specimen. Depth of cholangiocarcinoma invasion has also been shown to correlate with disease-specific and long-term survival and may be incorporated into a future AJCC staging system.[18] However, this technique cannot be used during preoperative evaluation and requires standardization of pathologic practice.

An alternative clinical staging system proposed by the Memorial Sloan Kettering Cancer Center (MSKCC) group incorporates clinical factors directly related to local tumor extent, including presence or absence of PV invasion and presence or absence of lobar atrophy.[19–21] The AJCC seventh edition T stage and MSKCC T stage are compared in **Table 1**. Recent data support the clinical application of the MSKCC staging in helping to predict resectability; in addition, early MSKCC stage (ie, T stage 1) has been associated with improved patient survival when compared with advanced stages.[21–23] A new staging system with goals of standardizing reporting and addressing

Table 1
Summary of the T classification of the AJCC (seventh edition) and MSKCC staging systems

	AJCC	MSKCC
T1	Confined to the bile duct	Involves biliary confluence; ± unilateral extension to second-order biliary radicals
T2	Invades beyond the wall of the bile duct to adjacent adipose (a) or hepatic parenchyma (b)	T1 ± ipsilateral PV involvement ± ipsilateral hepatic lobar atrophy
T3	Invades unilateral branches of PV or HA	Involves biliary confluence with bilateral extension to second-order radicles; or unilateral extension to second-order radicles with contralateral PV involvement or contralateral lobar atrophy; or main or bilateral PV involvement
T4	Invades main PV or its branches bilaterally; or CHA; or second-order biliary radicles bilaterally; or unilateral second-order biliary radicles with contralateral PV or HA	—

Abbreviations: CHA, common hepatic artery; HA, hepatic artery.
Adapted from Edge SB, Byrd DR, Compton CC, et al, editors. AJCC cancer staging manual. 7th edition. New York: Springer; 2010. p. 649; and Jarnagin WR, Fong Y, DeMatteo RP, et al. Staging, resectability, and outcome in 225 patients with hilar cholangiocarcinoma. Ann Surg 2001;234:507–17.

all aspects of perioperative care, including resectability, indications for transplantation, and prognosis, has been proposed; clinical application and validation of this system are yet to be published.[24]

PREOPERATIVE PATIENT SELECTION AND DIAGNOSTIC TECHNIQUES

Operative treatment of hilar cholangiocarcinoma continues to pose significant risk. Perioperative mortality ranges from 5% to 10%, and morbidity ranges from 30% to 60%. Only patients with clinical performance status of more than 50% of normal and without significant systemic comorbid disease (Eastern Cooperative Oncology Group grade ≤ 2) should be considered for curative resection or neoadjuvant therapy and liver transplantation.

Diagnosis of hilar cholangiocarcinoma can be elusive. However, before considering definitive treatment, diagnosis requires presence of a malignant appearing stricture and at least 1 of the following: (1) endoluminal biopsy or cytology positive for cholangiocarcinoma; (2) polysomy by fluorescent in situ hybridization; (3) mass lesion on cross-sectional imaging at the location of the malignant appearing stricture; or (4) CA 19-9 greater than 100.[11,25] Resection, but not transplantation, can be performed based on malignant appearing stricture alone, on an individual case-by-case basis.[11]

Almost all patients with hilar cholangiocarcinoma are initially evaluated for jaundice.[26,27] Initial imaging classically reveals intrahepatic, but not extrahepatic, biliary dilation. Biliary anatomy is evaluated with cholangiography. Cross-sectional imaging (either computed tomography [CT] or magnetic resonance [MR] imaging) and biliary imaging (endoscopic retrograde cholangiography [ERC] or MR cholangiography [MRC] or CT cholangiography) should be performed early during the evaluation process.[27–30] Choice of imaging modality varies with the clinician's preference and institutional experience. The goals of cross-sectional imaging are to evaluate for local, regional, and distal extent of disease. The 4 specific factors that must be assessed by preoperative imaging are: (1) metastatic disease, (2) ductal involvement, (3) vascular involvement, and (4) extent of hepatic atrophy. Positron emission tomography (PET) is not routinely used during diagnosis and staging of hilar cholangiocarcinoma. Sensitivity for the detection of regional and distant metastases is low. In addition, PET lacks specificity for evaluation of local tumor (particularly sclerosing variant) and nodal metastases.[31,32]

Distant metastases must be excluded before consideration of operative treatment. Nodal basins also need to be evaluated. Lymph node involvement in the regional nodal basin (hepatoduodenal ligament lymph nodes = N1) does not preclude resection but does preclude transplantation. Distant lymph node involvement (celiac or aortocaval nodes = N2) precludes both resection and transplantation. Local extent of disease should be ascertained both directly and indirectly. Cross-sectional imaging with vascular-timed contrast and cholangiography frequently identifies ductal involvement as well as tumor relationship to major vascular structures. Ipsilateral vascular involvement (either PV or hepatic artery) does not preclude resection; contralateral vascular involvement precludes resection but does not preclude transplantation. In cases in which a hilar mass cannot be identified, indirect signs of tumor extent such as vascular (arterial or venous) involvement or lobar atrophy can be ascertained.[33] Evidence of lobar atrophy (**Fig. 2**) must prompt a careful examination of ipsilateral vascular inflow, in particular PV. On occasion, lobar atrophy can develop from biliary obstruction alone, without vascular compromise.

Current cross-sectional techniques permit concomitant cholangiography either with MRC or CT (CT cholangiography and three-dimensional reconstruction) modalities.[29,34] Clear definition of the intrahepatic extension of cholangiocarcinoma is critical to resectability and operative approach. Such noninvasive cholangiography concomitantly with contrast-enhanced MR or CT angiography has excellent diagnostic and clinical efficacy. Despite noninvasive diagnostic techniques, most patients require an ERC to obtain an intraluminal specimen for histology or cytology and to provide preoperative biliary decompression. Patients with suspected hilar cholangiocarcinoma require an experienced endoscopist. Percutaneous transhepatic cholangiography (PTC) is reserved for patients who have an inadequate ERC (usually inadequate imaging to determine the extent of left or right duct involvement) or are

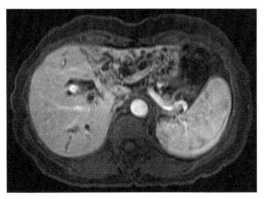

Fig. 2. MR imaging of Bismuth-Corlette type IIIB hilar cholangiocarcinoma with significant intrahepatic ductal dilatation of the left ductal system and left lobar atrophy.

not amenable to biliary decompression with endoscopy. PTC should be avoided whenever possible. Transperitoneal biopsy or fine-needle aspiration (FNA) of cholangiocarcinoma can lead to tumor seeding and has been associated with higher rates of postoperative recurrence.[35,36]

Imaging studies should be carefully interpreted by a multidisciplinary team. Individual images cannot be interpreted in isolation and a combination of cross-sectional images and dynamic biliary reconstructions is needed to appreciate tumor presence, location, and vascular involvement. Biliary stricture and corresponding proximal biliary dilatation can help delineate longitudinal extension of tumor along the duct. Viewing of both axial and coronal reconstructions helps to visualize the anatomic relationships between the tumor and vascular structures.

RESECTION AND TRANSPLANTATION CRITERIA

The following criteria for unresectability have been proposed:

1. Distant metastases
2. Lymph node metastases beyond hepatoduodenal ligament (ie, N2 lymph node involvement)
3. Bilateral ductal extension to the secondary (or segmental) biliary radicles
4. Encasement or occlusion of the main PV (or common hepatic artery) proximal to its bifurcation
5. Unilateral involvement of secondary (or segmental) biliary radicles with contralateral vascular involvement
6. Lobar atrophy with involvement of contralateral secondary (or segmental) biliary radicles
7. Lobar atrophy with involvement of contralateral PV or hepatic artery

Patients with unresectability criteria 3 to 7 are candidates for neoadjuvant chemoradiation and liver transplantation, if they have early stage (AJCC stage I or II) lymph node–negative disease.[11,37] Presence of distant metastases or any nodal metastases precludes liver transplantation.

Liver transplantation inclusion and exclusion criteria are designed to select those patients who are (1) unresectable, (2) least likely to develop metastatic disease, (3) most likely to respond to neoadjuvant chemoradiation, and (4) have the highest probability of survival after liver transplantation.[11] Liver resection and transplantation for hilar cholangiocarcinoma are mutually exclusive therapeutic pathways, without possibility for crossover. Patients found to have unresectable disease during exploration for resection do not do well with subsequent neoadjuvant therapy and liver transplantation. In our experience, operative exploration and subsequent neoadjuvant therapy increase the likelihood for recurrence after transplantation and technical difficulty with transplantation. Conversely, patients who fall out of the neoadjuvant therapy transplantation protocol cannot undergo liver resection even if they are believed to have potentially resectable disease. Neoadjuvant therapy causes widespread hilar biliary necrosis that would make resection and subsequent biliary reconstruction hazardous.

All patients included in the transplant protocol require a diagnosis of hilar cholangiocarcinoma based on presence of malignant appearing stricture and at least 1 of the 4 diagnostic criteria listed previously.[38] In addition, patients with PSC and cholangiocarcinoma are considered to have a field defect and are probably best treated by neoadjuvant therapy and liver transplantation rather than resection, even if they have otherwise potentially resectable tumors.

Candidates for transplantation should not have medical conditions that preclude transplantation and must not have active/uncontrolled infections. In addition, the following criteria preclude neoadjuvant therapy and transplantation[11,12,39]:

1. Intrahepatic, gallbladder, or distal cholangiocarcinoma (below the level of the cystic duct)
2. Primary tumor greater than 3 cm in radial diameter (perpendicular to the duct)
3. Any nodal or distant metastases
4. Any surgical attempt at exploration for resection or transperitoneal tumor biopsy or FNA, including endoscopic ultrasound-directed aspiration (EUS) of the tumor. Conversely, EUS/FNA of suspicious regional lymph nodes should be performed to exclude nodal metastases
5. Previous treatment with radiotherapy or chemotherapy that precludes full-dose neoadjuvant therapy
6. History of other malignancy within 5 years

PREOPERATIVE PATIENT PREPARATION
Resection

Cholangitis and any organ dysfunction must be addressed before resection of hilar cholangiocarcinoma, if possible.[40,41] Coagulopathy should be corrected with vitamin K. Systemic antibiotics and biliary drainage should be used before resection and reconstruction of biliary system to minimize perioperative risk of biliary sepsis and liver dysfunction. Biliary drainage of hepatic remnant is usually performed endoscopically when feasible and percutaneously among patients in whom endoscopic decompression cannot be achieved. Preoperative biliary drainage is particularly relevant for the remnant liver when preoperative contralateral PVE is required. Although there has been debate about the usefulness of biliary drainage overall, drainage is appropriate in patients with marked preoperative jaundice or cholangitis.[42] Current data do not support historically discussed risks of increased postoperative infections or tumor seeding with drainage alone; biliary drainage of hepatic remnant should be performed in symptomatic patients before resection.[43] However, drainage of the atrophic liver lobe is contraindicated because of the risk of persistent biliary infection if the tumor proves to be unresectable.

Choice of the extent of hepatic resection is highly dependent on institutional experience. Several high-volume centers routinely perform anatomic hemihepatectomy of the ipsilateral liver in conjunction with the bile duct resection and reconstruction.[1,2,21,44] However, others advocate for an extended hepatectomy to facilitate adequate resection.[1,45,46] Margin-negative resection is critical to achieving improved survival. Rates of margin-negative resection or survival have not differed between centers performing standard versus extended hepatectomy. Among patients selected for extended hepatectomy, PVE is frequently needed to optimize the functional liver remnant.[47] Combination of preoperative biliary drainage with PVE augments hepatic hypertrophy in preparation for resection.[48,49]

Transplantation

Neoadjuvant protocols differ by institution; however, in general, they consist of consecutive external-beam radiation (40–45 Gy) with concomitant 5-fluorouracil chemosensitization, followed by transcatheter radiation with iridium wires (brachytherapy 20–30 Gy). Brachytherapy wires are placed endoscopically, when possible, and via PTC, when an ERC approach fails. After brachytherapy, maintenance capecitabine is administered while patients await transplantation.[11,38]

The neoadjuvant protocol provides aggressive systemic and locoregional therapy and can result in significant toxicity. Recurrent cholangitis occurs in most, if not all, patients with various degrees of severity. Many patients, particularly those with PSC, can develop hepatic abscesses, requiring preoperative percutaneous drainage and prolonged antibiotic therapy. The patient dropout rate, largely because of tumor progression, after starting neoadjuvant therapy is approximately 11.5% per 3 months, and approaches 30% at 12 months among patients awaiting transplantation.[37,50] Independent factors associated with dropout from neoadjuvant protocol are initial CA 19-9 500 or greater, tumor 3 cm or greater, and MELD (Model for End-Stage Liver Disease) 20 or greater.[51] Routine pretransplant surveillance is performed every 3 months before transplantation as required by United Network for Organ Sharing/Organ Procurement and Transplantation Network policy for patients with malignancy awaiting liver transplantation. Evidence of disease progression or metastases while on the neoadjuvant protocol precludes transplantation.

OPERATIVE MANAGEMENT
Resection

After radiographic exclusion of distant and N2 metastases, diagnostic laparoscopy is performed. Occult liver or peritoneal metastases have been detected in up to 25% of laparoscopically explored patients, precluding the unnecessary morbidity of laparotomy among these patients.[52,53] During abdominal exploration, N2 lymph node basins are explored. If metastases are detected, resection is aborted. Intraoperative evaluation of local tumor extent and vascular involvement is essential for determining resectability. Gallbladder and cystic node are mobilized from the liver but left attached to the bile duct and hepatoduodenal ligament. The hepatoduodenal ligament is frequently thickened with dense desmoplasia and neural proliferation. In patients with Bismuth-Corlette type IIIa and IIIb tumors, the contralateral hilar plate is incised to evaluate proximal extent of the tumor. Careful and extensive hepatoduodenal ligament dissection is frequently necessary to evaluate resectability. Only patients in whom both arterial and portal inflow to the hepatic remnant can be preserved should proceed with resection. Individualized patients with limited vascular involvement of the inflow to the hepatic remnant, particularly involvement of the PV, are selected for concomitant resection and reconstruction at experienced and high-volume cholangiocarcinoma centers.[1,45,54] The role of arterial resection and reconstruction is controversial, and consistent success has been reported only at select high-volume centers.[1,55]

Complete tumor extirpation usually consists of complete hepatoduodenal ligament lymphadenectomy (including cystic, pericholedochal, periportal and retroportal, hepatic artery, hilar, and superior pancreaticoduodenal lymph nodes), resection of the entire extrahepatic bile duct from the hepatic hilus to the pancreas with the attached gallbladder, and concomitant liver resection of the ipsilateral hepatic lobe (**Fig. 3**). The biliary system is subsequently reconstructed using a Roux-en-Y hepaticojejunostomy.

Rare patients with Bismuth-Corlette type I cholangiocarcinoma do not require hepatic resection unless the tumor abuts hepatic parenchyma. Bismuth-Corlette type II cholangiocarcinoma is also rare but frequently shows tumor infiltration of segments I or IVB. Patients with Bismuth-Corlette type III lesions constitute most resectable patients and require concomitant ipsilateral hepatic resection to achieve a negative resection margin. Concomitant ipsilateral hepatectomy results in a margin-negative resection rate greater than 72% to 93% among patients selected for resection at high-volume centers. Tumor invasion of the proximal bile duct margin at the peripancreatic margin requires either bile duct re-excision (if technically feasible) or

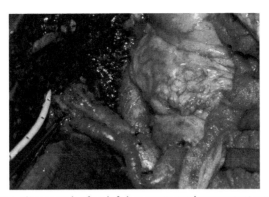

Fig. 3. Intraoperative photograph after left hepatectomy (segmentectomy I–IV) for type IIIB hilar cholangiocarcinoma. The extrahepatic biliary tree and all tissue from the hepatoduodenal ligament (including all nodal, neural, and desmoplastic tissue) have been resected with the tumor, with the exception of right hepatic artery and right PV. PTC tube exits right anterior ductal system; forceps overlying opening of right posterior ductal system.

consideration for pancreaticoduodenectomy. Type IV lesions are treated by neoadjuvant therapy and transplantation.

CAUDATE LOBECTOMY

Segment I ducts enter the hilus posteriorly at the confluence of the right and left hepatic ducts. Routine caudate lobectomy has been proposed for all patients with Bismuth III cholangiocarcinoma and selected patients with Bismuth II cholangiocarcinoma.[56,57] Pathologic extension of cholangiocarcinoma into a segment I duct has been confirmed in more than 40% of the patients. Early data suggested a 20% reduction in local recurrence rates with routine caudate lobectomy. Additional studies showed improvement in margin-negative resection and survival with addition of caudate lobectomy to hemihepatectomy.[40,57] Although caudate lobectomy is routinely performed in many hepatobiliary centers, select institutions do not perform routine segment I resection in patients with type II or IIIa cholangiocarcinoma with histologically negative segment I duct margin. The intraoperative histologic margin evaluation and surgical attempt at complete tumor extirpation with microscopically negative margin is the only known curative treatment of hilar cholangiocarcinoma.[58]

EXTENDED HEPATECTOMIES AND HILAR EN BLOC RESECTION

Extended hepatectomy and hilar en bloc "no-touch" techniques have been proposed to help improve margin-negative resection rate of hilar cholangiocarcinoma.[46,59] Theoretically, the extended hepatectomy approach is based on the branching anatomy of right and left hepatic arteries and confluence of the right and left hepatic ducts. Hilar cholangiocarcinoma is more likely to overly the right arterial system than the left hepatic artery. As such, the right hepatic artery is more likely to be infiltrated by tumor, precluding margin-negative resection of Bismuth-Corlette IIIb cholangiocarcinoma with a left hepatectomy.

Hence, select hepatobiliary centers have adopted extended hepatectomy (particularly right trisectionectomy) as the preferential resection approach for type III cholangiocarcinoma.[23,57] Preoperative right PVE with or without segment IV embolization is frequently performed to optimize function of the future liver remnant.[60] Resection of the extrahepatic bile duct and hepatoduodenal ligament are performed in a similar fashion; however, resection of Bismuth-Corlette III tumors is approached through a right trisectionectomy, with subsequent biliary reconstruction to segment II and III ducts. The margin-negative resection rate does not differ among centers selecting patients for hemihepatectomy versus extended hepatectomy, and the approaches seem to be driven by institutional experience.[1,2]

Hilar en bloc resection "no-touch" technique in combination with right trisectionectomy has been proposed as an aggressive resection strategy for patients with Bismuth-Corlette types I to IV cholangiocarcinoma.[46,59] The "no-touch" technique extends the application of the anatomic relationship of right and left hepatic arteries and ducts, emphasizing the site of the PV bifurcation posterior to the biliary confluence to avoid dissection in the vicinity of the cancer. The approach to the hepatoduodenal ligament differs significantly. The common hepatic artery is identified and the right hepatic artery is ligated immediately at its origin along the left border of the hepatoduodenal ligament. The main PV is divided proximal to bifurcation and the left PV is divided at the level of umbilical fissure. The parenchyma is then transected followed by transection of the left duct. The entire extrahepatic bile duct and biliary confluence to the level of the tumor-free left hepatic duct, right hepatic artery, PV bifurcation, hepatoduodenal ligament lymph nodes and liver segments IV to VIII and I are thus removed en bloc. Although extended left hepatectomies for resection of hilar cholangiocarcinoma have been performed, a similar en bloc "no-touch" approach with an extended left hepatectomy has not been proposed. Although the PV can be reconstructed with synthetic prosthetics or bioprosthetics, reconstruction of the right hepatic artery has precluded any substantive experience. Patients with left lobe atrophy or extension of cholangiocarcinoma to left biliary radicles are not candidates for hilar en bloc resection. In general, morbidity of extended resections can be significant, with up to 30% risk of hepatic insufficiency.[46] Comparative margin-negative resection rates and patient survival do not differ between high-volume centers with center-specific expertise with alternative operative approaches.

LIVER TRANSPLANTATION

Operative staging is essential before transplantation to exclude locally extensive disease and presence of nodal, peritoneal, and extrahepatic metastases.[11,12] When possible, operative staging is performed using hand-assisted laparoscopy. Operative staging involves a thorough intra-abdominal exploration and biopsy of any suspicious lesions, excision of the common hepatic artery lymph node overlying the hepatic artery at the takeoff of the gastroduodenal artery, and excision of the pericholedochal lymph node. Occasionally, patients are too sick to undergo a separate operation, and operative staging is performed when a donor liver becomes available.

Liver transplantation for hilar cholangiocarcinoma is performed similarly to transplantation for other acute and chronic liver diseases, with several technical considerations. Hilar dissection is avoided to prevent dissemination of the tumor. The bile duct is transected at the peripancreatic margin (as close to the pancreas as possible), and the margin is evaluated intraoperatively by frozen section. Similarly, the PV is transected as it emerges from the retropancreatic groove to excise most of the native vein present in the previously irradiated field. Marginal involvement has been limited to patients with underlying PSC, and has been observed in approximately 10% of patients with PSC. Operative management options include re-excision, if feasible, and pancreatoduodenectomy. Donor iliac artery jump graft from infrarenal aorta to the donor hepatic artery is used during deceased donor liver transplantation to avoid hepatic artery thrombosis, due to preoperative irradiation. This technique has not been successful with living donor liver transplantation because of the size mismatch between an iliac graft and a donor left or right hepatic artery. Arterial reconstruction with the irradiated recipient proper or common hepatic artery in living donor liver recipient is performed. These patients are subsequently monitored closely with Doppler ultrasonography during the postoperative period for any change in hepatic arterial flow.

The PV is reconstructed by a direct anastomosis between the donor and recipient PVs during deceased donor transplantation. A direct reconstruction is not possible for living donor liver recipients because of low division of the recipient PV. The gap between the recipient and donor PVs is reconstructed with a segment of deceased donor iliac vein as an interposition graft. Biliary reconstruction is performed with a Roux-en-Y choledochojejunostomy or hepaticojejunostomy. An external transjejunal cholangiocatheter is used routinely to obtain a cholangiogram during the early postoperative period with deceased donor transplantation; biliary reconstruction in a living donor transplant recipient is performed with an internal biliary stent.

MORBIDITY

Operative treatment of hilar cholangiocarcinoma carries higher perioperative mortality than any other elective operation. Perioperative mortality after hepatic resection at high-volume hepatobiliary centers and among multi-institutional series ranges between 5% and 10%.[21,45,61] Ninety-day mortality exceeds 10% in most series reporting 3 months follow-up.[59] Similarly, mortality is significant among patients enrolled in neoadjuvant therapy and liver transplantation protocols.[50]

Perioperative morbidity is also high and ranges from 30% to more than 60% in current reports. Infectious and biliary complications, such as wound infection, intraabdominal abscess, bile leak, and biloma, are most frequent. Rates of hepatic insufficiency have been reduced to approximately 10% to 20% with preoperative patient selection and use of PVE. Risk of PV thrombosis is low at experienced centers. Use of interposition grafts seems to increase rates of PV complications.[62] Complications from arterial resections are rarely reported from select high-volume centers with extensive experience.[1,55] However, recent meta-analyses have failed to show any survival benefit to routine PV resection for patients without tumor invasion into the resected vein. Moreover, greater morbidity and mortality for patients requiring arterial resections without improved survival were reported.[63] Most high-volume hepatobiliary centers do not perform hepatic artery resections and instead refer the patients for liver transplantation. Variability in treatment approaches to vascular invasion (particularly arterial involvement) might be rooted in the variability in donor liver availability for transplantation.

Vascular complications, however, are more common in liver transplant recipients. The higher rates of vascular complications after transplantation for hilar cholangiocarcinoma than for other liver diseases are attributable to high-dose neoadjuvant radiotherapy. These complications primarily occur with the reconstructed PV in both deceased and living donor recipients, and the reconstructed hepatic artery after living donor transplantation.[64] The overall rate of vascular complications after liver transplantation is approximately 40%: 20% for the hepatic artery (living donor recipients) and 20% for the PV (living and deceased donor recipients). Hepatic venous or caval outflow complications are rare and are comparable with noncholangiocarcinoma transplant recipients. Biliary complications after transplantation for hilar cholangiocarcinoma occur in approximately 30% of living donor liver recipients and 10% of deceased donor liver recipients.

RESECTION STATUS AND SURVIVAL

Success of treatment among patients with hilar cholangiocarcinoma is measured by rates of margin-negative resection and overall survival. Implicit in these metrics are data supporting predisposition for distant rather than local cancer recurrence after margin-negative resection.[65] Routine hemihepatectomy or extended hepatectomy during resection of hilar cholangiocarcinoma has significantly increased rates of margin-negative resection. Historically, margin-negative resection rate was less than 30% in a cohort of patients with a 20% rate of concomitant bile duct resection and hepatectomy.[66,67] As the rates of hemihepatectomy and extended hepatectomy increased to 85% to 100%, the margin-negative resection rate increased to 72% to 93%.[1,21,22,45,68] The extent of hepatectomy (hemihepatectomy vs extended hepatectomy) continues to depend on institutional preference. Central hepatectomy (segment IVB/V with caudate resection) has also been used with high margin-negative resection rate and low mortality.[69] Hepatectomy has increased 5-year overall survival rates up to 20% to 40% among patients with resected hilar cholangiocarcinoma, with some centers reporting more than 50% 5-year survival among margin-negative patients.[1,23,70]

Unresectable patients who complete neoadjuvant protocol and transplantation demonstrate up to 65% 5-year recurrence-free survival.[50] These patients report better health-related quality of life than liver transplant recipients receiving organs for diagnoses not related to cholangiocarcinoma.[71] However, up to 30% of transplant candidates drop out from the transplant protocol before transplantation.[37] Direct comparisons between resection and transplantation groups are not possible. Patient populations selected for each treatment arm are usually drastically different, without possibility for crossover.

ADJUVANT TREATMENT

To date, there are no convincing data to support use of adjuvant therapy among patients with resected hilar cholangiocarcinoma. Resected patients with node-negative disease (stages I and II) and margin-negative resection are not offered additional therapy. Select patients with node-positive or metastatic disease are usually treated within hepatobiliary trial parameters. The recent ABC-02 (Advanced Biliary Cancer phase 2) trial reported a benefit from a combination of cisplatin and gemcitabine compared with gemcitabine alone, among patients with locally advanced or metastatic and unresectable gallbladder or cholangiocarcinoma.[72,73] Other strategies include administration of 5-fluorouracil in combination with other cytotoxins, such as gemcitabine, leucovorin, mitomycin C, cisplatin, epirubicin, or interferon α.[74,75] Numerous trials comprising various cytotoxic agents (including FOLFIRINOX) as well as targeted molecular therapies are under investigation worldwide.[76] Significant palliation and rarely prolonged survival has been achieved with radiotherapy, occasionally with systemic radiosensitizers. External-beam radiotherapy and iridium brachytherapy, as well as newer local approaches, such as stereotactic body radiation therapy and photodynamic therapy, have all been shown to improve palliation.[77–79]

SUMMARY

Hilar cholangiocarcinoma is an aggressive primary biliary malignancy of the extrahepatic bile duct, requiring a multidisciplinary approach. Patients usually present with jaundice and dilatation of intrahepatic bile ducts. Multimodality imaging, including cross-sectional and cholangiographic examinations, is required for diagnosis and assessment of resectability. Endoscopic cholangiography is frequently needed to assist with diagnosis and temporary biliary drainage. Criteria for resection and transplantation need to be carefully evaluated for each individual patient before treatment recommendation. Concomitant hepatic resection must be performed for all patients with type III hilar cholangiocarcinoma, select patients with type I cholangiocarcinoma, and most patients with type II cholangiocarcinoma. Extended resections and major vascular resections can be safely performed. Only patients with tumor involvement of PV benefit from PV resection. Transplantation is a successful treatment strategy for patients with node-negative type IV cholangiocarcinoma. Oncologic success of transplantation depends on the adherence to neoadjuvant protocol and application of the inclusion and exclusion criteria before liver transplantation. Hepatic resection and transplantation for cholangiocarcinoma require significant institutional expertise and must be performed at high-volume hepatobiliary centers. Margin-negative tumor extirpation is the only known curative treatment of hilar cholangiocarcinoma.

REFERENCES

1. Nagino M, Ebata T, Yokoyama Y, et al. Evolution of surgical treatment for perihilar cholangiocarcinoma: a single-center 34-year review of 574 consecutive resections. Ann Surg 2013;258:129–40.
2. Nagorney DM, Kendrick ML. Hepatic resection in the treatment of hilar cholangiocarcinoma. Adv Surg 2006;40:159–71.
3. de Groen PC, Gores GJ, LaRusso NF, et al. Biliary tract cancers. N Engl J Med 1999;341:1368–78.
4. Bismuth H, Nakache R, Diamond T. Management strategies in resection for hilar cholangiocarcinoma. Ann Surg 1992;215:31–8.
5. Rea DJ, Heimbach JK, Rosen CB, et al. Liver transplantation with neoadjuvant chemoradiation is more effective than resection for hilar cholangiocarcinoma. Ann Surg 2005;242:451–8.
6. Hayashi S, Miyazaki M, Kondo Y, et al. Invasive growth patterns of hepatic hilar ductal carcinoma. A histologic analysis of 18 surgical cases. Cancer 1994;73:2922–9.
7. Sakamoto E, Nimura Y, Hayakawa N, et al. The pattern of infiltration at the proximal border of hilar bile duct carcinoma: a histologic analysis of 62 resected cases. Ann Surg 1998;227:405–11.
8. Jarnagin WR, Bowne W, Klimstra DS, et al. Papillary phenotype confers improved survival after resection of hilar cholangiocarcinoma. Ann Surg 2005; 241:703–12.
9. Bismuth H, Corlette MB. Intrahepatic cholangioenteric anastomosis in carcinoma of the hilus of the liver. Surg Gynecol Obstet 1975;140:170–8.
10. Heimbach JK, Gores GJ, Haddock MG, et al. Liver transplantation for unresectable perihilar cholangiocarcinoma. Semin Liver Dis 2004;24:201–7.
11. Rosen CB, Heimbach JK, Gores GJ. Liver transplantation for cholangiocarcinoma. Transpl Int 2010;23:692–7.
12. Rea DJ, Rosen CB, Nagorney DM, et al. Transplantation for cholangiocarcinoma: when and for whom? Surg Oncol Clin N Am 2009;18:325–37.
13. Lazaridis KN, Gores GJ. Primary sclerosing cholangitis and cholangiocarcinoma. Semin Liver Dis 2006;26:42–51.
14. Farley DR, Weaver AL, Nagorney DM. "Natural history" of unresected cholangiocarcinoma: patient outcome after noncurative intervention. Mayo Clin Proc 1995; 70:425–9.
15. Rosen CB, Nagorney DM, Wiesner RH, et al. Cholangiocarcinoma complicating primary sclerosing cholangitis. Ann Surg 1991;213:21–5.

16. Burak K, Angulo P, Pasha TM, et al. Incidence and risk factors for cholangio-carcinoma in primary sclerosing cholangitis. Am J Gastroenterol 2004;99: 523–6.

17. Edge SB, Byrd DR, Compton CC, et al. AJCC cancer staging manual. 7th edition. New York: Springer; 2010.

18. de Jong MC, Hong SM, Augustine MM, et al. Hilar cholangiocarcinoma: tumor depth as a predictor of outcome. Arch Surg 2011;146:697–703.

19. Burke EC, Jarnagin WR, Hochwald SN, et al. Hilar cholangiocarcinoma: patterns of spread, the importance of hepatic resection for curative operation, and a pre-surgical clinical staging system. Ann Surg 1998;228:385–94.

20. Jarnagin WR, Fong Y, DeMatteo RP, et al. Staging, resectability, and outcome in 225 patients with hilar cholangiocarcinoma. Ann Surg 2001;234:507–17.

21. Matsuo K, Rocha FG, Ito K, et al. The Blumgart preoperative staging system for hilar cholangiocarcinoma: analysis of resectability and outcomes in 380 patients. J Am Coll Surg 2012;215:343–55.

22. Zaydfudim VM, Clark CJ, Kendrick ML, et al. Correlation of staging systems to survival in patients with resected hilar cholangiocarcinoma. Am J Surg 2013; 206:159–65.

23. Hemming AW, Reed AI, Fujita S, et al. Surgical management of hilar cholangio-carcinoma. Ann Surg 2005;241:693–9.

24. DeOliveira ML, Schulick RD, Nimura Y, et al. New staging system and a registry for perihilar cholangiocarcinoma. Hepatology 2011;53:1363–71.

25. Blechacz B, Komuta M, Roskams T, et al. Clinical diagnosis and staging of chol-angiocarcinoma. Nat Rev Gastroenterol Hepatol 2011;8:512–22.

26. Khan SA, Davidson BR, Goldin R, et al. Guidelines for the diagnosis and treatment of cholangiocarcinoma: consensus document. Gut 2002;51(Suppl 6): VI1–9.

27. Khan SA, Davidson BR, Goldin RD, et al. Guidelines for the diagnosis and treatment of cholangiocarcinoma: an update. Gut 2012;61:1657–69.

28. Ruys AT, van Beem BE, Engelbrecht MR, et al. Radiological staging in patients with hilar cholangiocarcinoma: a systematic review and meta-analysis. Br J Radiol 2012;85:1255–62.

29. Hyodo T, Kumano S, Kushihata F, et al. CT and MR cholangiography: advantages and pitfalls in perioperative evaluation of biliary tree. Br J Radiol 2012; 85:887–96.

30. Masselli G, Gualdi G. Hilar cholangiocarcinoma: MRI/MRCP in staging and treatment planning. Abdom Imaging 2008;33:444–51.

31. Anderson CD, Rice MH, Pinson CW, et al. Fluorodeoxyglucose PET imaging in the evaluation of gallbladder carcinoma and cholangiocarcinoma. J Gastrointest Surg 2004;8:90–7.

32. Ruys AT, Bennink RJ, van Westreenen HL, et al. FDG-positron emission tomography/computed tomography and standardized uptake value in the primary diagnosis and staging of hilar cholangiocarcinoma. HPB (Oxford) 2011;13: 256–62.

33. Friesen BR, Gibson RN, Speer T, et al. Lobar and segmental liver atrophy associated with hilar cholangiocarcinoma and the impact of hilar biliary anatomical variants: a pictorial essay. Insights Imaging 2011;2:525–31.

34. Endo I, Shimada H, Sugita M, et al. Role of three-dimensional imaging in operative planning for hilar cholangiocarcinoma. Surgery 2007;142:666–75.

35. Chapman WC, Sharp KW, Weaver F, et al. Tumor seeding from percutaneous biliary catheters. Ann Surg 1989;209:708–13.

36. Sakata J, Shirai Y, Wakai T, et al. Catheter tract implantation metastases associated with percutaneous biliary drainage for extrahepatic cholangiocarcinoma. World J Gastroenterol 2005;11:7024–7.

37. Gores GJ, Darwish Murad S, Heimbach JK, et al. Liver transplantation for perihilar cholangiocarcinoma. Dig Dis 2013;31:126–9.

38. Gores GJ, Gish RG, Sudan D, et al. Model for end-stage liver disease (MELD) exception for cholangiocarcinoma or biliary dysplasia. Liver Transpl 2006;12: S95–7.

39. Heimbach JK, Sanchez W, Rosen CB, et al. Trans-peritoneal fine needle aspiration biopsy of hilar cholangiocarcinoma is associated with disease dissemination. HPB (Oxford) 2011;13:356–60.

40. Nimura Y, Kamiya J, Kondo S, et al. Aggressive preoperative management and extended surgery for hilar cholangiocarcinoma: Nagoya experience. J Hepatobiliary Pancreat Surg 2000;7:155–62.

41. Belghiti J, Ogata S. Preoperative optimization of the liver for resection in patients with hilar cholangiocarcinoma. HPB (Oxford) 2005;7:252–3.

42. Liu F, Li Y, Wei Y, et al. Preoperative biliary drainage before resection for hilar cholangiocarcinoma: whether or not? A systematic review. Dig Dis Sci 2011; 56:663–72.

43. Farges O, Regimbeau JM, Fuks D, et al. Multicentre European study of preoperative biliary drainage for hilar cholangiocarcinoma. Br J Surg 2013;100:274–83.

44. Rea DJ, Munoz-Juarez M, Farnell MB, et al. Major hepatic resection for hilar cholangiocarcinoma: analysis of 46 patients. Arch Surg 2004;139:514–23.

45. Hemming AW, Mekeel K, Khanna A, et al. Portal vein resection in management of hilar cholangiocarcinoma. J Am Coll Surg 2011;212:604–13.

46. Neuhaus P, Thelen A, Jonas S, et al. Oncological superiority of hilar en bloc resection for the treatment of hilar cholangiocarcinoma. Ann Surg Oncol 2012; 19:1602–8.

47. Makuuchi M, Thai BL, Takayasu K, et al. Preoperative portal embolization to increase safety of major hepatectomy for hilar bile duct carcinoma: a preliminary report. Surgery 1990;107:521–7.

48. Kubota K, Makuuchi M, Kusaka K, et al. Measurement of liver volume and hepatic functional reserve as a guide to decision-making in resectional surgery for hepatic tumors. Hepatology 1997;26:1176–81.

49. Seyama Y, Kubota K, Sano K, et al. Long-term outcome of extended hemihepatectomy for hilar bile duct cancer with no mortality and high survival rate. Ann Surg 2003;238:73–83.

50. Darwish Murad S, Kim WR, Harnois DM, et al. Efficacy of neoadjuvant chemoradiation, followed by liver transplantation, for perihilar cholangiocarcinoma at 12 US centers. Gastroenterology 2012;143:88–98.

51. Darwish Murad S, Kim WR, Therneau T, et al. Predictors of pretransplant dropout and posttransplant recurrence in patients with perihilar cholangiocarcinoma. Hepatology 2012;56:972–81.

52. Weber SM, DeMatteo RP, Fong Y, et al. Staging laparoscopy in patients with extrahepatic biliary carcinoma. Analysis of 100 patients. Ann Surg 2002;235: 392–9.

53. Joseph S, Connor S, Garden OJ. Staging laparoscopy for cholangiocarcinoma. HPB (Oxford) 2008;10:116–9.

54. de Jong MC, Marques H, Clary BM, et al. The impact of portal vein resection on outcomes for hilar cholangiocarcinoma: a multi-institutional analysis of 305 cases. Cancer 2012;118:4737–47.

55. Nagino M, Nimura Y, Nishio H, et al. Hepatectomy with simultaneous resection of the portal vein and hepatic artery for advanced perihilar cholangiocarcinoma: an audit of 50 consecutive cases. Ann Surg 2010;252:115–23.

56. Nimura Y, Hayakawa N, Kamiya J, et al. Hepatic segmentectomy with caudate lobe resection for bile duct carcinoma of the hepatic hilus. World J Surg 1990; 14:535–43.

57. Nagino M, Kamiya J, Arai T, et al. "Anatomic" right hepatic trisectionectomy (extended right hepatectomy) with caudate lobectomy for hilar cholangiocarcinoma. Ann Surg 2006;243:28–32.

58. Ribero D, Amisano M, Lo Tesoriere R, et al. Additional resection of an intraoperative margin-positive proximal bile duct improves survival in patients with hilar cholangiocarcinoma. Ann Surg 2011;254:776–81.

59. Neuhaus P, Jonas S, Bechstein WO, et al. Extended resections for hilar cholangiocarcinoma. Ann Surg 1999;230:808–18.

60. Nagino M, Kamiya J, Nishio H, et al. Two hundred forty consecutive portal vein embolizations before extended hepatectomy for biliary cancer: surgical outcome and long-term follow-up. Ann Surg 2006;243:364–72.

61. Nuzzo G, Giuliante F, Ardito F, et al. Improvement in perioperative and long-term outcome after surgical treatment of hilar cholangiocarcinoma: results of an Italian multicenter analysis of 440 patients. Arch Surg 2012;147:26–34.

62. Kondo S, Katoh H, Hirano S, et al. Portal vein resection and reconstruction prior to hepatic dissection during right hepatectomy and caudate lobectomy for hepatobiliary cancer. Br J Surg 2003;90:694–7.

63. Abbas S, Sandroussi C. Systematic review and meta-analysis of the role of vascular resection in the treatment of hilar cholangiocarcinoma. HPB (Oxford) 2013;15:492–503.

64. Mantel HT, Rosen CB, Heimbach JK, et al. Vascular complications after orthotopic liver transplantation after neoadjuvant therapy for hilar cholangiocarcinoma. Liver Transpl 2007;13:1372–81.

65. Kobayashi A, Miwa S, Nakata T, et al. Disease recurrence patterns after R0 resection of hilar cholangiocarcinoma. Br J Surg 2010;97:56–64.

66. Cameron JL, Pitt HA, Zinner MJ, et al. Management of proximal cholangiocarcinomas by surgical resection and radiotherapy. Am J Surg 1990;159:91–7.

67. Tsao JI, Nimura Y, Kamiya J, et al. Management of hilar cholangiocarcinoma: comparison of an American and a Japanese experience. Ann Surg 2000;232: 166–74.

68. Sano T, Shimada K, Sakamoto Y, et al. One hundred two consecutive hepatobiliary resections for perihilar cholangiocarcinoma with zero mortality. Ann Surg 2006;244:240–7.

69. Chen XP, Lau WY, Huang ZY, et al. Extent of liver resection for hilar cholangiocarcinoma. Br J Surg 2009;96:1167–75.

70. Igami T, Nishio H, Ebata T, et al. Surgical treatment of hilar cholangiocarcinoma in the "new era": the Nagoya University experience. J Hepatobiliary Pancreat Sci 2010;17:449–54.

71. Darwish Murad S, Heimbach JK, Gores GJ, et al. Excellent quality of life after liver transplantation for patients with perihilar cholangiocarcinoma who have undergone neoadjuvant chemoradiation. Liver Transpl 2013;19:521–8.

72. Valle JW, Wasan H, Johnson P, et al. Gemcitabine alone or in combination with cisplatin in patients with advanced or metastatic cholangiocarcinomas or other biliary tract tumours: a multicentre randomised phase II study–the UK ABC-01 study. Br J Cancer 2009;101:621–7.

73. Valle J, Wasan H, Palmer DH, et al. Cisplatin plus gemcitabine versus gemcitabine for biliary tract cancer. N Engl J Med 2010;362:1273–81.
74. Todoroki T. Chemotherapy for bile duct carcinoma in the light of adjuvant chemotherapy to surgery. Hepatogastroenterology 2000;47:644–9.
75. Nakeeb A, Pitt HA. Radiation therapy, chemotherapy and chemoradiation in hilar cholangiocarcinoma. HPB (Oxford) 2005;7:278–82.
76. Geynisman DM, Catenacci DV. Toward personalized treatment of advanced biliary tract cancers. Discov Med 2012;14:41–57.
77. Kuvshinoff BW, Armstrong JG, Fong Y, et al. Palliation of irresectable hilar cholangiocarcinoma with biliary drainage and radiotherapy. Br J Surg 1995;82:1522–5.
78. Gerhards MF, van Gulik TM, Gonzalez Gonzalez D, et al. Results of postoperative radiotherapy for resectable hilar cholangiocarcinoma. World J Surg 2003;27:173–9.
79. Barney BM, Olivier KR, Miller RC, et al. Clinical outcomes and toxicity using stereotactic body radiotherapy (SBRT) for advanced cholangiocarcinoma. Radiat Oncol 2012;7:67.

Distal Cholangiocarcinoma

Neha Lad, MD, David A. Kooby, MD*

KEYWORDS

- Distal cholangiocarcinoma • Nodal dissection • Neoadjuvant therapy
- Surgical resection

KEY POINTS

- Distal cholangiocarcinoma is an uncommon malignancy, and early diagnosis remains a challenge.
- More accurate diagnostic modalities for early-stage diagnosis are needed.
- Advances in medical therapy and neoadjuvant treatment may aid surgery and further improve postoperative outcomes.
- Margin-negative resection in conjunction with thorough nodal dissection is the strongest prognostic factor.
- Surgical resection coupled with adjuvant therapy provides the most favorable outcome.
- Future efforts should be aimed at reducing surgical complications and improving medical therapy, with overall improvement in perioperative and long-term outcomes for patients with distal cholangiocarcinoma.

INCIDENCE

Worldwide cholangiocarcinoma (CC) is a relatively uncommon cancer accounting for approximately 3% of all diagnosed gastrointestinal malignancies,[1] comprising tumors arising anywhere in the biliary tree. The incidence of CC is rising, and it is estimated that more than 10,000 cases of extrahepatic CC and gallbladder carcinoma combined will be diagnosed in the United States in 2013.[2] Distal cholangiocarcinoma (DCC) is defined as CC of the common bile duct (from the cystic duct to the ampulla of Vater), and represents 20% to 40% of the total.[3–5]

CLASSIFICATION

CC has been conventionally classified according to anatomic location as intrahepatic (ICC), perihilar (PCC), and distal (DCC). The perihilar and distal subtypes are together

Funding: Ann & Paul Hastings Scholarship for Excellence in Surgical Oncology and Patient Care.
Disclosures/Conflict of Interest: None.
Division of Surgical Oncology, Department of Surgery, Winship Cancer Institute, Emory University School of Medicine, 1365C Clifton Road, Northeast, Atlanta, GA 30322, USA
* Corresponding author. 1365C Clifton Road, Northeast, Building C, 2nd Floor, Atlanta, GA 30322.
E-mail address: dkooby@emory.edu

Surg Oncol Clin N Am 23 (2014) 265–287
http://dx.doi.org/10.1016/j.soc.2013.11.001
1055-3207/14/$ – see front matter © 2014 Elsevier Inc. All rights reserved.

classified as extrahepatic cholangiocarcinoma (ECC). Tumors arising in the upper third of extrahepatic bile duct (ie, above the confluence of cystic and common hepatic duct) are called perihilar tumors. Mid–bile duct tumors arise between the confluence of cystic duct and common bile duct and the upper border of the duodenum. Distal bile duct tumors arise in the duodenal and intrapancreatic portion of bile duct up to papilla of Vater; however, they are distinct from ampullary carcinoma.[6] The mid–bile duct group of tumors is uncommon, and is often included within discussions of DCC. When amenable, DCCs are usually managed with pancreaticoduodenectomy (PD).[4,7]

ETIOLOGY

Most cases of CC are sporadic and occur de novo without any identifiable risk factors. Approximately 10% of CCs are known to occur in the presence of chronic inflammation within the biliary tract and injury to ductal epithelium, causing a compensatory increase in mitotic activity, thereby increasing the likelihood of mutation and dysplasia.[1,8] Many of the following described conditions create such a chronic inflammatory state within the biliary tree.

Primary Sclerosing Cholangitis

Primary sclerosing cholangitis (PSC) is thought to be an autoimmune disease with an increased prevalence of human leukocyte antigen (HLA) alleles A1, B8, and DR3,[9] resulting in cholestatic liver disease characterized by diffuse inflammation and fibrosis of the intrahepatic and extrahepatic bile ducts. Patients with PSC are at a significantly higher risk than the general population of developing CC.[10] Incidence of CC in PSC is roughly 15%,[11] and nearly half of the patients with CC are detected at the same time or within a year of the diagnosis of patients harboring PSC.[12,13] The presence of occult CC has been found to be as high as 40% in autopsy specimens of PSC patients.[14,15] In prospectively assessed population studies, the risk of developing CC appears to be 1% per year in patients with PSC.[10,12]

Patients with PSC and concomitant inflammatory bowel disease (ulcerative colitis and Crohn disease) are at a significantly increased risk of developing CC,[14,16] with ECC being more commonly associated with Crohn disease.[17] Medical and surgical therapy does not appear to alter the risk of CC in this subset of patients.[3,13]

The incidence of DCC is approximately 13% in the setting of PSC.[18] Chronic inflammation leads to dysplastic changes in the epithelium and subsequent malignant transformation in the distal bile duct.[8] The coexistence of PSC and CC may confuse and delay the diagnosis, which may ultimately increase in the number of patients with unresectable tumors at presentation.[12,14,19]

Choledochal Cyst

Choledochal cyst disease represents congenital or acquired ectasia of the biliary tree, presumably caused by malunion of the pancreatic duct and common bile duct (CBD). The pancreatic duct joins the CBD proximal to the sphincter complex of Oddi, causing reflux and stasis of pancreatic enzymes proximally into the bile duct, which may be an important factor leading to carcinogenesis in choledochal cysts.[8,20,21]

Although congenital choledochal cysts are more commonly found in girls in the first decade of life,[22] recent series suggest that the number of adults presenting with choledochal cyst disease is increasing.[23,24] Adults harboring choledochal cysts tend to have an increased incidence of biliary carcinoma, which can be explained by an increasing rate of intestinal metaplasia in the wall of choledochal cysts with advancing age.[25,26] Complete cyst excision is the standard of care in these patients, owing to an increased lifetime risk of development of CC in untreated patients.[27]

Parasitic Infestation

The liver flukes, *Clonorchis sinensis* and *Opisthorchis viverrini*, are proven carcinogenic agents for CC, especially in the endemic regions of East Asia.[28–30] The global estimate of *C sinensis* infection is 35 million persons, of whom 15 million are estimated to be in China,[31] whereas that of *O viverrini* is 10 million, of whom 8 million are in Thailand.[32] These food-borne trematodes chronically infect the bile ducts, cause oxidative DNA damage of the biliary epithelium, and induce malignant transformation.[30] There is a 5-fold increase over that of general population for developing CC with either clonorchiasis or opisthorciasis infection.[33] The annual incidence of CC attributed to liver flukes in Thailand is nearly 5000 persons,[34] whereas the annual global incidence ranges between 8000 to 10,000 individuals.[33] Praziquantel (Bayer HealthCare Pharmaceuticals, Germany), an antihelminth, is the mainstay of treatment. Improvements in sanitation and educational campaigns can help reduce the incidence of infection by these helminths.

Cholelithiasis

Incidence of chronic cholelithiasis and hepatolithiasis has been reported as a risk factor for development of ECC.[35,36] The occurrence of CC appears to decline with time after cholecystectomy.[36–38] Large population-based studies have failed to establish a direct causal relationship between CC and choledocholithiasis.[39]

Toxins used for a variety of reasons can induce CC. One such toxin is thorotrast, which was used as a radiologic contrast agent in the early and mid-1900s and was found to be associated with an increased incidence of CC, and was thus banned.[40,41] The estimated latency from exposure to diagnosis of malignancy ranges between 16 and 45 years.[40,41] A large series from Germany reported an increased mortality resulting from toxin exposure, which is corroborated by findings in other work.[42]

Biliary papillomatosis is a rare disease characterized by the presence of multiple papillary adenomas lining the mucosa of the biliary tract. This premalignant condition has high malignant potential. The incidence of carcinoma can be as high as 83% in patients harboring multifocal papillary adenomas. The mucin-producing variant has been associated with poorer outcome in comparison with non–mucin-producing biliary papillomatosis.[43]

Smoking appears to carry a weak association with ECC development,[17] and may contribute to an increased incidence of CC in patients with PSC.[40,44]

Alcohol consumption, alcoholic liver disease, and nonspecific cirrhosis are reported have strong associations with ECC in various hospital-based case-control studies.[17,40,45] Although moderate alcohol consumption is not clearly linked, heavy alcohol use may be associated with a 2- to 15-fold increase in the risk of developing CC.[40]

Other factors that may be associated with the development of CC include hepatitis viruses B and C, although the existing data are scarce and too inconclusive to establish a direct association with CC.[17,40,45–47]

Diabetes mellitus,[36] chronic pancreatitis,[17] and thyrotoxicosis[17] are reported to be associated with a higher risk of ECC. Obesity was not recognized to be directly associated with ECC[17]; however, data are too limited to draw any conclusions. Rare associations of papillitis and cytomegalovirus inclusions have been reported in patients diagnosed with DCC.[48] A comprehensive list of various known risk factors is given in **Table 1**.

Table 1	
Etiology of distal cholangiocarcinoma	
Stronger Risk Factors	**Weaker Risk Factors**
Primary sclerosing cholangitis	Hepatitis viruses B, C
Choledochal cyst	Smoking
Parasite: liver flukes	Diabetes mellitus
Toxins: thorotrast	Chronic pancreatitis
Biliary papillomatosis	Thyrotoxicosis
Heavy alcohol consumption	

PATHOLOGY

Grossly, CC is classified into sclerosing, nodular, and papillary subtypes. Sclerosing (schirrhous) tumors, which comprise more than 80% of CCs, are associated with intense desmoplasia and longitudinal infiltration along the ducts, with a low resectability rate. These tumors tend to be highly invasive and are more commonly found in hilar rather than distal bile ducts. Nodular tumors are characterized by a firm, irregular masses projecting into the lumen. Sometimes nodular tumors appear to be constricting annular lesions, and are frequently described as nodular-sclerosing. The papillary variant forms nearly 10% of all CCs, presents as a bulky exophytic mass, often arises from a well-defined stalk projecting into the bile duct lumen, and is more commonly found in the distal bile ducts.[49,50] The papillary subtype is more often resectable in comparison with the other variants, and has a more favorable prognosis.[3,15]

Microscopically, greater than 90% of CCs are well-differentiated and mucin-producing adenocarcinomas.[3,49] Other rare histologic types include squamous cell carcinoma, adenosquamous carcinoma, small-cell carcinoma, and clear-cell carcinoma.

Two types of precursor lesions have been proposed in the carcinogenesis of CC: intraductal papillary neoplasm of the bile duct (IPNB) and biliary intraepithelial neoplasia (BilIN). BilIN is a microscopic premalignant, noninvasive neoplastic lesion that can progress to tubular adenocarcinoma against a background of chronic inflammation via grades BilIN-1, BilIN-2, and BilIN-3, based on the degree of cellular atypia.[51,52] IPNB is a macroscopic papillary growth of atypical biliary epithelium, which occurs in association with chronic inflammatory conditions and produces mucin. It has been characterized as IPNB-1 (premalignant or borderline) and IPNB-2 (carcinoma in situ) using the World Health Organization criteria for pancreatic intraductal papillary mucinous neoplasms.[53] IPNB can progress to either mucinous carcinoma or tubular adenocarcinoma. The biological behavior and prognosis of mucinous carcinoma are considerably more favorable than those of tubular adenocarcinoma.[51,54]

Tumors arising in intra-ampullary segments of the CBD are now classified as ampullary-ductal carcinomas by the American Joint Committee on Cancer (AJCC)/ Union for International Cancer Control.[7]

MOLECULAR PATHOGENESIS

The mechanism of cholangiocarcinogenesis is a multistep process that evolves from normal biliary epithelial cells through chronic inflammation and cellular damage, ultimately leading to malignant transformation of cholangiocytes.[55] The following are the main cell-cycle pathways implicated in cholangiocarcinogenesis:

- Interleukin-6, against the background of chronic inflammation, has mitogenic effects on malignant cholangiocytes and decreases the expression of p21, a cell-cycle controller protein.[56,57]
- The JAK/STAT pathway is one of the key signaling cascades that imparts resistance toward apoptosis for CC cells, and has been found to responsive to sorafenib in animal models.[58]
- Transforming growth factor (TGF)-β, a cytokine, and Smad-4, a tumor suppressor gene downstream of TGF-β signaling, disrupt the cell cycle and are involved in tumor progression.[59,60]
- ErbB-2 proto-oncogene coded receptor tyrosine kinase ErbB-2 is overexpressed in malignant cholangiocytes and plays a major role in the progression of disease.[61]
- Cyclooxygenase-2 (COX-2), the inducible isoform of the enzyme cyclooxygenase, is increased in the presence of inflammation and is upregulated in CC, especially in patients affected with PSC.[61,62] Inducible nitric oxide synthase has also been implicated in biliary tract carcinogenesis by damaging the DNA repair system, causing oxidative DNA damage, and stimulating COX-2 expression.[63–65]
- Malignant cells are known to have a higher threshold to the antiapoptotic protein, Bcl-2, which is overexpressed.[66]
- Vascular endothelial growth factor mediates adaptive proliferative response to cholestasis in cholangiocytes.[67]

CLINICAL PRESENTATION

CC has overlapping clinical features with other perihilar and periampullary tumors. Adenocarcinoma of the pancreatic head may present in similar fashion to DCC and may pose a diagnostic dilemma, as medical therapy for these 2 cancer types differs.[68–70] Both tumor types typically present with painless jaundice, abdominal pain, and weight loss.[71] Other symptoms of cholestasis, such as pruritus, clay-colored stools, malabsorption, and cholangitis, may occur.[72] Although in the United States fever is uncommon in DCC and is seen more commonly in PCC,[4,5] it is commonly associated with cholangitis, abdominal pain, and jaundice in Thailand.[73] Some patients may present with intermittent jaundice, which is often found in papillary subtypes. The papillary growth obstructs the bile flow and then sheds off portions of the tumor, relieving the cholestatic symptoms. DCC and PCC can usually be distinguished from ICC, which more commonly presents as vague abdominal discomfort and relatively delayed onset of cholestatic symptoms.

A suspicion of CC should prompt regular diagnostic workup including complete blood count, electrolytes, liver function tests, and tumor markers, besides imaging and other invasive diagnostic tests. Common hepatic duct or common bile duct obstruction leads to an increase in direct bilirubin and alkaline phosphatase (ALP) accompanied by γ-glutamyltransferase (GGT), indicating biliary origin. The clinical picture and laboratory workup may mimic choledocholithiasis or benign strictures, but total bilirubin greater than 10 mg/dL and ALP values higher than 5 times normal should raise suspicion for a malignant cause, although these values are not specific enough for diagnosis.[73,74] Distal tumors are typically in close proximity to major vascular structures and organs, and thereby tend to spread earlier to nearby anatomy. Even benign biliary strictures can simulate the symptoms of malignant obstruction, but appropriate past medical history may help in the diagnosis. However, taking into consideration that 5% to 15% of the biliary strictures are benign and there is no reliable diagnostic modality that can accurately distinguish the benign from the malignant lesion, surgeons need to be cautious under these circumstances.[75]

DIFFERENTIAL DIAGNOSIS

A wide range of abnormalities can present in a similar way to DCC, making definitive diagnosis challenging. Alternative abnormalities that should be considered include pancreatic head masses (adenocarcinoma, benign or premalignant cysts, intraductal papillary mucinous neoplasm, and so forth), ampullary neoplasms, duodenal tumors, benign biliary stricture, and PSC.

PREOPERATIVE EVALUATION

Ultrasonography (US) alone has limited utility in diagnosing DCC. With a suspicion of biliary dilation and reliable history, US helps exclude gallstones. It may miss small tumors and cannot accurately define tumor extent. US is highly operator-dependent, and along with color Doppler it may help diagnose tumor-induced compression or vascular thrombosis.[76] US may be more helpful for the diagnosis and analysis of ICC and PCC.[77,78]

Contrast-enhanced high-resolution computed tomography (CT) helps by providing good views of the tumor, dilated ducts, lymphadenopathy, and metastases. Abdominal lymphadenopathy is common in PSC and does not necessarily indicate metastatic disease.[76] Multislice 3-dimensional CT has been found to be superior to conventional CT, US, and endoscopic retrograde cholangiopancreatography (ERCP) in the diagnosis of ECC.[79]

Magnetic resonance imaging (MRI) is an optimal preoperative imaging technique used to determine tumor resectability, invasion into periductal tissues, and nodal and extrahepatic metastases commonly seen in the subperitoneal space of the hepatoduodenal ligament. The tumor is usually visualized as a short stricture or a polypoid mass, which appears hypovascular and has low signal intensity on T1-weighted fat-suppressed MRI. These lesions have low signal intensity relative to adjacent normal pancreatic parenchyma on immediate postgadolinium T1-weighted images, and often show a thin rim of peripheral enhancement on 2-minute postgadolinium fat-suppressed images.[80]

MRI can be coupled with magnetic resonance cholangiopancreatography (MRCP) as a noninvasive alternative to ERCP or percutaneous transhepatic cholangioscopy (PTC) to obtain a cholangiogram. MRCP has been shown to have sensitivity of 90% in the evaluation of ECC at the nonicteric stage.[81] ERCP can be used as an initial modality when biliary obstruction exists, owing to both its diagnostic and therapeutic nature[82]; however, it is useful to perform axial CT or MRI before stenting when possible.

ERCP has the advantage over MRCP as a diagnostic imaging modality for biliary strictures because of its ability to obtain tissue samples and for the therapeutic options it provides, such as stent placement. Supplementing ERCP with intraductal US (IDUS) gives more reliable and precise information about differentiation of malignant versus benign lesions than MRCP without additional imaging sequences.[83,84] The sensitivity of brush cytology obtained through ERCP in detecting CC varies widely between 23% and 80%, but the specificity remains close to 100%.[85–90] Use of forceps biopsy or fine-needle aspiration as adjuncts to brush cytology significantly improves the sensitivity of brush cytology.[89,91]

Endoscopic US provides views of the extrahepatic biliary tract, gallbladder, regional lymph nodes, and mesenteric vasculature. Fine-needle aspiration of distal biliary, pancreatic, and ampullary lesions, along with associated peripancreatic nodes, enhances the sensitivity of DCC detection. Although there may a small risk of tumor seeding with biopsy, the likelihood of this remains unclear.[76]

Positron emission tomography (PET) and PET/CT may have a potential role in preoperative staging but needs to be validated. Maximum standardized uptake values from early and delayed PET/CT may be useful parameters in the differentiation of malignant and benign extrahepatic biliary disease without any added benefit of delayed PET/CT in suspicious cases of ECC.[92]

Transpapillary cholangioscopy (TC) involves passage of a scope (10F diameter) through a therapeutic endoscope channel to obtain direct visualization of the intraductal mucosa. In a prospective multicenter study, TC showed an increased ability to distinguish between benign and malignant strictures when compared with ERCP alone, and facilitated targeted biopsy.[93] TC also carries a higher sensitivity in detecting bile duct carcinoma.[82] PTC involves insertion of a cholangioscope through a percutaneous tract, and is an excellent procedure for obtaining target biopsies. Although this has higher sensitivity and is relatively easier, it requires an invasive technique, in contrast to the transpapillary approach.[82] PTC may be attempted if ERCP is unsuccessful or technically unfeasible.[94]

Fluorescence in situ hybridization (FISH) detects chromosomal polysomy, improves the diagnostic yield and accuracy of indeterminate biliary strictures, and increases the sensitivity of brush cytology. FISH has been proposed as a routine test in evaluation of indeterminate pancreaticobiliary strictures.[76,95] Digitized image analysis (DIA) detects the presence of aneuploidy in DNA, and can be used in cases of negative brush cytology and forceps biopsy to improve their sensitivity.[82] However, DIA has not been found to be an independent predictor of malignancy.[95] A DNA-methylation assay consisting of a 5-gene panel may be useful in detecting ECC and may help in increasing the sensitivity of preoperative diagnosis.[96]

IDUS involves introduction of a high-frequency miniprobe over a guide wire into the biliary system. It can be used to assess vascular invasion, especially in the right hepatic artery and portal vein, as well as depth of invasion and the longitudinal extension patterns of cancer along the bile duct. IDUS may be used to identify tumor invasion within the hepatoduodenal ligament, but assessment of nodal metastases can be challenging with this modality.[82] IDUS in combination with endoscopic transpapillary biopsy may improve tumor diagnosis in the case of ampullary lesions.[97]

Low-coherence enhanced back-scattering spectroscopy (LEBS) uses infrared light to produce cross-sectional images.[80] This novel light-scattering technology takes the advantage of the field effect of carcinogenesis to detect various cancers of the lung, esophagus, colon, pancreas, and biliary tract. LEBS is a promising modality, as it is less invasive and potentially a more sensitive diagnostic tool for diagnosis. The application of LEBS in biliary tumors is being evaluated in the periampullary duodenum for signals suggestive of malignancy.[80]

Tumor Markers

Carbohydrate antigen (CA)19-9 is the most commonly used tumor marker for biliary cancers, with sensitivity of 53% to 92%, specificity of 45% to 80%, and positive predictive value of 16% to 40% depending on the cutoff values for malignant biliary obstruction.[98–101] C-reactive protein has been proposed as a useful correction factor to improve the diagnostic value of CA19-9 in patients with malignant biliary obstruction.[98] In patients with PSC, CA19-9 has limited value in detecting CC because of its low specificity.[102] However, CA19-9 as an adjunct to cross-sectional imaging has showed sensitivity of 91% to 100% in detecting CC in patients with PSC.[103] The usual cutoff value for diagnosing CC is 100 U/mL, which is lowered in patients with PSC.

Carcinoembryonic antigen (CEA) has diagnostic yield inferior to that of CA19-9 in detecting CC, with sensitivity of 38% to 53% and sensitivity of 86% to 100%.[101,104,105] An index score of 400U using the formula CA19-9 + (CEA × 40) had an accuracy of 86% in diagnosing CC in PSC.[104] CA19-9 and CEA in conjunction with brush cytology and DNA analysis has sensitivity and specificity of 88% and 80%, respectively, and in PSC patients with CC 100% and 85%, respectively.[106] Though not useful for screening, as diagnostic markers CA19-9 and CEA, as with most tumor markers, can be monitored in patients following surgical resection to detect recurrence or metastasis.

Immunoglobulin G fraction 4 (IgG4) can be measured in PSC patients or if a benign cause of biliary stricture is suspected. IgG4-related sclerosing cholangitis is a characteristic type of cholangitis of unknown etiology that is associated with high serum IgG4 levels[107,108] and dense infiltration of IgG4-positive plasma cells with extensive fibrosis of the bile duct wall.[108,109] It is often associated with autoimmune pancreatitis, and responds to steroid therapy.[108,110,111] IgG4 commonly presents as obstructive jaundice and mimics malignant biliary obstruction. Serum IgG4 levels greater than 135 mg/dL are considered diagnostic of IgG4-scleroscing cholangitis. Combined with imaging showing narrowing and thickening of bile ducts with coexistence of autoimmune pancreatitis, characteristic histologic examination or response to steroid therapy should clinch the diagnosis of IgG4-sclerosing cholangitis.[110] It is important to exclude other causes such as CC, PSC, pancreatic cancer, and secondary sclerosing cholangitis.

Human equilibrative nucleoside transporter 1 (hENT-1) is another molecular marker expressed highly in biliary tract malignancies. hENT-1 may be associated with improved survival, and may be useful as a prognostic marker to help guide chemotherapy regimens.[112]

HER-3, a protein from the tyrosine kinase receptor family, is overexpressed in ECC, especially in nodular and infiltrative subtypes, and the overexpression is correlated with decreased survival.[113] This target could be a potential candidate for molecular therapy.

PREOPERATIVE STENT

The precise advantage of preoperative biliary drainage is controversial. In patients with symptomatic malignant obstruction, biliary drainage improves symptoms of jaundice, pruritus, loss of appetite, and nausea. If patients are scheduled to undergo chemotherapy, biliary drainage is essential to reduce hepatotoxic damage from chemotherapeutic agents; however, if the patient is asymptomatic and surgical resection is anticipated within 1 to 2 weeks, drainage is usually not advised. Avoiding preoperative biliary drainage for these patients may lower rates of complications such as cholangitis, pancreatitis, and perforation, which may delay surgery.[114,115] Absence of preoperative biliary drainage may result in an increase in rates of postoperative fistula, as anastomotic leaks may be more prevalent.[116] If the surgery is to be undertaken more than 3 weeks or later, or if the disease is unresectable and the patient is symptomatic, preoperative biliary drainage should be considered.[117]

STAGING

Staging of DCC according to the current AJCC-7 guidelines is presented in **Table 2**.

Table 2
AJCC guidelines for distal cholangiocarcinoma staging

Primary Tumor (T)			
Tx	Primary tumor cannot be assessed		
T0	No evidence of primary tumor		
Tis	Carcinoma in situ		
T1	Tumor confined to bile duct histologically		
T2	Tumor invades beyond the wall of bile duct		
T3	Tumor invades the gallbladder, pancreas, duodenum, or other adjacent organs without involvement of celiac axis or superior mesenteric artery (SMA)		
T4	Tumor invades celiac axis or SMA		
Regional Lymph Nodes (N)			
Nx	Regional lymph nodes cannot be assessed		
N0	No regional lymph node metastasis		
N1	Regional lymph node metastasis		
Distant Metastasis (M)			
M0	No distant metastasis		
M1	Distant metastasis		
Anatomic Stage			
Stage 0	Tis	N0	M0
Stage IA	T1	N0	M0
Stage IB	T2	N0	M0
Stage IIA	T3	N0	M0
Stage IIB	T1	N1	M0
	T2	N1	M0
	T3	N1	M0
Stage III	T4	Any N	M0
Stage IV	Any T	Any N	Any M

From Edge SB, Byrd DR, Compton CC, et al, editors. AJCC cancer staging manual. 7th edition. New York: Springer; 2010; with permission.

CRITERIA FOR UNRESECTABILITY

The criteria for unresectability in patients with DCC include medically unfit patients; those with distant metastases (liver + other organs); those with distant lymph node metastases (beyond portal, hepatic, peripancreatic; ie, celiac and superior mesenteric nodes); and those with major vascular involvement (major portal vein or superior mesenteric vein involvement, superior mesenteric artery or celiac axis involvement).[118]

SURGICAL MANAGEMENT

Surgical resection is the main treatment option for resectable DCC, which is typically addressed via PD, similarly to carcinoma of the pancreatic head, ampulla of Vater, or second portion of the duodenum. A subset of small tumors (2%–8%),[119,120] in the mid-portion of the CBD may be tackled with bile duct resection (BDR) followed by biliary reconstruction, usually with Roux-en-Y hepaticojejunostomy. Portal and retropancreatic node dissection helps to enhance pathologic staging. A series from Memorial Sloan-Kettering has shown that for optimal nodal assessment, a total lymph node count 11 lymph nodes is recommended to prevent understaging of DCC.[121]

Perioperative Outcomes

A recent large published series focusing on surgical outcomes of CC from the National Surgical Quality Improvement Program database included 243 patients who underwent pancreatectomy for DCC from 2005 to 2009 across several institutes in United States.[122] The postoperative morbidity rate was reported to be 47.1% with an observed to expected (O/E) morbidity index of 1.1. The most frequent complications were sepsis (16%), followed by surgical-site infection (9.1%) and pneumonia (3.3%). Risk factors found to be significantly associated with postoperative morbidity in DCC were transfusion of more than 7 units of packed red blood cells, underweight body habitus (body mass index less than 18.5 kg/m^2), longer operative time (>5 hours), preoperative hyperbilirubinemia greater than 3 mg/dL, and history of chronic obstructive pulmonary disease with dyspnea. The postoperative mortality was reported to be only 1.2% with an O/E mortality ratio of 0.4.[122]

Another large series from The Johns Hopkins Hospital included 239 patients spanning 3 decades from 1973 to 2004 diagnosed with DCC,[5] 96% of whom underwent resection via PD or BDR and lymphadenectomy. The perioperative mortality was the least in DCC patients (3%) in comparison with ICC and PCC patients. The most common postoperative complications were pancreatic leak (13%), wound infection (11%), and delayed gastric emptying (10%). The median overall survival was 18 months. Compared with resected ICC and PCC, resected DCC had intermediate 5-year survival of 23%, versus 40% in ICC and 10% in PCC. Margin status, nodal status, tumor size, and tumor differentiation were independently associated with survival.[5] This report was an updated series showing similar results for patients with resected DCC from the same institution.[4]

Role of Hepatopancreaticoduodenectomy

A major hepatectomy along with PD in the presence of a positive proximal bile duct margin extending to only one hemi-liver is called hepatopancreaticoduodenectomy. This aggressive procedure increases the rate of R0 resection, which is one of the most important prognostic factors. Taking into account the high rates of morbidity and mortality associated with this procedure, its role is controversial. It should be reserved for fit patients with no evidence of regional disease, in centers with adequate expertise and acceptable mortality rates only for achieving R0 resection.[123]

Role of Portal Vein Resection

Surgery with intent of complete resection is the only potentially curative treatment for CC. Vascular involvement is associated with decreased survival.[124] Hence, resection of the portal vein and/or superior mesenteric vein is recommended for complete tumor extirpation, when feasible and necessary. This scenario is more commonly observed with pancreatic adenocarcinoma than with DCC.

Role of Diagnostic Laparoscopy

A smaller series by Vollmer and colleagues[125] studied the role of staging laparoscopy (SL) and laparoscopic ultrasonography (LUS) in different subsets of periampullary and gallbladder cancer. In cases of ECC, SL and LUS were found to increase the rate of resection, but no definitive utility could be established. It has been recommended, as a current standard of management, that SL and LUS should be performed before resection in higher-risk individuals (poor performance status or suggestion of peritoneal or hepatic metastases) to prevent unnecessary laparotomy in up to 30% patients with CC.[126]

Surgical Resection in Recurrent CC

A large Korean series demonstrated that surgical resection of metastases in patients with CC prolonged survival, and adjuvant therapy coupled with surgical resection in patients with recurrence did not impart any survival advantage.[127] The survival of patients with recurrence who did not undergo resection was not affected by adjuvant therapy. Of the 474 patients with ECC 35% developed recurrent disease, of whom 8% underwent metastasectomy. Current data validating the role of metastasectomy for recurrent CC are insufficient, but surgical resection may be considered based on the individual patient profile. The main indicator of benefit for this approach is a prolonged disease-free interval from the time of the original resection to that of the recurrence (at least a year, perhaps longer). The recurrence must be amenable to margin-negative resection without excessively high risk to the patient for this approach to be considered appropriate.

PATHOLOGIC PROGNOSTIC FACTORS
Resection Margin Status

The pathologic features of DCC and their influences on survival after resection are shown in **Table 3**. The presence of microscopic and macroscopic disease at the surgical margin is one of the important predictors of survival for CC. A microscopic-positive (R1) margin was shown to be an independent factor associated with worse overall survival by Murakami and colleagues ($P = .019$)[128] and Fernanadez-Ruiz and colleagues ($P = .005$).[129] R0 resection was associated with significantly improved 5-year survival in patients (27% vs 0%, $P = .001$[5] and 44% vs 0%, $P = .04$[130]). Surgery conferred survival advantage only in those patients with R0 resection, whereas patients in the R1/R2 resection group had survival similar to those who were palliated with photodynamic therapy, with 1-year survival rates of 87%, 55%, and 51%, respectively (R0 vs R1/R2 or photodynamic therapy [PDT], $P<.001$).[124] Although most studies reported margin status to be an independent predictor of survival, Noji and colleagues[131] (N = 228, including 118 DCC) did not find margin status to be prognostic for ECC ($P = .714$). These findings could be confounded by the presence of other adverse pathologic factors such as nodal metastasis and poorly differentiated tumors.

Nodal Metastasis

Nodal metastasis increases a patient's risk for recurrence after resection of DCC. Several studies have reported positive nodes to be an independent prognostic factor for poor survival.[5,128,131–134] Metastasis in up to 2 nodes is associated with improved survival, and involvement of 3 or more nodes is associated with worse survival ($P = .003$, hazard ratio 7.502, 95% confidence interval 1.98–28.31).[130] Murakami and colleagues[132] reported that patients with 2 or fewer positive nodes had significantly higher 5-year survival, 83% versus 0% ($P<.001$). The cohort with 3 or more positive nodes had a significantly higher rate of distant metastasis ($P<.001$).[132] In addition, patients with nodal spread exhibit a significantly higher rate of postoperative recurrence ($P = .008$).[132] Lymph node metastases are also associated with a significantly higher likelihood of bone metastasis in ECC.[135]

Table 3
Pathologic prognostic factors and survival in distal cholangiocarcinoma

Study, Year	Resected DCC (n)	Survival (%)			Prognostic Factors						
		1 y	3 y	5 y	R0 Margin	Differentiation	LN (+)	PNI	LVI	Size	pT Stage
Tompkins et al,[6] 1981	18	63	28	28	—	—	—	—	—	—	—
Nakeeb et al,[4] 1996	80	70	31	28	NS	P<.04	P<.02	—	—	NS	—
Yoshida et al,[130] 2002	27	65	37	37	P = .04	NS	P = .003[a]	NS	NS	—	—
DeOliveira et al,[5] 2007	229	—	—	23	P = .001	P = .007	P = .001	—	—	P = .001	—
Woo et al,[134] 2007	91	—	—	54	—	NS	P = .012	—	—	—	—
Murakami et al,[128] 2007	43	72	53	44	P = .019	NS	P = .042	NS	—	—	—
Shimizu et al,[137] 2008	29	—	—	45	—	NS	NS	P≤.05	—	—	—
Fernandez-Ruiz et al,[129] 2009	68[b] (31 DCC)	21	7	2	P = .005[c]	—	NS[c]	—	—	—	—
Qiao et al,[133] 2011	122	83	49	33	NS	—	P = .036	—	—	—	NS
Matull et al,[124] 2011	31	48	25	21	—	—	—	—	—	—	—
Noji et al,[131] 2012	118 (228 ECC)	—	—	40	NS[c]	NS[c]	P<.0001[c]	NS[c]	NS[c]	—	NS[c]
Pattanathein et al,[156] 2013	58[b]	62	22	11	NS[c]	NS[c]	P = .007[c]	—	NS[c]	—	—

Abbreviations: DCC, distal cholangiocarcinoma; ECC, extrahepatic cholangiocarcinoma; LN, lymph nodes; LVI, lymphovascular invasion; NS, not significant; PNI, perineural invasion.
[a] Involvement of ≥3 LN.
[b] ECC.
[c] P values for ECC.

As the presence of nodal metastases and positive resection margins is the most important prognostic factor associated with poor survival after surgical resection, aggressive resection, when feasible, along with adequate lymph node dissection, may lead to improved survival.

Perineural Invasion

Perineural invasion (PNI) is associated with a 3-fold decrease in 5-year survival for all periampullary adenocarcinoma sites (16% vs 37.8%, P = .02),[136] but did not reach significance when analyzed for DCC alone.[136] PNI has been reported to be an independent prognostic factor (P<.05) that is associated with an increased risk of recurrence.[137] More studies need to be done to evaluate the definitive association of PNI with surgical outcomes in DCC.

Extracapsular Lymph Node Invasion

Extracapsular lymph node invasion involves extension of cancer cells through the nodal capsule into the perinodal fatty tissue. Compared with PCC, in DCC the presence of extracapsular invasion is found to be significantly higher (9.8% vs 36.8%).[131] Data evaluating extracapsular extension to establish any conclusion regarding outcomes for patients with cancer are scarce.

MEDICAL MANAGEMENT
Neoadjuvant Therapy

Considering the similarities between DCC and pancreatic head adenocarcinoma in their anatomic location, prognosis, immunohistochemical patterns, response to chemotherapy (gemcitabine or 5-fluorouracil [5-FU]), and nature of surgical resection (PD), neoadjuvant chemoradiation has been proposed as a treatment strategy for DCC, taking into account its effectiveness in pancreatic adenocarcinoma.[138] McMasters and colleagues[139] reported that of the 9 patients with ECC (5 PCC, 4 DCC) who received preoperative chemoradiation, 100% had R0 resections, and 3 of 9 patients (33%) had complete pathologic response. Furthermore, 6 patients (67%) who were deemed unresectable at presentation were successfully downstaged and ultimately had margin-negative resections. There was no increase in morbidity in patients who underwent neoadjuvant therapy in comparison with those who did not.

Nelson and colleagues[140] reported a significantly improved 5-year survival in 12 patients who underwent neoadjuvant treatment compared with adjuvant treatment (53% vs 23%), with similar surgical morbidity. Although there are insufficient existing data to establish a standard of care, preoperative therapy may play a role in the future and for patients at higher risk of positive margins, positive nodes, and early recurrence.

Adjuvant Therapy

Chemotherapy

5-FU given as a single chemotherapeutic agent showed a response rate of 10%,[141] but in combination with leucovorin and cisplatin showed improved response rates of up to 32% and survival.[142,143] In more recent studies, gemcitabine and oxaliplatin in combination with radiation therapy (RT) has been found to have promising results (overall survival 17 months) for patients with advanced, unresectable disease.[144] A phase II study showed that cetuximab along with gemcitabine and oxaliplatin was reported to have a response rate of 63% and complete response in 10%, and one-third of the patients underwent subsequent resection.[145] Efficacy of other target inhibitor drugs (eg, bevacizumab, erlotinib, and capecitabine) regarding their antitumor potential is also being scrutinized.

Radiation Therapy

Data regarding addition of RT in the adjuvant setting remains conflicting.[130,146] Schoenthaler and colleagues[147] reported an improvement in survival after postoperative RT in patients with microscopic residual disease following resection. More recent data showed that the patients receiving adjuvant chemoradiation had 5-year survival, disease-free survival, metastasis-free survival, and locoregional control rates of 33%, 37%, 42%, and 78%, respectively.[140] A large population-based analysis of ECC from the Surveillance, Epidemiology, and End Results database showed that surgery alone or surgery along with RT showed evidence of improved survival, whereas RT alone was associated with survival decrement.[148] External beam RT in unresectable ECC including 21 DCC patients showed overall survival and local control rates at 1 year to be 59% and 90%, respectively, and 22% and 71% at 2 years.[149]

PALLIATION

Most patients are inoperable at the time of diagnosis, and providing an improved quality of life in their short survival span is the primary goal. Biliary decompression is required to relieve symptoms of jaundice, pain, and pruritus, and prevention of cholestatic liver failure and cholangitis. This goal can be achieved by endoscopic or percutaneous drainage or surgical bypass. Nonsurgical biliary stenting is the first choice in patients with short life expectancy.[150] Endoscopic stenting is associated with fewer early treatment-related complications in comparison with palliative surgery, with no difference in survival in patients with malignant distant biliary obstruction.[151] Endoscopic metal stents have outcomes similar to those with plastic stents, but with improved patency rates.[152] Percutaneous transhepatic biliary drainage is often performed when ERCP has failed, whereas surgery is usually reserved for relief of dual obstructions of the bile duct and duodenum.[117] Covered and uncovered self-expandable metal stents (SEMS) have been shown to have similar patency rates and overall survival, but a significantly higher rate of stent migration and pancreatitis was observed in patients with covered SEMS, and tumor ingrowth with recurrent obstruction was noted in those with uncovered SEMS.[153] Surgical bypass may be reconsidered in patients with a good estimated life expectancy if stenting has failed.[76]

Photodynamic Therapy

This novel technique involves injection of a nontoxic photosensitizer, commonly sodium porfimer, which is preferentially retained by tumor cells and exposed to light via cholangioscopy. The light is absorbed by a photosensitizer and transferred to oxygen, which results in highly reactive oxygen intermediates, in turn resulting in tumor cell death. In a prospective observational pilot study, cholangioscopy-guided PDT showed a significant tumor ablation in 55% patients, and appears to be a safe alternative in select patients with inoperable ECC.[154] PDT in addition to stenting improved survival, biliary drainage, and quality of life in patients with unresectable CC.[155] PDT, which is usually given to unresectable patients, was also found to have survival similar to that those with R1/R2 resection.[124] However, it is not recommended for routine use.[76]

SUMMARY

DCC is an uncommon malignancy, and early diagnosis remains a challenge. More accurate diagnostic modalities for early-stage diagnosis are needed. Advances in medical therapy and neoadjuvant treatment may aid surgery and further improve postoperative outcomes. Margin-negative resection in conjunction with thorough nodal dissection appears to be the strongest prognostic factor. Surgical resection coupled with adjuvant therapy provides the most favorable outcome. Future efforts should be aimed at reducing surgical complications and improving medical therapy, leading to overall improvement in perioperative and long-term outcomes for patients with this disorder.

REFERENCES

1. Shaib Y, El-Serag HB. The epidemiology of cholangiocarcinoma. Semin Liver Dis 2004;24:115–25.
2. Siegel R, Naishadham D, Jemal A. Cancer statistics, 2013. CA Cancer J Clin 2013;63:11–30.
3. Jarnagin WR. Cholangiocarcinoma of the extrahepatic bile ducts. Semin Surg Oncol 2000;19:156–76.
4. Nakeeb A, Pitt HA, Sohn TA, et al. Cholangiocarcinoma. A spectrum of intrahepatic, perihilar, and distal tumors. Ann Surg 1996;224:463–73 [discussion: 473–5].
5. DeOliveira ML, Cunningham SC, Cameron JL, et al. Cholangiocarcinoma: thirty-one-year experience with 564 patients at a single institution. Ann Surg 2007;245: 755–62.
6. Tompkins RK, Thomas D, Wile A, et al. Prognostic factors in bile duct carcinoma: analysis of 96 cases. Ann Surg 1981;194:447–57.
7. Adsay NV, Bagci P, Tajiri T, et al. Pathologic staging of pancreatic, ampullary, biliary, and gallbladder cancers: pitfalls and practical limitations of the current AJCC/UICC TNM staging system and opportunities for improvement. Semin Diagn Pathol 2012;29:127–41.
8. Veillette G, Castillo CF. Distal biliary malignancy. Surg Clin North Am 2008;88: 1429–47, xi.
9. Charatcharoenwitthaya P, Lindor KD. Primary sclerosing cholangitis: diagnosis and management. Curr Gastroenterol Rep 2006;8:75–82.
10. Burak K, Angulo P, Pasha TM, et al. Incidence and risk factors for cholangiocarcinoma in primary sclerosing cholangitis. Am J Gastroenterol 2004;99: 523–6.
11. Talwalkar JA, Lindor KD. Primary sclerosing cholangitis. Inflamm Bowel Dis 2005;11:62–72.
12. Fevery J, Verslype C. An update on cholangiocarcinoma associated with primary sclerosing cholangitis. Curr Opin Gastroenterol 2010;26:236–45.
13. Ahrendt SA, Pitt HA, Nakeeb A, et al. Diagnosis and management of cholangiocarcinoma in primary sclerosing cholangitis. J Gastrointest Surg 1999;3:357–67 [discussion: 367–8].
14. Broome U, Olsson R, Loof L, et al. Natural history and prognostic factors in 305 Swedish patients with primary sclerosing cholangitis. Gut 1996;38:610–5.
15. Pitt HA, Dooley WC, Yeo CJ, et al. Malignancies of the biliary tree. Curr Probl Surg 1995;32:1–90.
16. Broome U, Lofberg R, Veress B, et al. Primary sclerosing cholangitis and ulcerative colitis: evidence for increased neoplastic potential. Hepatology 1995;22: 1404–8.
17. Welzel TM, Graubard BI, El-Serag HB, et al. Risk factors for intrahepatic and extrahepatic cholangiocarcinoma in the United States: a population-based case-control study. Clin Gastroenterol Hepatol 2007;5:1221–8.

18. Rosen CB, Nagorney DM, Wiesner RH, et al. Cholangiocarcinoma complicating primary sclerosing cholangitis. Ann Surg 1991;213:21–5.

19. Bergquist A, Ekbom A, Olsson R, et al. Hepatic and extrahepatic malignancies in primary sclerosing cholangitis. J Hepatol 2002;36:321–7.

20. Komi N, Tamura T, Miyoshi Y, et al. Histochemical and immunohistochemical studies on development of biliary carcinoma in forty-seven patients with choledochal cyst—special reference to intestinal metaplasia in the biliary duct. Jpn J Surg 1985;15:273–8.

21. Tanaka K, Ikoma A, Hamada N, et al. Biliary tract cancer accompanied by anomalous junction of pancreaticobiliary ductal system in adults. Am J Surg 1998;175:218–20.

22. Yamaguchi M. Congenital choledochal cyst. Analysis of 1,433 patients in the Japanese literature. Am J Surg 1980;140:653–7.

23. Edil BH, Cameron JL, Reddy S, et al. Choledochal cyst disease in children and adults: a 30-year single-institution experience. J Am Coll Surg 2008;206:1000–5 [discussion: 1005–8].

24. Soreide K, Korner H, Havnen J, et al. Bile duct cysts in adults. Br J Surg 2004; 91:1538–48.

25. Komi N, Tamura T, Tsuge S, et al. Relation of patient age to premalignant alterations in choledochal cyst epithelium: histochemical and immunohistochemical studies. J Pediatr Surg 1986;21:430–3.

26. Komi N, Tamura T, Miyoshi Y, et al. Nationwide survey of cases of choledochal cyst. Analysis of coexistent anomalies, complications and surgical treatment in 645 cases. Surg Gastroenterol 1984;3:69–73.

27. Nicholl M, Pitt HA, Wolf P, et al. Choledochal cysts in western adults: complexities compared to children. J Gastrointest Surg 2004;8:245–52.

28. Infection with liver flukes (*Opisthorchis viverrini, Opisthorchis felineus* and *Clonorchis sinensis*). IARC Monogr Eval Carcinog Risks Hum 1994;61:121–75.

29. Bouvard V, Baan R, Straif K, et al. A review of human carcinogens—Part B: biological agents. Lancet Oncol 2009;10:321–2.

30. Shin HR, Oh JK, Masuyer E, et al. Epidemiology of cholangiocarcinoma: an update focusing on risk factors. Cancer Sci 2010;101:579–85.

31. Lun ZR, Gasser RB, Lai DH, et al. Clonorchiasis: a key foodborne zoonosis in China. Lancet Infect Dis 2005;5:31–41.

32. Andrews RH, Sithithaworn P, Petney TN. *Opisthorchis viverrini*: an underestimated parasite in world health. Trends Parasitol 2008;24:497–501.

33. Furst T, Keiser J, Utzinger J. Global burden of human food-borne trematodiasis: a systematic review and meta-analysis. Lancet Infect Dis 2012;12:210–21.

34. Sripa B, Bethony JM, Sithithaworn P, et al. Opisthorchiasis and Opisthorchis-associated cholangiocarcinoma in Thailand and Laos. Acta Trop 2011; 120(Suppl 1):S158–68.

35. Cai WK, Sima H, Chen BD, et al. Risk factors for hilar cholangiocarcinoma: a case-control study in China. World J Gastroenterol 2011;17:249–53.

36. Wu Q, He XD, Yu L, et al. The metabolic syndrome and risk factors for biliary tract cancer: a case-control study in China. Asian Pac J Cancer Prev 2012;13:1963–9.

37. Kimura W, Shimada H, Kuroda A, et al. Carcinoma of the gallbladder and extrahepatic bile duct in autopsy cases of the aged, with special reference to its relationship to gallstones. Am J Gastroenterol 1989;84:386–90.

38. Nordenstedt H, Mattsson F, El-Serag H, et al. Gallstones and cholecystectomy in relation to risk of intra- and extrahepatic cholangiocarcinoma. Br J Cancer 2012; 106:1011–5.

39. Nishimura M, Naka S, Hanazawa K, et al. Cholangiocarcinoma in the distal bile duct: a probable etiologic association with choledocholithiasis. Dig Dis Sci 2005;50:2153–8.

40. Tyson GL, El-Serag HB. Risk factors for cholangiocarcinoma. Hepatology 2011; 54:173–84.

41. Lipshutz GS, Brennan TV, Warren RS. Thorotrast-induced liver neoplasia: a collective review. J Am Coll Surg 2002;195:713–8.

42. Becker N, Liebermann D, Wesch H, et al. Mortality among Thorotrast-exposed patients and an unexposed comparison group in the German Thorotrast study. Eur J Cancer 2008;44:1259–68.

43. Lee SS, Kim MH, Lee SK, et al. Clinicopathologic review of 58 patients with biliary papillomatosis. Cancer 2004;100:783–93.

44. Chalasani N, Baluyut A, Ismail A, et al. Cholangiocarcinoma in patients with primary sclerosing cholangitis: a multicenter case-control study. Hepatology 2000; 31:7–11.

45. Shaib YH, El-Serag HB, Nooka AK, et al. Risk factors for intrahepatic and extrahepatic cholangiocarcinoma: a hospital-based case-control study. Am J Gastroenterol 2007;102:1016–21.

46. El-Serag HB, Engels EA, Landgren O, et al. Risk of hepatobiliary and pancreatic cancers after hepatitis C virus infection: a population-based study of U.S. veterans. Hepatology 2009;49:116–23.

47. Barusrux S, Nanok C, Puthisawas W, et al. Viral hepatitis B, C infection and genotype distribution among cholangiocarcinoma patients in northeast Thailand. Asian Pac J Cancer Prev 2012;13(Suppl):83–7.

48. Ruiz-Tovar J, Martin-Perez E, Gamallo-Amat C. Distal cholangiocarcinoma associated with papillitis with viral CMV inclusions. Dig Surg 2005;22:464–6.

49. Weinbren K, Mutum SS. Pathological aspects of cholangiocarcinoma. J Pathol 1983;139:217–38.

50. Zografos GN, Farfaras A, Zagouri F, et al. Cholangiocarcinoma: principles and current trends. Hepatobiliary Pancreat Dis Int 2011;10:10–20.

51. Bickenbach K, Galka E, Roggin KK. Molecular mechanisms of cholangiocarcinogenesis: are biliary intraepithelial neoplasia and intraductal papillary neoplasms of the bile duct precursors to cholangiocarcinoma? Surg Oncol Clin N Am 2009;18:215–24, vii.

52. Zen Y, Adsay NV, Bardadin K, et al. Biliary intraepithelial neoplasia: an international interobserver agreement study and proposal for diagnostic criteria. Mod Pathol 2007;20:701–9.

53. Nakanishi Y, Zen Y, Kondo S, et al. Expression of cell cycle-related molecules in biliary premalignant lesions: biliary intraepithelial neoplasia and biliary intraductal papillary neoplasm. Hum Pathol 2008;39:1153–61.

54. Zen Y, Sasaki M, Fujii T, et al. Different expression patterns of mucin core proteins and cytokeratins during intrahepatic cholangiocarcinogenesis from biliary intraepithelial neoplasia and intraductal papillary neoplasm of the bile duct—an immunohistochemical study of 110 cases of hepatolithiasis. J Hepatol 2006;44:350–8.

55. Fava G, Lorenzini I. Molecular pathogenesis of cholangiocarcinoma. Int J Hepatol 2012;2012:630543.

56. Okada K, Shimizu Y, Nambu S, et al. Interleukin-6 functions as an autocrine growth factor in a cholangiocarcinoma cell line. J Gastroenterol Hepatol 1994;9:462–7.

57. Tadlock L, Patel T. Involvement of p38 mitogen-activated protein kinase signaling in transformed growth of a cholangiocarcinoma cell line. Hepatology 2001;33:43–51.

58. Blechacz BR, Smoot RL, Bronk SF, et al. Sorafenib inhibits signal transducer and activator of transcription-3 signaling in cholangiocarcinoma cells by activating the phosphatase shatterproof 2. Hepatology 2009;50:1861–70.

59. Zen Y, Harada K, Sasaki M, et al. Intrahepatic cholangiocarcinoma escapes from growth inhibitory effect of transforming growth factor-beta1 by overexpression of cyclin D1. Lab Invest 2005;85:572–81.

60. Xu X, Kobayashi S, Qiao W, et al. Induction of intrahepatic cholangiocellular carcinoma by liver-specific disruption of Smad4 and Pten in mice. J Clin Invest 2006;116:1843–52.

61. Endo K, Yoon BI, Pairojkul C, et al. ERBB-2 overexpression and cyclooxygenase-2 up-regulation in human cholangiocarcinoma and risk conditions. Hepatology 2002;36:439–50.

62. Sirica AE, Lai GH, Endo K, et al. Cyclooxygenase-2 and ERBB-2 in cholangiocarcinoma: potential therapeutic targets. Semin Liver Dis 2002;22:303–13.

63. Ishimura N, Bronk SF, Gores GJ. Inducible nitric oxide synthase upregulates cyclooxygenase-2 in mouse cholangiocytes promoting cell growth. Am J Physiol Gastrointest Liver Physiol 2004;287:G88–95.

64. Jaiswal M, LaRusso NF, Gores GJ. Nitric oxide in gastrointestinal epithelial cell carcinogenesis: linking inflammation to oncogenesis. Am J Physiol Gastrointest Liver Physiol 2001;281:G626–34.

65. Okuda K, Nakanuma Y, Miyazaki M. Cholangiocarcinoma: recent progress. Part 2: molecular pathology and treatment. J Gastroenterol Hepatol 2002;17: 1056–63.

66. Harnois DM, Que FG, Celli A, et al. Bcl-2 is overexpressed and alters the threshold for apoptosis in a cholangiocarcinoma cell line. Hepatology 1997; 26:884–90.

67. Gaudio E, Barbaro B, Alvaro D, et al. Vascular endothelial growth factor stimulates rat cholangiocyte proliferation via an autocrine mechanism. Gastroenterology 2006;130:1270–82.

68. Valle JW, Wasan H, Johnson P, et al. Gemcitabine alone or in combination with cisplatin in patients with advanced or metastatic cholangiocarcinomas or other biliary tract tumours: a multicentre randomised phase II study—the UK ABC-01 Study. Br J Cancer 2009;101:621–7.

69. Valle J, Wasan H, Palmer DH, et al. Cisplatin plus gemcitabine versus gemcitabine for biliary tract cancer. N Engl J Med 2010;362:1273–81.

70. Conroy T, Desseigne F, Ychou M, et al. FOLFIRINOX versus gemcitabine for metastatic pancreatic cancer. N Engl J Med 2011;364:1817–25.

71. Johnson SR, Kelly BS, Pennington LJ, et al. A single center experience with extrahepatic cholangiocarcinomas. Surgery 2001;130:584–90 [discussion: 590–2].

72. Lee M, Banerjee S, Posner MC, et al. Distal extrahepatic cholangiocarcinoma presenting as cholangitis. Dig Dis Sci 2010;55:1852–5.

73. Wiwanitkit V. Clinical findings among 62 Thais with cholangiocarcinoma. Trop Med Int Health 2003;8:228–30.

74. Pellegrini CA, Thomas MJ, Way LW. Bilirubin and alkaline phosphatase values before and after surgery for biliary obstruction. Am J Surg 1982;143:67–73.

75. Bennett JJ, Green RH. Malignant masquerade: dilemmas in diagnosing biliary obstruction. Surg Oncol Clin N Am 2009;18:207–14, vii.

76. Khan SA, Davidson BR, Goldin RD, et al. Guidelines for the diagnosis and treatment of cholangiocarcinoma: an update. Gut 2012;61:1657–69.

77. Hann L, Fong Y, Shriver C, et al. Malignant hepatic hilar tumors: can ultrasonography be used as an alternative to angiography with CT arterial portography for determination of resectability? J Ultrasound Med 1996;15:37–45.
78. Hann L, Greatrex K, Bach A, et al. Cholangiocarcinoma at the hepatic hilus: sonographic findings. AJR Am J Roentgenol 1997;168:985–9.
79. Xu AM, Cheng HY, Jiang WB, et al. Multi-slice three-dimensional spiral CT cholangiography: a new technique for diagnosis of biliary diseases. Hepatobiliary Pancreat Dis Int 2002;1:595–603.
80. Marsh Rde W, Alonzo M, Bajaj S, et al. Comprehensive review of the diagnosis and treatment of biliary tract cancer 2012. Part I: diagnosis—clinical staging and pathology. J Surg Oncol 2012;106:332–8.
81. Sai JK, Suyama M, Kubokawa Y, et al. Early detection of extrahepatic bile-duct carcinomas in the nonicteric stage by using MRCP followed by EUS. Gastrointest Endosc 2009;70:29–36.
82. Tamada K, Ushio J, Sugano K. Endoscopic diagnosis of extrahepatic bile duct carcinoma: advances and current limitations. World J Clin Oncol 2011;2:203–16.
83. Domagk D, Wessling J, Reimer P, et al. Endoscopic retrograde cholangiopancreatography, intraductal ultrasonography, and magnetic resonance cholangiopancreatography in bile duct strictures: a prospective comparison of imaging diagnostics with histopathological correlation. Am J Gastroenterol 2004;99:1684–9.
84. Farrell RJ, Agarwal B, Brandwein SL, et al. Intraductal US is a useful adjunct to ERCP for distinguishing malignant from benign biliary strictures. Gastrointest Endosc 2002;56:681–7.
85. Venu RP, Geenen JE, Kini M, et al. Endoscopic retrograde brush cytology. A new technique. Gastroenterology 1990;99:1475–9.
86. Ponchon T, Gagnon P, Berger F, et al. Value of endobiliary brush cytology and biopsies for the diagnosis of malignant bile duct stenosis: results of a prospective study. Gastrointest Endosc 1995;42:565–72.
87. Stewart CJ, Mills PR, Carter R, et al. Brush cytology in the assessment of pancreatico-biliary strictures: a review of 406 cases. J Clin Pathol 2001;54:449–55.
88. Domagk D, Poremba C, Dietl KH, et al. Endoscopic transpapillary biopsies and intraductal ultrasonography in the diagnostics of bile duct strictures: a prospective study. Gut 2002;51:240–4.
89. Schoefl R, Haefner M, Wrba F, et al. Forceps biopsy and brush cytology during endoscopic retrograde cholangiopancreatography for the diagnosis of biliary stenoses. Scand J Gastroenterol 1997;32:363–8.
90. Jailwala J, Fogel EL, Sherman S, et al. Triple-tissue sampling at ERCP in malignant biliary obstruction. Gastrointest Endosc 2000;51:383–90.
91. Farrell RJ, Jain AK, Brandwein SL, et al. The combination of stricture dilation, endoscopic needle aspiration, and biliary brushings significantly improves diagnostic yield from malignant bile duct strictures. Gastrointest Endosc 2001;54:587–94.
92. Choi EK, Yoo Ie R, Kim SH, et al. The clinical value of dual-time point ^{18}F-FDG PET/CT for differentiating extrahepatic cholangiocarcinoma from benign disease. Clin Nucl Med 2013;38:e106–11.
93. Chen YK, Parsi MA, Binmoeller KF, et al. Single-operator cholangioscopy in patients requiring evaluation of bile duct disease or therapy of biliary stones (with videos). Gastrointest Endosc 2011;74:805–14.

94. Razumilava N, Gores GJ. Classification, diagnosis, and management of cholangiocarcinoma. Clin Gastroenterol Hepatol 2013;11:13–21.e11 [quiz: e13–4].

95. Fritcher EG, Kipp BR, Halling KC, et al. A multivariable model using advanced cytologic methods for the evaluation of indeterminate pancreatobiliary strictures. Gastroenterology 2009;136:2180–6.

96. Shin SH, Lee K, Kim BH, et al. Bile-based detection of extrahepatic cholangiocarcinoma with quantitative DNA methylation markers and its high sensitivity. J Mol Diagn 2012;14:256–63.

97. Heinzow HS, Lenz P, Lallier S, et al. Ampulla of Vater tumors: impact of intraductal ultrasound and transpapillary endoscopic biopsies on diagnostic accuracy and therapy. Acta Gastroenterol Belg 2011;74:509–15.

98. La Greca G, Sofia M, Lombardo R, et al. Adjusting CA19-9 values to predict malignancy in obstructive jaundice: influence of bilirubin and C-reactive protein. World J Gastroenterol 2012;18:4150–5.

99. Patel AH, Harnois DM, Klee GG, et al. The utility of CA 19-9 in the diagnoses of cholangiocarcinoma in patients without primary sclerosing cholangitis. Am J Gastroenterol 2000;95:204–7.

100. Gores GJ. Early detection and treatment of cholangiocarcinoma. Liver Transpl 2000;6:S30–4.

101. Buffet C, Fourre C, Altman C, et al. Bile levels of carcino-embryonic antigen in patients with hepatopancreatobiliary disease. Eur J Gastroenterol Hepatol 1996;8:131–4.

102. Hultcrantz R, Olsson R, Danielsson A, et al. A 3-year prospective study on serum tumor markers used for detecting cholangiocarcinoma in patients with primary sclerosing cholangitis. J Hepatol 1999;30:669–73.

103. Charatcharoenwitthaya P, Enders FB, Halling KC, et al. Utility of serum tumor markers, imaging, and biliary cytology for detecting cholangiocarcinoma in primary sclerosing cholangitis. Hepatology 2008;48:1106–17.

104. Ramage JK, Donaghy A, Farrant JM, et al. Serum tumor markers for the diagnosis of cholangiocarcinoma in primary sclerosing cholangitis. Gastroenterology 1995;108:865–9.

105. Nichols JC, Gores GJ, LaRusso NF, et al. Diagnostic role of serum CA 19-9 for cholangiocarcinoma in patients with primary sclerosing cholangitis. Mayo Clin Proc 1993;68:874–9.

106. Lindberg B, Arnelo U, Bergquist A, et al. Diagnosis of biliary strictures in conjunction with endoscopic retrograde cholangiopancreaticography, with special reference to patients with primary sclerosing cholangitis. Endoscopy 2002; 34:909–16.

107. Hamano H, Kawa S, Horiuchi A, et al. High serum IgG4 concentrations in patients with sclerosing pancreatitis. N Engl J Med 2001;344:732–8.

108. Nishino T, Oyama H, Hashimoto E, et al. Clinicopathological differentiation between sclerosing cholangitis with autoimmune pancreatitis and primary sclerosing cholangitis. J Gastroenterol 2007;42:550–9.

109. Zen Y, Harada K, Sasaki M, et al. IgG4-related sclerosing cholangitis with and without hepatic inflammatory pseudotumor, and sclerosing pancreatitis-associated sclerosing cholangitis: do they belong to a spectrum of sclerosing pancreatitis? Am J Surg Pathol 2004;28:1193–203.

110. Ohara H, Okazaki K, Tsubouchi H, et al. Clinical diagnostic criteria of IgG4-related sclerosing cholangitis 2012. J Hepatobiliary Pancreat Sci 2012;19: 536–42.

111. Ghazale A, Chari ST, Zhang L, et al. Immunoglobulin G4-associated cholangitis: clinical profile and response to therapy. Gastroenterology 2008;134:706–15.

112. Fisher SB, Fisher KE, Patel SH, et al. Excision repair cross-complementing gene-1, ribonucleotide reductase subunit M1, ribonucleotide reductase subunit M2, and human equilibrative nucleoside transporter-1 expression and prognostic value in biliary tract malignancy. Cancer 2013;119:454–62.

113. Lee HJ, Chung JY, Hewitt SM, et al. HER3 overexpression is a prognostic indicator of extrahepatic cholangiocarcinoma. Virchows Arch 2012;461:521–30.

114. Iacono C, Ruzzenente A, Campagnaro T, et al. Role of preoperative biliary drainage in jaundiced patients who are candidates for pancreatoduodenectomy or hepatic resection: highlights and drawbacks. Ann Surg 2013;257: 191–204.

115. Povoski SP, Karpeh MS Jr, Conlon KC, et al. Association of preoperative biliary drainage with postoperative outcome following pancreaticoduodenectomy. Ann Surg 1999;230:131–42.

116. Sohn TA, Yeo CJ, Cameron JL, et al. Do preoperative biliary stents increase postpancreaticoduodenectomy complications? J Gastrointest Surg 2000;4: 258–67 [discussion: 267–8].

117. Lee JH. Self-expandable metal stents for malignant distal biliary strictures. Gastrointest Endosc Clin N Am 2011;21:463–80, viii–ix.

118. Schulick RD. Criteria of unresectability and the decision-making process. HPB (Oxford) 2008;10:122–5.

119. Fong Y, Blumgart LH, Lin E, et al. Outcome of treatment for distal bile duct cancer. Br J Surg 1996;83:1712–5.

120. Wade TP, Prasad CN, Virgo KS, et al. Experience with distal bile duct cancers in U.S. Veterans Affairs hospitals: 1987-1991. J Surg Oncol 1997;64:242–5.

121. Ito K, Ito H, Allen PJ, et al. Adequate lymph node assessment for extrahepatic bile duct adenocarcinoma. Ann Surg 2010;251:675–81.

122. Loehrer AP, House MG, Nakeeb A, et al. Cholangiocarcinoma: are North American surgical outcomes optimal? J Am Coll Surg 2013;216:192–200.

123. DeOliveira ML, Kambakamba P, Clavien PA. Advances in liver surgery for cholangiocarcinoma. Curr Opin Gastroenterol 2013;29:293–8.

124. Matull WR, Dhar DK, Ayaru L, et al. R0 but not R1/R2 resection is associated with better survival than palliative photodynamic therapy in biliary tract cancer. Liver Int 2011;31:99–107.

125. Vollmer CM, Drebin JA, Middleton WD, et al. Utility of staging laparoscopy in subsets of peripancreatic and biliary malignancies. Ann Surg 2002;235:1–7.

126. Joseph S, Connor S, Garden OJ. Staging laparoscopy for cholangiocarcinoma. HPB (Oxford) 2008;10:116–9.

127. Song SC, Heo JS, Choi DW, et al. Survival benefits of surgical resection in recurrent cholangiocarcinoma. J Korean Surg Soc 2011;81:187–94.

128. Murakami Y, Uemura K, Hayashidani Y, et al. Prognostic significance of lymph node metastasis and surgical margin status for distal cholangiocarcinoma. J Surg Oncol 2007;95:207–12.

129. Fernandez-Ruiz M, Guerra-Vales JM, Colina-Ruizdelgado F. Comorbidity negatively influences prognosis in patients with extrahepatic cholangiocarcinoma. World J Gastroenterol 2009;15:5279–86.

130. Yoshida T, Matsumoto T, Sasaki A, et al. Prognostic factors after pancreatoduodenectomy with extended lymphadenectomy for distal bile duct cancer. Arch Surg 2002;137:69–73.

131. Noji T, Miyamoto M, Kubota KC, et al. Evaluation of extra capsular lymph node involvement in patients with extra-hepatic bile duct cancer. World J Surg Oncol 2012;10:106.

132. Murakami Y, Uemura K, Hayashidani Y, et al. Pancreatoduodenectomy for distal cholangiocarcinoma: prognostic impact of lymph node metastasis. World J Gastroenterol 2007;31:337–42 [discussion: 343–4].

133. Qiao QL, Zhang TP, Guo JC, et al. Prognostic factors after pancreatoduodenectomy for distal bile duct cancer. Am Surg 2011;77:1445–8.

134. Woo S, Ryu J, Lee S, et al. Recurrence and prognostic factors of ampullary carcinoma after radical resection: comparison with distal extrahepatic cholangiocarcinoma. Ann Surg Oncol 2007;14:3195–201.

135. Katayose Y, Nakagawa K, Yamamoto K, et al. Lymph nodes metastasis is a risk factor for bone metastasis from extrahepatic cholangiocarcinoma. Hepatogastroenterology 2012;59:1758–60.

136. Hatzaras I, George N, Muscarella P, et al. Predictors of survival in periampullary cancers following pancreaticoduodenectomy. Ann Surg Oncol 2010;17: 991–7.

137. Shimizu Y, Kimura F, Shimizu H, et al. The morbidity, mortality, and prognostic factors for ampullary carcinoma and distal cholangiocarcinoma. Hepatogastroenterology 2008;55:699–703.

138. Turaga KK, Tsai S, Wiebe LA, et al. Novel multimodality treatment sequencing for extrahepatic (mid and distal) cholangiocarcinoma. Ann Surg Oncol 2013; 20:1230–9.

139. McMasters KM, Tuttle TM, Leach SD, et al. Neoadjuvant chemoradiation for extrahepatic cholangiocarcinoma. Am J Surg 1997;174:605–8 [discussion: 608–9].

140. Nelson JW, Ghafoori AP, Willett CG, et al. Concurrent chemoradiotherapy in resected extrahepatic cholangiocarcinoma. Int J Radiat Oncol Biol Phys 2009;73: 148–53.

141. Glimelius B, Hoffman K, Sjoden PO, et al. Chemotherapy improves survival and quality of life in advanced pancreatic and biliary cancer. Ann Oncol 1996;7: 593–600.

142. Choi CW, Choi IK, Seo JH, et al. Effects of 5-fluorouracil and leucovorin in the treatment of pancreatic-biliary tract adenocarcinomas. Am J Clin Oncol 2000; 23:425–8.

143. Ducreux M, Rougier P, Fandi A, et al. Effective treatment of advanced biliary tract carcinoma using 5-fluorouracil continuous infusion with cisplatin. Ann Oncol 1998;9:653–6.

144. Laurent S, Monsaert E, Boterberg T, et al. Feasibility of radiotherapy with concomitant gemcitabine and oxaliplatin in locally advanced pancreatic cancer and distal cholangiocarcinoma: a prospective dose finding phase I-II study. Ann Oncol 2009;20:1369–74.

145. Gruenberger B, Schueller J, Heubrandtner U, et al. Cetuximab, gemcitabine, and oxaliplatin in patients with unresectable advanced or metastatic biliary tract cancer: a phase 2 study. Lancet Oncol 2010;11:1142–8.

146. Alden ME, Waterman FM, Topham AK, et al. Cholangiocarcinoma: clinical significance of tumor location along the extrahepatic bile duct. Radiology 1995;197: 511–6.

147. Schoenthaler R, Phillips TL, Castro J, et al. Carcinoma of the extrahepatic bile ducts. The University of California at San Francisco experience. Ann Surg 1994;219:267–74.

148. Fuller CD, Wang SJ, Choi M, et al. Multimodality therapy for locoregional extra-hepatic cholangiocarcinoma: a population-based analysis. Cancer 2009;115: 5175–83.
149. Ghafoori AP, Nelson JW, Willett CG, et al. Radiotherapy in the treatment of patients with unresectable extrahepatic cholangiocarcinoma. Int J Radiat Oncol Biol Phys 2011;81:654–9.
150. Witzigmann H, Lang H, Lauer H. Guidelines for palliative surgery of cholangio-carcinoma. HPB (Oxford) 2008;10:154–60.
151. Smith AC, Dowsett JF, Russell RC, et al. Randomised trial of endoscopic stent-ing versus surgical bypass in malignant low bile duct obstruction. Lancet 1994; 344:1655–60.
152. Moss AC, Morris E, Leyden J, et al. Malignant distal biliary obstruction: a systematic review and meta-analysis of endoscopic and surgical bypass results. Cancer Treat Rev 2007;33:213–21.
153. Lee JH, Krishna SG, Singh A, et al. Comparison of the utility of covered metal stents versus uncovered metal stents in the management of malignant biliary strictures in 749 patients. Gastrointest Endosc 2013;78(2):312–24. http://dx. doi.org/10.1016/j.gie.2013.02.032.
154. Choi HJ, Moon JH, Ko BM, et al. Clinical feasibility of direct peroral cholangioscopy-guided photodynamic therapy for inoperable cholangiocarci-noma performed by using an ultra-slim upper endoscope (with videos). Gastrointest Endosc 2011;73:808–13.
155. Ortner ME, Caca K, Berr F, et al. Successful photodynamic therapy for nonre-sectable cholangiocarcinoma: a randomized prospective study. Gastroenter-ology 2003;125:1355–63.
156. Pattanathien P, Khuntikeo N, Promthet S, et al. Survival rate of extrahepatic chol-angiocarcinoma patients after surgical treatment in Thailand. Asian Pac J Cancer Prev 2013;14(1):321–4.

Hepatocellular Carcinoma
Diagnosis, Management, and Prognosis

Andrew J. Page, MD[a], David C. Cosgrove, MD[b],
Benjamin Philosophe, MD[a], Timothy M. Pawlik, MD, MPH, PhD[c],*

KEYWORDS

- Hepatocellular carcinoma • Transplantation • Locoregional therapy
- Transarterial chemoembolization (TACE) • Sorafenib

KEY POINTS

- The progress made in the diagnosis and management of hepatocellular carcinoma (HCC) represents one of the growing successes in surgical oncology.
- Despite advances in HCC diagnosis and management, the incidence of HCC is still increasing, and HCC represents the fifth most common cancer and the third most common cause of cancer death worldwide.
- Over the last 20 years alone, advances have been made to elucidate the mechanisms of carcinogenesis, to diagnose disease at an earlier stage, and to improve local and systemic treatment of HCC.

INTRODUCTION

The progress made in the diagnosis and management of hepatocellular carcinoma (HCC) represents one of the growing successes in surgical oncology. Despite these advances, the incidence of HCC is still increasing, and HCC represents the fifth most common cancer and the third most common cause of cancer death worldwide.[1] Over the last 20 years alone, advances have been made to elucidate the mechanisms of carcinogenesis, to diagnose disease at an earlier stage, and to improve local and systemic treatment of HCC.

Conflicts of Interest: The authors declare no conflicts of interest with respect to the authorship and/or publication of this article.
Funding: The authors received no financial support for the research and/or authorship of this article.
[a] Department of Surgery, Johns Hopkins Hospital, 600 North Wolfe Street, Baltimore, MD 21287, USA; [b] Department of Medical Oncology, Johns Hopkins Hospital, 600 North Wolfe Street, Baltimore, MD 21287, USA; [c] Division of Surgical Oncology, Department of Surgery, Johns Hopkins Hospital, 600 North Wolfe Street, Blalock 688, Baltimore, MD 21287, USA
* Corresponding author.
E-mail address: tpawlik1@jhmi.edu

CARCINOGENESIS AND DIAGNOSIS
Genetics

As technology has improved, the mechanisms for the generation of cirrhosis and subsequent HCC behave become better understood. The well-known environmental risk factors that may lead to underlying cirrhosis include hepatitis B virus (HBV), hepatitis C virus (HCV), exposure to toxins such as aflatoxin, and alcohol intake. For each of these causes of HCC, specific genetic mutations have been isolated.[2] In HCV-related HCC, mutations have been identified in p53, in the disintegrin and metalloproteinase domain–containing protein 22 (ADAM22), in the Janus kinase/signal transducer and activator of transcription (JAK) pathway, in the beta-catenin gene CTNNB1, in the transport protein particle (TRAPP), in the never in mitosis A–related kinase 8 (NEK8) gene, and in the AT-rich interactive domain 2 (ARID2) gene.[3] HBV-related HCC is associated with p53 mutations but also with exclusive mutations in ATPase family AAA domain–containing 2 (ATAD2) and interferon regulatory factor 2 (IRF2) genes. Although there is some overlap in the genetic mutations responsible for HCC in the background of HBV versus HCV, there are notable differences, with HCV being associated with increased CTNNB1 mutations and fewer p53 mutations.[4] Alcohol consumption has shown a correlation to mutations in the chromatin remodelers, which predispose to dysregulation and the development of HCC.[5] The mechanism for the development of aflatoxin-induced HCC has been genetically described by specific base substitutions, which can lead to HCC in the absence of any underlying liver disease.[6]

From a population-based perspective, specific patient polymorphisms have also recently been identified as potential risk factors for the development of chronic hepatitis and cirrhosis. Using genome-wide association analyses and single-nucleotide polymorphisms, subsets of patients have been identified at a specifically higher risk for the development of HCC, independent of the well-established external exposures.[7]

Molecular Mechanisms

The downstream pathways in which HBV and HCV promote HCC are becoming better understood. One such pathway is through promoting stem-cell activity,[8] which has been shown by the upregulation of the well-known stemness-associated marker epithelial cell adhesion molecule (EpCAM) and beta-catenin.[9] Other more recent markers to show stem cell–like properties in HCC include the NANOG transcription factor, octamer-binding transcription factor 4 (OCT4), sex-determining region Y box 2 (SOX2), and Kruppel-like factor 4.[9–11]

Another newly uncovered mechanism of HCC carcinogenesis is secondary to the relative hypoxia and subsequent angiogenesis incurred by the cirrhotic liver. At the macroscopic level, nodular cirrhosis leads to a decrease in hepatic vasculature, which is followed by a hypoxic environment. In the setting of hypoxia, there is upregulation of hypoxia inducible factor 1 alpha (H1F1α). Stimulation of this factor leads to upregulation of vascular endothelial growth factor (VEGF), cyclo-oxygenase 2, angiopoietin 2, and several matrix metalloproteinases.[12–14] These inappropriately upregulated angiogenic and inflammatory signals predispose the underlying parenchyma to damage, inhibition of regeneration, and subsequent HCC.[8] Specific mechanisms have also shown that both HBV and HCV have unique upregulation of the transcription factor HIF1α at the genetic level.[15] The downstream activation of these proangiogenic growth signals has shown promise in the systemic management of HCC, because some of these factors may be targeted and blocked with agents like sorafenib.[16]

HBV and HCV have also been shown to self-inhibit their viral clearance from infected liver cells. This phenomenon of avoiding clearance is multifaceted. First, immune cell types and their reactive dysfunction from HBV and HCV can include dendritic cells that are made defective, regulatory T cells that are inappropriately induced, and CD8+ effector T cells that are downregulated.[17–19] The innate immune response and cytokines are also disrupted with HCV and HBV, with interferon decreased, and natural killer cells and polymorphonuclear cells upregulated. This immune imbalance leads to unregulated inflammation and an environment for the establishment of cirrhosis and subsequent cancer.[20,21]

Tumor Markers and Screening

Screening for HCC has been studied in many trials and suggested in numerous guidelines. The most accepted and updated guidelines are available from the American Association for the Study of Liver Diseases (AASLD).[22] One of the notable recent changes from prior algorithms is the decreased use of serum levels of alfa-fetoprotein (AFP), and the increased reliance on surveillance ultrasound imaging of the liver every 6 months. When a lesion is suspected on ultrasound, contrast enhanced dynamic imaging is indicated. The hallmark radiologic signs of HCC include intense arterial uptake followed by washout of contrast in the venous phase (**Fig. 1**).[22] If the lesion does not have these characteristics, a biopsy should be considered. If the lesion is less than 1 cm it is more difficult to make a definitive diagnosis of HCC versus a regenerative nodule; as such, the lesion should, at a minimum, be closely followed with surveillance imaging every 3 to 6 months.

Although AFP has been used in the past as a serum tumor marker for HCC, its sensitivity and specificity are limited.[22,23] Factors that influence the usefulness of AFP include the disadvantage that AFP is increased in patients with hepatitis and chronic liver disease without HCC, and the finding that AFP is correlated with tumor size (ie, small tumors are less likely to have increased AFP).[24] To address the problem of poor specificity for HCC, focus has been dedicated on differentiating specific AFPs based on the degree of glycosylation and correlation with disease state.[25,26] One of the first markers examined has been the fucosylation variant lectin (*Lens culinaris* agglutinin) fraction of AFP (AFP-L3), which has been shown to be highly specific for HCC.[27,28] The relative percentage of AFP-L3 to AFP has also been shown to be an indicator of poor prognosis on multivariate analysis for patients with HCC.[29]

Another tumor marker being adopted into practice is Des-gamma-carboxy-prothrombin (DCP), a protein secreted in the setting of abnormal hepatocellular

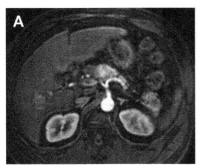
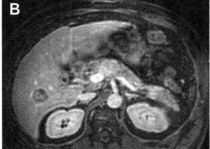

Fig. 1. (*A*) Magnetic resonance imaging (MRI) of HCC with characteristic arterial enhancement. (*B*) MRI of HCC with characteristic washout of contrast on venous phase.

function. Sensitivities and specificities for DCP range from 28% to 89% and 87% to 96%, respectively.[30–32] Like AFP-L3, DCP has shown promise to correlate with HCC stage, portal vein invasion, and prognosis; furthermore, DCP does not seem to be increased in the setting of chronic liver disease.[32–34]

AFP, AFP-L3, and DCP have shown no relationship to each other. As such, attempts have been made to improve screening accuracy of patients with cirrhosis using all three markers in an additive fashion. Tateishi and colleagues,[35] using AFP greater than 200 ng/mL, DCP greater than 40 mAU/mL, and AFP-L3 greater than 15%, found that the accuracy of these tumor markers in combination was higher than that of any test in isolation. However, one of the greatest hindrances to developing an accurate combinatorial test is standardizing assays and cutoff values. Despite better serologic markers becoming available, some groups have recommended abandoning serologic markers and relying on screening ultrasound.[23] Our practice has been to not abandon AFP, but to use it while also recognizing that a normal AFP cannot be relied on to exclude HCC.

Biomarkers have also shown promise as potential indicators of developing HCC in the setting of cirrhosis. Their role in screening protocols and staging guidelines is still in development. Some of these biomarkers are listed in **Table 1**.[36–45]

SURGICAL THERAPY

Once the diagnosis of HCC is suspected, therapeutic options include surgical resection, transplant, systemic chemotherapy, or locoregional therapies (eg, ablation, transarterial chemoembolization [TACE]). The factors that determine which treatment plan is most appropriate include tumor burden, underlying liver function, and patient performance status.

Resection

The perioperative mortality for HCC surgical resection is higher (4%–4.7%) than for resection for benign disease or colorectal liver metastasis, which is likely a reflection of the burden of chronic liver disease in patients with HCC. Therefore, patient selection

Table 1
Potential biomarkers used in the management of hepatocellular cancer

Marker	Level	Mechanism	Usefulness
Osteopontin[36–38]	>156 ng/mL	Upregulated phosphoprotein in setting of tumor invasion, progression, or metastasis	When combined with AFP cutoff of 20 ng/mL, sensitivity and specificity were 95% and 96% in diagnosing HCC
Vascular endothelial growth factor[39–41]	>245 pg/mL; >450 pg/mL	Marker of angiogenesis	Predicts overall and cancer-free survival
Hepatocyte growth factor[42–44]	>0.6 ng/mL	Nonspecific growth factor	In patients with HCV, increased levels correlated with diagnosis of HCC
Insulinlike growth factor 1[45]	Reduction of serum levels	Endocrine, paracrine, and mitogenic role	Decreasing insulinlike growth factor 1 levels preceded development of HCC

is especially critical in the evaluation of patients with HCC for surgical resection.[46,47] The best candidates for surgical resection of HCC are those with early stage, minimal, or well-compensated cirrhosis, and good performance status.[22,48] Adequate cross-sectional contrast-enhanced imaging is one of the first tests in diagnosing HCC. If clinical suspicion is high (by history and increased serum markers), combined with improved imaging, there is no indication for biopsy. Imaging is also critical in determining suitability for resection because as it provides insight into tumor burden for staging, presence of vascular invasion of the primary tumor, presence of cirrhosis, and information for predicting the future liver remnant (FLR). Factors that could exclude appropriate resection are multiple tumors in multiple segments, vascular invasion, evidence of severe cirrhosis, or an FLR that is too small (**Fig. 2**).

In order to evaluate FLR, both the function and the volume of the liver need consideration. For assessing volume, both computed tomography (CT) and magnetic resonance imaging (MRI) volumetrics have been used.[49,50] Data by Kubota and colleagues[51] were instrumental in establishing early guidelines for extent of resection and FLR prediction. This group was able to correlate preoperative volumetric CT imaging and liver function with guidelines for the extent of safe resection of HCC. From their assessments and the adoption by others, hepatectomy with a remnant of 20% to 30% is considered safe for patients with normal liver, 30% to 40% for patients with chronic hepatitis, and 40% to 50% for cirrhotics.[51,52]

To assess function, Child-Pugh classification has historically been the assessment of choice. This score is based on 3 biochemical parameters (bilirubin, albumin, and prothrombin time) as well as 2 clinical parameters (ascites and encephalopathy). The Child-Pugh score correlates with morbidity and mortality after hepatectomy.[53,54] More recently, native Model for End-Stage Liver Disease (MELD) score has also been shown to be helpful in identifying patients at highest risk of morbidity, mortality, and specifically postoperative liver failure.[55,56] Delis and colleagues[57] retrospectively examined a population of 69 patients with HCC and cirrhosis and showed that, along with American Society of Anesthesiologists (ASA) score, MELD scores ($\leq$9) were independent predictors of perioperative mortality (7.2% vs 19%; $P<.02$) and overall morbidity (36.23% vs 48%; $P<.02$).

Functional tools to assess liver function include measurement of indocyanine green clearance, galactose elimination capacity, lidocaine metabolism, and ratios of arterial body ketones.[58] Although these tools have shown promise in predicting perioperative outcomes after hepatectomy with patients with HCC, they are still limited in that they measure global liver function.[59] To more accurately assess more focal liver function, nuclear imaging techniques like [99]mTc-galactosyl serum albumin scintigraphy and

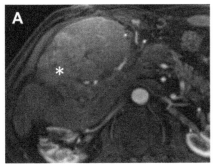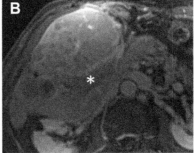

Fig. 2. (A) Infiltrative HCC involving most of the right hemiliver (*asterisk*). (B) Infiltrative HCC with evidence of tumor thrombus in the right portal vein (*asterisk*).

[99]mTc-mebrofenin hepatobiliary scintigraphy have been used and show promise for clinical application.[59]

Some patients with inadequate FLR should be considered for portal vein embolization (PVE). PVE causes atrophy of the ipsilateral lobe of the liver, which is embolized with contralateral lobar hypertrophy, thereby increasing the FLR. Access to selective PVE is typically performed percutaneously and the portal vein is occluded with coils, gel foam, or glue. Prospective trials and mechanistic studies have supported the application of PVE in the management of HCC.[60–62] Ribero and colleagues[63] described the safety of PVE and its efficacy for growing the FLR. These investigators showed that patients with an adequate FLR were at lower risk of postoperative morbidity and liver insufficiency. Furthermore, they noted that the degree/rate of liver hypertrophy was equally, or more, important as the absolute final FLR volume after PVE. These investigators reported that a degree of hypertrophy less than 5% had a sensitivity of 80% and specificity of 94% in predicting hepatic dysfunction. Minimal hypertrophy after PVE was associated with a greater risk for longer hospital stays and 90-day mortality.

If patients are deemed appropriate candidates, they may undergo resection. Outcomes from surgical resection are variable, with 5-year survival rates ranging from 20% to 70%.[64–67] Explanations for this variability are attributed to the heterogeneity of the population of patients who are resected. This variability includes small tumors (<5 cm), tumors in the setting of multinodular disease, large tumors (>5–10 cm), and tumors with major vascular invasion (MVI). Many groups report outcomes of resection for tumors that would not be considered for liver transplantation, and the outcomes among these patients are associated with earlier recurrence and shorter survival compared with patients with more limited disease.

Many groups have characterized the best outcomes after hepatic resection for small (<5 cm tumors). Poon and colleagues[68] examined a series of Child-Pugh class A patients with HCC with solitary tumors less than 5 cm, fewer than 3 tumors less than 3 cm, and tumors without MVI, and showed excellent 5-year survival (68%). Shi and colleagues[69] showed similar extended survival after resection in this subset of patients, and additionally reported 5-year survival for tumors less than 2 cm at 100%. In a recent review by Nathan and colleagues,[70] examining a 10-year era of the Surveillance Epidemiology and End Results (SEER) database, the investigators reported that, among patients with small tumors, outcomes were excellent and that surgery may even have been underused in this group that would benefit from resection.

In the past, multinodular HCC has represented a subset of patients who have had poor perioperative and long-term outcomes following resection, with 5-year survival rates as low as 25% to 30%.[71–73] However, secondary to advances in diagnosis, surgical techniques, and perioperative care, recent data have shown markedly better outcomes in this cohort of high-risk patients. Ishizawa and colleagues[74] showed that resection of multinodular HCC had an improved 5-year overall survival of 58%. Although transplantation should be considered the mainstay of therapy for these patients, up to 20% of patients with multinodular disease progress and do not make it to transplant. As such, some investigators have argued that resection of HCC in the setting of multinodular disease should not be considered an absolute contraindication to resection.[75]

Large tumors (>5–10 cm) pose unique prognostic and treatment challenges for resection as well.[76–78] As with multinodular disease, the 5-year overall survival after resection for large tumors in the past has been poor, ranging from 16% to 33%.[79–82] However, more recently, with the advent of better techniques and therapies, specifically PVE, the outcomes for resection of large tumors has improved.

Vauthey and colleagues[83] examined outcomes after resection of large HCC (or multinodular) tumors and found an overall 5-year survival of 39%. In a separate study, Yang and colleagues[84] similarly noted a 5-year overall survival of 38.5% among patients with large HCC, with an acceptable perioperative morbidity and mortality.

Major vascular invasion represents one of the most important poor prognostic factors after resection, with 5-year survival approximately 60% without MVI, and 10% with MVI; worse survival correlates with more proximal and extensive invasion of the portal veins.[85] For patients with proximal MVI, hepatic resection is generally contraindicated. However, if MVI is not extensive and involves only sectorial branches, then hepatic resection should be considered in the setting of adequate FLR, potentially after treating with locoregional therapies. In a multicenter study, Pawlik and colleagues[66] showed that resection of HCC with MVI improved median survival and that 5-year survival was improved from 5% to 23% depending on the presence of minimal or no liver fibrosis ($P = .001$). However, perioperative mortality in these patients needs to be carefully considered because it may be as high as 7%.

TRANSPLANTATION

Liver transplantation is the only treatment modality that offers the potential to both treat the HCC and cure the underlying liver disease. Throughout most of the 1980s, transplantation for HCC had recurrence rates of greater than 50%. Survival was also disappointing, with 5-year survival rates ranging from 10% to 35%.[86] From these early data, it became evident that the successes and prognosis of transplantation for HCC relied on the biology of the tumor (size, number of nodules, vascular invasion).

In 1996, Mazzaferro and colleagues[76] published their seminal study, which showed that patients with a solitary tumor of less than 5 cm, or those with a maximum of 3 nodules less than or equal to 3 cm, without vascular invasion or extrahepatic spread, had improved recurrence (5%–15%) and survival (>70%). Since the adoption of the Milan criteria, other groups have validated the success of this prioritization tool for transplantation.[87–89] The United Network of Organ Sharing (UNOS) has since standardized liver allocation in the United States for patients with HCC who meet the Milan criteria, automatically appointing them 22 MELD points in an effort to prioritize them. Given the reported successes of the criteria, other centers have questioned how far the Milan criteria can be expanded without affecting transplantation outcomes. The best known expanded criteria are probably those proposed by the University of California, San Francisco (UCSF). The UCSF Criteria are more inclusive than the Milan criteria: 1 tumor less than 6.5 cm, or 2 or 3 nodules less than 4.5 cm with a total tumor diameter less than 8 cm.[90] The UCSF group published results showing that transplant using these expanded criteria can lead to results comparable with those obtained with the Milan criteria.[91] Other groups have similarly reported reasonable long-term results with expanded criteria, particularly in the context of adjuvant locoregional therapies for patients awaiting transplant (eg Kyoto, Dallas, Pamplona, Asian, Edmonton, Shanghai, Hangzhou, and Chengdu) (Table 2).[92–97]

With more accumulated data for patients now being transplanted outside the Milan criteria, the overall 5-year survival for patients within and outside the Milan criteria do not seem comparable. This concept of the further the distance, the further the price has been named the Metroticket concept and shows that the farther patients stray from the Milan criteria after transplantation, the more their 5-year survival also decreases.[98,99]

Table 2
Expanded criteria and survival with transplant for HCC

	Total Patients	Patients by Milan	Patients by Expanded	1-y Survival by Milan (%)	1-y Survival by Expanded (%)	5-y Survival by Milan (%)	5-y Survival by Expanded (%)
Yao et al,[92] 2002	70	46	24	91	71	72	57
Leung et al,[93] 2004	144	74	14	86	NA	51	NA
Todo and Furukawa,[94] 2004	316	138	171	81	75	78	60
Decaens et al,[95] 2006	479	279	188	80	78	60	46
Onaca et al,[97] 2007	1206	631	575	85	67	62	43
Duffy et al,[96] 2007	467	173	294	91	88	79	64

Abbreviation: NA, not available.

In the subset of patients with well-compensated cirrhosis and early stage HCC, transplantation still offers the best disease-free and overall survival compared with resection.[100,101] Bellavance and colleagues,[100] in a comparison of transplant and resection for early stage HCC, showed a 66% 5-year survival for transplantation versus 46% for matched resections. Despite the general overall better outcomes with transplantation, the scarcity of organs remains an issue. While patients are on the waiting list for transplants, greater than 20% of patients with HCC may progress or have other medical issues causing them to be removed from the list.[88,102] The main risk factors associated with an increased likelihood of being removed from the transplant list include increased AFP, initial tumor size, multinodularity, and increased MELD. Strategies designed to improve access to transplants and decrease progression of disease include increasing the pool of donors through living donor liver transplantation (LDLT), treatment with locoregional therapy, or resection while on the waiting list.[103,104]

There is a growing body of literature with inconsistent data regarding the role of LDLT for patients both inside and outside the Milan criteria. Outcomes for LDLT inside the Milan criteria are similar to deceased liver transplants.[94,105–107] Although this may increase the donor liver availability, donor safety for LDLT remains a concern. Approximately 40% of donors experience a complication (most being minor) and mortality is 0.5% to 1%.[108] When considering the usefulness of LDLT, Sarasin and colleagues[109] showed that LDLT is cost-effective when the expected waiting time exceeds 7 months, similar to considering locoregional therapies.

Locoregional therapies can be used for bridging and downstaging. Bridging refers to the use of locoregional therapy for patients within transplant criteria who are awaiting transplant. In contrast, downstaging pertains to patients who are not within transplantable criteria; the locoregional therapy is designed to treat the tumor to an extent that patients are subsequently deemed appropriate for transplantation. To date, there are no prospective data to indicate that the use of locoregional therapies to bridge tumors within transplant criteria improves posttransplant survival or decreases dropout from the transplant list.[110–113] There are also no data to suggest that any specific locoregional therapy (eg, ablation, TACE) has a preferential benefit compared with the others.[114,115]

Despite the paucity of prospective data on bridging therapy, this approach makes some intuitive sense because data show tumor response and improved survival in nonsurgical patients treated with locoregional therapy.[116,117] One study of bridge therapy in an intention-to-treat analysis suggested that patients in need of transplant derive a benefit when waiting times are longer than 6 months.[118]

Several consensus guidelines for bridging and downstaging patients have been developed.[103,114] These guidelines state that the type of treatment or therapy (eg, ablation vs TACE) should be based on the extent of disease. Ablation is more effective for tumors less than 5 cm, whereas intra-arterial therapy is more applicable for larger lesions.

The role of liver resection as a bridging therapy to transplantation is also controversial. The greatest advantage of liver resection as a bridge therapy is that transplantation may be avoided for select patients with small tumors and low MELD scores.[88,119] Resection also offers accurate staging and insight into the biology of the tumor before potential transplantation. Nathan and colleagues[120] showed the usefulness of pathology review of the tumor with regard to prognosis. Examining the primary tumors after resection, the investigators noted a variable 5-year survival of 29% to 55%, and tumor size, multifocality, and vascular invasion were independent predictors of survival. Although there may be benefits of bridging therapy with resection, there are downsides that include increasing the operative risk of eventual liver transplantation and potentially causing liver decompensation.[87,121]

LOCOREGIONAL THERAPIES

There are circumstances in which the patient is not an appropriate operative candidate, or the degree of underlying liver disease precludes resection or transplantation. For these patients, locoregional therapies are available and include ablation (radiofrequency, microwave), percutaneous ethanol injection (PEI), transarterial radioembolization (TARE), drug-eluting beads (DEBs), and TACE.

Ablative Therapies

These treatment modalities work by destroying liver cells through direct chemical toxicity or by modifying neoplastic cell temperature with laser, microwaves, radiofrequency, or cryoablation. These ablative therapies can be approached through percutaneous, laparoscopic, or open laparotomies. Modalities in common use include PEI, radiofrequency ablation (RFA), microwave ablation, irreversible electroporation (IRE), and light-activated drug therapy. With PEI, the distribution of toxic ethanol may be blocked by tumor septae and capsulation, which tends to make ethanol injection less effective in tumors larger than 2 cm. In contrast, the thermal energy with RFA is not limited by tumor septae, and creates a necrotic rim around the tumor, potentially eliminating satellite lesions.[122] Microwave ablation heats the water in tumor cells and induces cell death through coagulative necrosis.[123] Irreversible electroporation is a newer ablative therapy. This treatment disrupts the cell membrane integrity by altering the cell membrane potential, directly causing cell death.[124] Light-activated drug therapy works through creation of toxic oxygen singlets created with injection of talaporfin sodium. The talaporfin is injected intravenously, and light focused on the tumor focally activates the talaporfin, which destroys all cells in that field.[125]

The data for these treatment outcomes have grown as the acceptance of this technology has increased. For tumors smaller than 3 cm, treatment with these modalities has resulted in 5-year survival approaching as high as 80%. For tumors between 3 cm and 5 cm, 5-year survival rates are reported to range from 40% to 70%.[126–128] Several studies have prospectively compared PEI with RFA.[129–131] Two meta-analyses have summarized these conclusions, finding that RFA had fewer treatment sessions, shorter hospitalizations, improved local recurrence, better tumor necrosis, and improved progression-free survival and overall survival.[122,126,127]

There is growing evidence around the use of microwave ablation and IRE. Shibata and colleagues,[132] in a randomized controlled study, compared RFA with microwave ablation and found no difference in complication rates or the incidence of developing residual disease. However, the follow-up was limited to 6 to 27 months, the assessment of residual disease was not standardized, and the microwave technology used was only first generation.[133] To date, there are no published trials examining outcomes for IRE or light-activated drug therapies.[124]

Current recommendations support using RFA or microwave ablation rather than PEI for HCC. RFA or microwave ablation should be specifically considered for patients with HCC less than 3 cm or for HCC less than 5 cm who are not candidates for resection or transplant. However, PEI should be considered when RFA or microwave ablation is not technically appropriate, as with lesions near the hepatic hilum when there is concern for damage secondary to peritumor necrosis.[22] The application of newer modalities like IRE and light-activated drug therapy remains to be determined.

TACE

HCC can also be treated using a transarterial approach. TACE relies on the phenomenon that HCC is typically supplied by the hepatic arteries. Treatment strategies can exploit this finding. With a catheter-based approach, chemotherapy (mitomycin C, doxorubicin, cisplatin) mixed in a lipiodol emulsion can be injected directly into the artery feeding the tumor, and subsequently the hepatic artery terminating in the tumor can be embolized. The lipiodol creates an emulsion that helps retain chemotherapy within the tumor, maximizing exposure of the tumor to the chemotherapy and minimizing normal parenchymal toxicity.[122,134] However, there are no strong clinical data to support that lipiodol improves delivery systems, and it may inhibit accurate CT assessment of tumor vascularity after treatment given its hyperdense appearance on CT.[122]

The outcomes reported for TACE have been variable in several randomized controlled trials. In one of the earliest studies examining TACE, the Groupe d'Etude et de Traitement du Carcinome Hépatocellulaire reported that TACE for unresectable HCC resulted in reduced tumor growth but did not significantly improve survival.[135] In contrast, Lo and colleagues[117] reported improved tumor response and survival for patients with unresectable HCC, with an improved 3-year survival of 26% in the treated arm versus 3% in the control/untreated arm ($P = .002$), with a relative risk (RR) of death of 0.49 (95% confidence interval, 0.29–0.81; $P = .006$).

One difficulty in evaluating the efficacy and standardization of TACE relates to assessing tumor response following therapy. Evaluating the response to locoregional therapies is critical to measuring the effects of treatment and applying that response to prognosis. Different criteria have been developed to objectively define tumor response. These assessments include the World Health Organization (WHO) and the Response Evaluation Criteria in Solid Tumors (RECIST) criteria, both of which evaluate unidimensional and bidimensional tumor measurements in response to therapy. In contrast, the European Association for the Study of the Liver (EASL) criteria examine the degree of necrosis in response to therapy.[122,136] The modified RECIST (mRECIST) assesses not just size of the tumor but also the decrease in arterial enhancement of the targeted lesion (**Fig. 3**).[137] Even more recently, others have suggested the use of diffusion-weighted MRI.[138] Notwithstanding the difficulty in assessing tumor response, 2 meta-analyses have investigated the efficacy of transarterial therapies in the treatment of unresectable HCC.[139,140] Using RECIST criteria, complete and partial responses were noted among 35% of treated patients. With regard to survival, 2-year survival following TACE was 41% versus 27% in the non-TACE–treated group. The survival benefit of intra-arterial

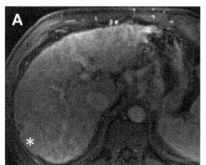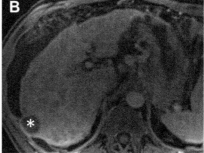

Fig. 3. (A) MRI of pre-TACE HCC lesion (*asterisk*). (B) MRI 4 months following TACE; note that the tumor is now necrotic and avascular (*asterisk*), signifying an excellent result.

therapy was only noted in those studies that used chemotherapy embolization (TACE) and not those that simply used bland embolization (TAE).

In addition to the lipiodol-based approach, transarterial chemotherapy can also be given with drug delivery systems using polymeric microspheres/beads ionically bound with chemotherapy agents: so-called DEB-TACE. Preclinical studies have shown that the beads improve focal tumor delivery, and chemotherapy is released at a more gradual rate, thereby decreasing normal liver and systemic toxicity.[141–144] There have been a few trials that have compared standard TACE with DEB-TACE. In the PRECISION V study, Lammer and colleagues[145] prospectively showed that DEB-TACE showed no difference in response rates compared with standard TACE. However, on subset analysis, DEB-TACE did offer a benefit for patients with more advanced disease. DEB-TACE may be better tolerated. As shown in the PRECISION trial, 25% of patients in the TACE arm manifested toxic side effects, versus only 16.1% in the DEB-TACE arm. More specifically, the DEB-TACE group had fewer liver toxicity events ($P<.001$) and decreased difference in change from baseline cardiac function ($P = .018$).[146]

TARE

TARE is another locoregional therapy used for unresectable HCC. TARE treats the tumor using an intra-arterial approach, but, instead of delivering chemotherapy via the feeding hepatic artery, isolated radiation is delivered to the tumor. The most common delivery modality for TARE is with yttrium-90 (^{90}Y). ^{90}Y is loaded onto microspheres of glass or resin and, when injected into tumor-feeding arteries, delivers high-energy radiation with a short half-life and a short tissue penetration.[147] This mechanism of radiotherapy avoids damaging the normal liver parenchyma.[148] Data have shown that ^{90}Y is safe and has efficacy in controlling tumor progression.[22,148] Mazzaferro and colleagues[149] completed a phase 2 study with ^{90}Y therapy and noted an objective tumor response (40.4%) and complete response (9.6%) using EASL criteria. The use of ^{90}Y may be particularly applicable for patients with portal vein thrombosis because there is growing evidence that TARE does not cause macroscopic arterial embolization, and the risk of ischemia and subsequent necrosis is less than with TACE.[150] At present, there is a phase III trial (TRACE) comparing TARE with TACE.[151]

SYSTEMIC THERAPY FOR HCC
Cytotoxic Therapy

There are clinical scenarios in which locoregional therapies, resection, and transplantation are not appropriate or have been exhausted and systemic chemotherapy is indicated. Cytotoxic chemotherapy has in the past provided no clinically meaningful benefit to patients with advanced HCC, and the literature describes many clinical trials showing low response rates and no improvement in survival.[152,153] Most classes of chemotherapeutic agents have been investigated, either as single agents or in combinations, often with initial promise in early phase trials, but disappointing outcomes in the more rigorous phase 3 setting. Doxorubicin is probably the most widely used cytotoxic agent in this population in the United States, although the data in support of that use are limited. The response rates in early phase trials of doxorubicin were 10% to 20%, and median survival was 3 to 4 months. It is a testament to the paucity of alternative choices that these data were enough to make this agent an accepted standard of care for patients with advanced HCC.

Several investigators thought that response rates could be improved with combination chemotherapy. One of the most discussed combinations was cisplatin, interferon, doxorubicin, and 5-fluorouracil (the PIAF regimen), which resulted in significant anti-tumor activity in a phase 2 study of 50 patients. This study led to a randomized study comparing PIAF with single-agent doxorubicin in patients with unresectable or metastatic HCC. PIAF led to an increased response rate (20.9% vs 10.5%) but no significant improvement in overall survival.[153]

In recent years, other cytotoxic combinations have been investigated in select subsets of patients with HCC, including gemcitabine with oxaliplatin in patients with nonalcoholic liver disease, which yielded a disease control rate of 76% with an acceptable toxicity profile.[154] However, at this time, treatment guidelines indicate that no cytotoxic therapy, either single agent or combination, should be used in patients with HCC outside the context of a clinical trial.

Targeted Therapy

As noted earlier, a plethora of molecular mechanistic pathways underlying HCC tumorigenesis and proliferation have been elucidated in recent years, and interest has turned to targeting key components of these pathways. Sorafenib, a multitargeted kinase inhibitor, showed a significant overall survival benefit in patients with advanced or metastatic HCC compared with placebo in 2 separate phase 3 trials. In the landmark Sorafenib HCC Assessment Randomized Protocol (SHARP), performed mostly in Europe, more than 600 patients with advanced HCC, intact liver function (Child-Pugh class A), and good performance status were randomized to sorafenib or placebo.[16] The study was stopped at the second planned interim analysis because of a significant difference in overall survival favoring the sorafenib arm, with median survival of 10.7 months and 7.9 months for sorafenib and placebo respectively (hazard ratio [HR], 0.69 [0.55–0.87]; $P<.001$). The response rate was only 2% in the sorafenib arm (and 1% in the placebo arm), with most of the clinical and survival benefit gleaned by patients with stable disease. This finding is in keeping with other studies of tyrosine kinases in a variety of diseases, because the mechanism of action of most of these agents does not lead to cytotoxicity, but to a reduction in proliferation and growth. A similar overall survival benefit from sorafenib was noted in a second phase 3 trial, performed in the Asia-Pacific region, with similar entry criteria and treatment plan. In this study of more than 200 patients, those in the sorafenib arm had a median survival of 6.5 months, compared with 4.2 months for those on placebo. The HR of 0.68 (0.50–0.93; $P<.14$) was almost identical to that seen in the SHARP trial, although the absolute survival was lower, likely because of an enrolled subject pool with more advanced disease (radiographically and biochemically) and a slightly worse performance status as a whole.[155]

These studies led to US Food and Drug Administration approval of sorafenib in late 2007 for patients with unresectable or untransplantable HCC and preserved liver function (Child-Pugh class A or B). Although most patients on the phase 3 trials had excellent liver function (Child-Pugh class A), several smaller trials have reported no significant difference in tolerability or pharmacokinetic profile of the drug in patients with Child-Pugh class B cirrhosis.[156]

The observed toxicity profiles in the clinical trials were minor, with hand-foot syndrome, fatigue, and diarrhea reported as the most frequent adverse events. In practice, especially in the United States, these toxicities have proved more prevalent and problematic, and many patients are unable to tolerate the recommended dose of 400 mg twice daily. GIDEON (Global Investigation of therapeutic decisions in hepatocellular carcinoma and of its treatment with sorafenib), a large, multinational, prospective noninterventional study assessing real-world use of sorafenib in patients with HCC, has revealed marked differences in prescribing patterns, dosing strategies and patient tolerance in different geographic regions.[157]

The approval of sorafenib for the treatment of advanced HCC marked a major advance for patients with HCC and gave way to numerous subsequent studies of targeted agents in this setting, with hope of better outcomes than those observed with the chemotherapy trials of the last 2 decades. However, despite a wide range of therapeutic targets, including angiogenic pathways (VEGF), various growth factor pathways (Epidermal growth factor [EGFR], Platelet derived growth factor receptor [PDGFR], Fibroblast growth factor receptor [FGFR]), mammalian target of rapamycin (mTOR) signaling, and the mitogen-activated protein (MAP) kinase pathway (Rat sarcoma [RAS]/Rapidly accelerated fibrosarcoma [RAF]/Mitogen extracellular kinase [MEK]), no systemic agent has yet shown additional benefit in a phase 3 trial. Notable failures include sunitinib (a potent angiogenesis inhibitor, which was compared directly with sorafenib in a first-line trial, but proved more toxic, thus prompting study closure at interim analysis). Brivanib (a more narrowly targeted agent, focused on VEGF receptor and FGFR), which had preclinical evidence of enhanced activity in the setting of prior sorafenib failure and revealed early promise in both first-line and second-line settings, ultimately failed to meet the primary survival end point in a phase 3 trial. Everolimus (an mTOR inhibitor, with a long record in other diseases), which had reasonable efficacy signals in early phase trials for patients with prior sorafenib exposure, was similarly recently shown not to have met its primary end point in a multicenter phase 3 study.[158,159] These disappointments will not discourage further clinical development, but should focus efforts on robust biomarker development and rational sequencing or combination of systemic treatments in individual patients. More recently designed trials have included a priori assessment of a gene or protein of interest to preferentially deliver therapy to those patients most likely to benefit, with encouraging data on mesenchymal-epithelial transition targeted agents.[160]

Combined Locoregional and Systemic Therapies

Since the advent of these targeted therapies in HCC, an area that has held promise is their integration with locoregional approaches, such as TACE or TARE. The rationale for such combinations is the documented upregulation of progrowth pathways in response to the embolic therapies, specifically an acute increase in HIF1α, leading to increased VEGF activity, as well as other angiogenic stimuli. The use of antiangiogenic agents in combination with embolization could thus minimize the risk of posttreatment tumor expansion, potentially increasing disease-free and overall survival. A phase 2 study of sorafenib in conjunction with DEB-TACE revealed an acceptable toxicity profile and promising efficacy data, reporting overall survival of almost 2 years in a cohort of patients with Barcelona clinic liver cancer (BCLC) class B and C disease. Another trial of bevacizumab in combination with conventional TACE also reported encouraging results with an objective response rate of 60% and no unexpected toxicity.[161] These data show that combination therapy may be a fertile area for further development. It is hoped that rational therapy sequences, biomarker-driven combinations, and novel targets will provide incremental improvements in the systemic treatment of patients with advanced HCC.

SUMMARY

The management of HCC has evolved significantly over the past 20 years, and the mechanisms of carcinogenesis and disease progression are better understood. The current state and the future success of the treatment of HCC will continue to rely on a multidisciplinary approach.

REFERENCES

1. El-Serag HB, Rudolph KL. Hepatocellular carcinoma: epidemiology and molecular carcinogenesis. Gastroenterology 2007;132(7):2557–76.
2. Nishida N, Kudo M. Recent advancements in comprehensive genetic analyses for human hepatocellular carcinoma. Oncology 2013;84(Suppl 1):93–7.
3. Totoki Y, Tatsuno K, Yamamoto S, et al. High-resolution characterization of a hepatocellular carcinoma genome. Nat Genet 2011;43(5):464–9.
4. Li M, Zhao H, Zhang X, et al. Inactivating mutations of the chromatin remodeling gene ARID2 in hepatocellular carcinoma. Nat Genet 2011;43(9):828–9.
5. Guichard C, Amaddeo G, Imbeaud S, et al. Integrated analysis of somatic mutations and focal copy-number changes identifies key genes and pathways in hepatocellular carcinoma. Nat Genet 2012;44(6):694–8.
6. Huang J, Deng Q, Wang Q, et al. Exome sequencing of hepatitis B virus-associated hepatocellular carcinoma. Nat Genet 2012;44(10):1117–21.
7. Hoshida Y, Fuchs BC, Tanabe KK. Genomic risk of hepatitis C-related hepatocellular carcinoma. J Hepatol 2012;56(3):729–30.
8. Arzumanyan A, Reis HM, Feitelson MA. Pathogenic mechanisms in HBV- and HCV-associated hepatocellular carcinoma. Nat Rev Cancer 2013;13(2):123–35.
9. Yamashita T, Budhu A, Forgues M, et al. Activation of hepatic stem cell marker EpCAM by Wnt-β-catenin signaling in hepatocellular carcinoma. Cancer Res 2007;67(22):10831–9.
10. Monk M, Holding C. Human embryonic genes re-expressed in cancer cells. Oncogene 2001;20(56):8085–91.
11. Zhao RC, Zhu YS, Shi Y. New hope for cancer treatment: exploring the distinction between normal adult stem cells and cancer stem cells. Pharmacol Ther 2008;119(1):74–82.
12. Vrancken K, Paeshuyse J, Liekens S. Angiogenic activity of hepatitis B and C viruses. Antivir Chem Chemother 2012;22(4):159–70.
13. Sanz-Cameno P, Martín-Vílchez S, Lara-Pezzi E, et al. Hepatitis B virus promotes angiopoietin-2 expression in liver tissue: role of HBV x protein. Am J Pathol 2006;169(4):1215–22.
14. Abe M, Koga H, Yoshida T, et al. Hepatitis C virus core protein upregulates the expression of vascular endothelial growth factor via the nuclear factor-κB/hypoxia-inducible factor-1α axis under hypoxic conditions. Hepatol Res 2012; 42(6):591–600.
15. Keith B, Simon MC. Hypoxia-inducible factors, stem cells, and cancer. Cell 2007;129(3):465–72.
16. Llovet JM, Ricci S, Mazzaferro V, et al. Sorafenib in advanced hepatocellular carcinoma. N Engl J Med 2008;359(4):378–90.
17. van der Molen RG, Sprengers D, Binda RS, et al. Functional impairmont of myeloid and plasmacytoid dendritic cells of patients with chronic hepatitis B. Hepatology 2004;40(3):738–46.
18. Yoo Y, Ueda H, Park K, et al. Regulation of transforming growth factor-beta 1 expression by the hepatitis B virus (HBV) X transactivator. Role in HBV pathogenesis. J Clin Invest 1996;97(2):388.
19. Lopes AR, Kellam P, Das A, et al. Bim-mediated deletion of antigen-specific CD8+ T cells in patients unable to control HBV infection. J Clin Invest 2008; 118(5):1835.
20. Guidotti LG, Chisari FV. Immunobiology and pathogenesis of viral hepatitis. Annu Rev Pathol 2006;1:23–61.

21. Fazle Akbar S, Inaba K, Onji M. Upregulation of MHC class II antigen on dendritic cells from hepatitis B virus transgenic mice by interferon-γ: abrogation of immune response defect to a T-cell-dependent antigen. Immunology 1996;87(4):519–27.

22. Bruix J, Sherman M. Management of hepatocellular carcinoma: an update. Hepatology 2011;53(3):1020–2.

23. Sherman M. Serological surveillance for hepatocellular carcinoma: time to quit. J Hepatol 2010;52(4):614–5.

24. Sherman M. Screening for hepatocellular carcinoma. Hepatol Res 2007;37(s2): S152–65.

25. Yuen MF, Lai CL. Serological markers of liver cancer. Best Pract Res Clin Gastroenterol 2005;19(1):91–9.

26. Li D, Mallory T, Satomura S. AFP-L3: a new generation of tumor marker for hepatocellular carcinoma. Clin Chim Acta 2001;313(1):15–9.

27. Staden LV, Bukofzer S, Kew MC, et al. Differential lectin reactivities of α-fetoprotein in hepatocellular carcinoma: diagnostic value when serum α-fetoprotein levels are slightly raised. J Gastroenterol Hepatol 1992;7(3):260–5.

28. Yamashita F, Tanaka M, Satomura S, et al. Prognostic significance of Lens culinaris agglutinin A-reactive alpha-fetoprotein in small hepatocellular carcinomas. Gastroenterology 1996;111(4):996–1001.

29. Toyoda H, Kumada T, Tada T, et al. Clinical utility of highly sensitive Lens culinaris agglutinin-reactive alpha-fetoprotein in hepatocellular carcinoma patients with alpha-fetoprotein <20 ng/mL. Cancer Sci 2011;102(5):1025–31.

30. Aoyagi Y, Oguro M, Yanagi M, et al. Clinical significance of simultaneous determinations of alpha-fetoprotein and des-gamma-carboxy prothrombin in monitoring recurrence in patients with hepatocellular carcinoma. Cancer 1996;77(9):1781–6.

31. Marrero JA, Su GL, Wei W, et al. Des-gamma carboxyprothrombin can differentiate hepatocellular carcinoma from nonmalignant chronic liver disease in American patients. Hepatology 2003;37(5):1114–21.

32. Ikoma J, Kaito M, Ishihara T, et al. Early diagnosis of hepatocellular carcinoma using a sensitive assay for serum des-γ-carboxy prothrombin: a prospective study. Hepatogastroenterology 2002;49(43):235–8.

33. Hamamura K, Shiratori Y, Shiina S, et al. Unique clinical characteristics of patients with hepatocellular carcinoma who present with high plasma des-γ-carboxy prothrombin and low serum α-fetoprotein. Cancer 2000;88(7):1557–64.

34. Koike Y, Shiratori Y, Sato S, et al. Des-γ-carboxy prothrombin as a useful predisposing factor for the development of portal venous invasion in patients with hepatocellular carcinoma. Cancer 2001;91(3):561–9.

35. Tateishi R, Yoshida H, Matsuyama Y, et al. Diagnostic accuracy of tumor markers for hepatocellular carcinoma: a systematic review 2008;2(1):17–30.

36. Anborgh PH, Mutrie JC, Tuck AB, et al. Role of the metastasis-promoting protein osteopontin in the tumour microenvironment. J Cell Mol Med 2010;14(8):2037–44.

37. Ye QH, Qin LX, Forgues M, et al. Predicting hepatitis B virus–positive metastatic hepatocellular carcinomas using gene expression profiling and supervised machine learning. Nat Med 2003;9(4):416–23.

38. Shang S, Plymoth A, Ge S, et al. Identification of osteopontin as a novel marker for early hepatocellular carcinoma. Hepatology 2012;55(2):483–90.

39. Moon WS, Rhyu KH, Kang MJ, et al. Overexpression of VEGF and angiopoietin 2: a key to high vascularity of hepatocellular carcinoma? Mod Pathol 2003;16(6):552–7.

40. Poon R, Ho J, Tong C, et al. Prognostic significance of serum vascular endothelial growth factor and endostatin in patients with hepatocellular carcinoma. Br J Surg 2004;91(10):1354–60.

41. Kaseb AO, Morris JS, Hassan MM, et al. Clinical and prognostic implications of plasma insulin-like growth factor-1 and vascular endothelial growth factor in patients with hepatocellular carcinoma. J Clin Oncol 2011;29(29):3892–9.

42. Nakatsura T, Yoshitake Y, Senju S, et al. Glypican-3, overexpressed specifically in human hepatocellular carcinoma, is a novel tumor marker. Biochem Biophys Res Commun 2003;306(1):16–25.

43. Nakamura T. Structure and function of hepatocyte growth factor. Prog Growth Factor Res 1991;3(1):67–85.

44. Yamagamim H, Moriyama M, Matsumura H, et al. Serum concentrations of human hepatocyte growth factor is a useful indicator for predicting the occurrence of hepatocellular carcinomas in C-viral chronic liver diseases. Cancer 2002; 95(4):824–34.

45. Mazziotti G, Sorvillo F, Morisco F, et al. Serum insulin-like growth factor I evaluation as a useful tool for predicting the risk of developing hepatocellular carcinoma in patients with hepatitis C virus-related cirrhosis. Cancer 2002;95(12): 2539–45.

46. Asiyanbola B, Chang D, Gleisner AL, et al. Operative mortality after hepatic resection: are literature-based rates broadly applicable? J Gastrointest Surg 2008;12(5):842–51.

47. Parikh AA, Gentner B, Wu TT, et al. Perioperative complications in patients undergoing major liver resection with or without neoadjuvant chemotherapy. J Gastrointest Surg 2003;7(8):1082–8.

48. Joh JW, Johnson PJ, Monden M, et al. Biology of hepatocellular carcinoma. Ann Surg Oncol 2008;15(4):962–71.

49. Brouquet A, Andreou A, Shindoh J, et al. Methods to improve resectability of hepatocellular carcinoma. Multidisciplinary treatment of hepatocellular carcinoma. Springer; 2013. p. 57–67.

50. Chun YS, Ribero D, Abdalla EK, et al. Comparison of two methods of future liver remnant volume measurement. J Gastrointest Surg 2008;12(1):123–8.

51. Kubota K, Makuuchi M, Kusaka K, et al. Measurement of liver volume and hepatic functional reserve as a guide to decision-making in resectional surgery for hepatic tumors. Hepatology 1997;26(5):1176–81.

52. Manizate F, Hiotis SP, Labow D, et al. Liver functional reserve estimation: state of the art and relevance to local treatments. Oncology 2010;78(Suppl. 1):131–4.

53. Pugh R, Murray-Lyon I, Dawson J, et al. Transection of the oesophagus for bleeding oesophageal varices. Br J Surg 1973;60(8):646–9.

54. Santambrogio R, Kluger MD, Costa M, et al. Hepatic resection for hepatocellular carcinoma in patients with Child-Pugh's A cirrhosis: is clinical evidence of portal hypertension a contraindication? HPB (Oxford) 2013;15(1):78–84.

55. Cucchetti A, Ercolani G, Vivarelli M, et al. Impact of model for end-stage liver disease (MELD) score on prognosis after hepatectomy for hepatocellular carcinoma on cirrhosis. Liver Transpl 2006;12(6):966–71.

56. Delis SG, Bakoyiannis A, Biliatis I, et al. Model for end-stage liver disease (MELD) score, as a prognostic factor for post-operative morbidity and mortality in cirrhotic patients, undergoing hepatectomy for hepatocellular carcinoma. HPB (Oxford) 2009;11(4):351–7.

57. Delis SG, Bakoyiannis A, Dervenis C, et al. Perioperative risk assessment for hepatocellular carcinoma by using the MELD score. J Gastrointest Surg 2009; 13(12):2268–75.

58. Wong T, Lo CM. Resection strategies for hepatocellular carcinoma. Semin Liver Dis 2013;33:273–81 Thieme.

59. Hoekstra LT, de Graaf W, Nibourg GA, et al. Physiological and biochemical basis of clinical liver function tests: a review. Ann Surg 2013;257(1):27–36.

60. Hemming AW, Reed AI, Howard RJ, et al. Preoperative portal vein embolization for extended hepatectomy. Ann Surg 2003;237(5):686.

61. Farges O, Belghiti J, Kianmanesh R, et al. Portal vein embolization before right hepatectomy: prospective clinical trial. Ann Surg 2003;237(2):208.

62. Abdalla EK, Barnett CC, Doherty D, et al. Extended hepatectomy in patients with hepatobiliary malignancies with and without preoperative portal vein embolization. Arch Surg 2002;137(6):675.

63. Ribero D, Abdalla E, Madoff D, et al. Portal vein embolization before major hepatectomy and its effects on regeneration, resectability and outcome. Br J Surg 2007;94(11):1386–94.

64. Lee KK, Kim DG, Moon IS, et al. Liver transplantation versus liver resection for the treatment of hepatocellular carcinoma. J Surg Oncol 2010;101(1):47–53.

65. Zhou XD, Tang ZY, Yang BH, et al. Experience of 1000 patients who underwent hepatectomy for small hepatocellular carcinoma. Cancer 2001;91(8):1479–86.

66. Pawlik TM, Poon RT, Abdalla EK, et al. Hepatectomy for hepatocellular carcinoma with major portal or hepatic vein invasion: results of a multicenter study. Surgery 2005;137(4):403–10.

67. Yamashita Y, Taketomi A, Itoh S, et al. Longterm favorable results of limited hepatic resections for patients with hepatocellular carcinoma: 20 years of experience. J Am Coll Surg 2007;205(1):19–26.

68. Poon RT, Fan ST, Lo CM, et al. Long-term survival and pattern of recurrence after resection of small hepatocellular carcinoma in patients with preserved liver function: implications for a strategy of salvage transplantation. Ann Surg 2002;235(3):373.

69. Shi M, Guo RP, Lin XJ, et al. Partial hepatectomy with wide versus narrow resection margin for solitary hepatocellular carcinoma: a prospective randomized trial. Ann Surg 2007;245(1):36.

70. Nathan H, Hyder O, Mayo SC, et al. Surgical therapy for early hepatocellular carcinoma in the modern era. Ann Surg 2013. [Epub ahead of print].

71. Pawlik TM, Delman KA, Vauthey JN, et al. Tumor size predicts vascular invasion and histologic grade: implications for selection of surgical treatment for hepatocellular carcinoma. Liver Transpl 2005;11(9):1086–92.

72. Nagasue N, Kohno H, Chang YC, et al. Liver resection for hepatocellular carcinoma. Results of 229 consecutive patients during 11 years. Ann Surg 1993;217(4):375.

73. Wang BW, Mok KT, Liu SI, et al. Is hepatectomy beneficial in the treatment of multinodular hepatocellular carcinoma? J Formos Med Assoc 2008;107(8):616–26.

74. Ishizawa T, Hasegawa K, Aoki T, et al. Neither multiple tumors nor portal hypertension are surgical contraindications for hepatocellular carcinoma. Gastroenterology 2008;134(7):1908–16.

75. Truty MJ, Vauthey JN. Surgical resection of high-risk hepatocellular carcinoma: patient selection, preoperative considerations, and operative technique. Ann Surg Oncol 2010;17(5):1219–25.

76. Mazzaferro V, Regalia E, Doci R, et al. Liver transplantation for the treatment of small hepatocellular carcinomas in patients with cirrhosis. N Engl J Med 1996;334(11):693–700.

77. Lai EC, Ng IO, Ng MM, et al. Long-term results of resection for large hepatocellular carcinoma: a multivariate analysis of clinicopathological features. Hepatology 1990;11(5):815–8.

78. Wu CC, Ho YZ, Ho WL, et al. Preoperative transcatheter arterial chemoemboli-zation for resectable large hepatocellular carcinoma: a reappraisal. Br J Surg 1995;82(1):122–6.
79. Régimbeau JM, Farges O, Shen BY, et al. Is surgery for large hepatocellular carcinoma justified? J Hepatol 1999;31(6):1062–8.
80. Hanazaki K, Kajikawa S, Shimozawa N, et al. Hepatic resection for large hepatocellular carcinoma. Am J Surg 2001;181(4):347–53.
81. Fong Y, Sun RL, Jarnagin W, et al. An analysis of 412 cases of hepatocellular carcinoma at a Western center. Ann Surg 1999;229(6):790.
82. Poon RT, Fan ST, Wong J. Selection criteria for hepatic resection in patients with large hepatocellular carcinoma larger than 10 cm in diameter. J Am Coll Surg 2002;194(5):592–602.
83. Vauthey JN, Pawlik TM, Lauwers GY, et al. Is hepatic resection for large or multi-nodular hepatocellular carcinoma justified? Results from a multi-institutional database. Ann Surg Oncol 2005;12(5):364–73.
84. Yang LY, Fang F, Ou DP, et al. Solitary large hepatocellular carcinoma: a specific subtype of hepatocellular carcinoma with good outcome after hepatic resection. Ann Surg 2009;249(1):118–23.
85. Ikai I, Yamamoto Y, Yamamoto N, et al. Results of hepatic resection for hepatocellular carcinoma invading major portal and/or hepatic veins. Surg Oncol Clin N Am 2003;12(1):65–75.
86. Iwatsuki S, Gordon RD, Shaw BW Jr, et al. Role of liver transplantation in cancer therapy. Ann Surg 1985;202(4):401.
87. Adam R, Azoulay D, Castaing D, et al. Liver resection as a bridge to transplantation for hepatocellular carcinoma on cirrhosis: a reasonable strategy? Ann Surg 2003;238(4):508.
88. Llovet JM, Fuster J, Bruix J. Intention-to-treat analysis of surgical treatment for early hepatocellular carcinoma: resection versus transplantation. Hepatology 1999;30(6):1434–40.
89. Bruix J, Sherman M. Management of hepatocellular carcinoma. Hepatology 2005;42(5):1208–36.
90. Yao FY, Ferrell L, Bass NM, et al. Liver transplantation for hepatocellular carcinoma: comparison of the proposed UCSF criteria with the Milan criteria and the Pittsburgh modified TNM criteria. Liver Transpl 2002;8(9):765–74.
91. Yao FY, Ferrell L, Bass NM, et al. Liver transplantation for hepatocellular carcinoma: expansion of the tumor size limits does not adversely impact survival. Hepatology 2001;33(6):1394–403.
92. Yao FY, Bass NM, Nikolai B, et al. Liver transplantation for hepatocellular carcinoma: analysis of survival according to the intention-to-treat principle and dropout from the waiting list. Liver Transpl 2002;8(10):873–83.
93. Leung JY, Zhu AX, Gordon FD, et al. Liver transplantation outcomes for early-stage hepatocellular carcinoma: results of a multicenter study. Liver Transpl 2004;10(11):1343–54.
94. Todo S, Furukawa H. Living donor liver transplantation for adult patients with hepatocellular carcinoma: experience in Japan. Ann Surg 2004;240(3):451.
95. Decaens T, Roudot-Thoraval F, Hadni-Bresson S, et al. Impact of UCSF criteria according to pre-and post-OLT tumor features: analysis of 479 patients listed for HCC with a short waiting time. Liver Transpl 2006;12(12):1761–9.
96. Duffy JP, Vardanian A, Benjamin E, et al. Liver transplantation criteria for hepatocellular carcinoma should be expanded: a 22-year experience with 467 patients at UCLA. Ann Surg 2007;246(3):502.

97. Onaca N, Davis GL, Goldstein RM, et al. Expanded criteria for liver transplantation in patients with hepatocellular carcinoma: a report from the International Registry of Hepatic Tumors in Liver Transplantation. Liver Transpl 2007;13(3):391–9.

98. Llovet JM, Schwartz M, Mazzaferro V. Resection and liver transplantation for hepatocellular carcinoma. Semin Liver Dis 2005;25:181–200 New York: Thieme-Stratton; c1981.

99. Mazzaferro V, Llovet JM, Miceli R, et al. Predicting survival after liver transplantation in patients with hepatocellular carcinoma beyond the Milan criteria: a retrospective, exploratory analysis. Lancet Oncol 2009;10(1):35–43.

100. Bellavance EC, Lumpkins KM, Mentha G, et al. Surgical management of early-stage hepatocellular carcinoma: resection or transplantation? J Gastrointest Surg 2008;12(10):1699–708.

101. Earl TM, Chapman WC. Hepatocellular carcinoma: resection versus transplantation. Semin Liver Dis 2013;33:282–92 Thieme Medical Publishers.

102. Yao FY, Bass NM, Nikolai B, et al. A follow-up analysis of the pattern and predictors of dropout from the waiting list for liver transplantation in patients with hepatocellular carcinoma: implications for the current organ allocation policy. Liver Transpl 2003;9(7):684–92.

103. Cescon M, Cucchetti A, Ravaioli M, et al. Hepatocellular carcinoma locoregional therapies for patients in the waiting list. Impact on transplantability and recurrence rate. J Hepatol 2013;58(3):609–18.

104. de Lope CR, Tremosini S, Forner A, et al. Management of HCC. J Hepatol 2012; 56:S75–87.

105. Kaihara S, Kiuchi T, Ueda M, et al. Living-donor liver transplantation for hepatocellular carcinoma. Transplantation 2003;75(3):S37–40.

106. Gondolesi GE, Roayaie S, Muñoz L, et al. Adult living donor liver transplantation for patients with hepatocellular carcinoma: extending UNOS priority criteria. Ann Surg 2004;239(2):142.

107. Fisher R, Kulik L, Freise C, et al. Hepatocellular carcinoma recurrence and death following living and deceased donor liver transplantation. Am J Transplant 2007; 7(6):1601–8.

108. Ghobrial RM, Freise CE, Trotter JF, et al. Donor morbidity after living donation for liver transplantation. Gastroenterology 2008;135(2):468–76.

109. Sarasin FP, Majno PE, Llovet JM, et al. Living donor liver transplantation for early hepatocellular carcinoma: a life-expectancy and cost-effectiveness perspective. Hepatology 2001;33(5):1073–9.

110. Majno PE, Adam R, Bismuth H, et al. Influence of preoperative transarterial lipiodol chemoembolization on resection and transplantation for hepatocellular carcinoma in patients with cirrhosis. Ann Surg 1997;226(6):688.

111. Porrett PM, Peterman H, Rosen M, et al. Lack of benefit of pre-transplant locoregional hepatic therapy for hepatocellular cancer in the current MELD era. Liver Transpl 2006;12(4):665–73.

112. Decaens T, Roudot-Thoraval F, Bresson-Hadni S, et al. Impact of pretransplantation transarterial chemoembolization on survival and recurrence after liver transplantation for hepatocellular carcinoma. Liver Transpl 2005;11(7):767–75.

113. Pelletier SJ, Fu S, Thyagarajan V, et al. An intention-to-treat analysis of liver transplantation for hepatocellular carcinoma using organ procurement transplant network data. Liver Transpl 2009;15(8):859–68.

114. Clavien PA, Lesurtel M, Bossuyt PM, et al. Recommendations for liver transplantation for hepatocellular carcinoma: an international consensus conference report. Lancet Oncol 2012;13(1):e11–22.

115. Jarnagin W, Chapman WC, Curley S, et al. Surgical treatment of hepatocellular carcinoma: expert consensus statement. HPB (Oxford) 2010;12(5):302–10.
116. Llovet JM, Real MI, Montaña X, et al. Arterial embolisation or chemoembolisation versus symptomatic treatment in patients with unresectable hepatocellular carcinoma: a randomised controlled trial. Lancet 2002;359(9319):1734–9.
117. Lo CM, Ngan H, Tso WK, et al. Randomized controlled trial of transarterial lipiodol chemoembolization for unresectable hepatocellular carcinoma. Hepatology 2002;35(5):1164–71.
118. Llovet J, Mas X, Aponte J, et al. Cost effectiveness of adjuvant therapy for hepatocellular carcinoma during the waiting list for liver transplantation. Gut 2002;50(1):123–8.
119. Teh SH, Christein J, Donohue J, et al. Hepatic resection of hepatocellular carcinoma in patients with cirrhosis: model of end-stage liver disease (MELD) score predicts perioperative mortality. J Gastrointest Surg 2005;9(9):1207–15.
120. Nathan H, Schulick RD, Choti MA, et al. Predictors of survival after resection of early hepatocellular carcinoma. Ann Surg 2009;249(5):799–805.
121. Belghiti J, Cortes A, Abdalla EK, et al. Resection prior to liver transplantation for hepatocellular carcinoma. Ann Surg 2003;238(6):885.
122. Meza-Junco J, Montano-Loza AJ, Liu DM, et al. Locoregional radiological treatment for hepatocellular carcinoma; Which, when and how? Cancer Treat Rev 2012;38(1):54–62.
123. Simon CJ, Dupuy DE, Mayo-Smith WW. Microwave ablation: principles and applications. Radiographics 2005;25(Suppl 1):S69–83.
124. Lencioni R, Cioni D, Della Pina C, et al. Hepatocellular carcinoma: new options for image-guided ablation. J Hepatobiliary Pancreat Sci 2010;17(4):399–403.
125. Wang S, Keltner L, Winship J, et al. A phase I/II safety and efficacy study of intratumoral light-activated drug therapy using talaporfin sodium in patients with inoperable hepatocellular carcinoma. J Clin Oncol (Meeting Abstracts) 2009; 2009:e15684.
126. Bouza C, López-Cuadrado T, Alcázar R, et al. Meta-analysis of percutaneous radiofrequency ablation versus ethanol injection in hepatocellular carcinoma. BMC Gastroenterol 2009;9(1):31.
127. Orlando A, Leandro G, Olivo M, et al. Radiofrequency thermal ablation vs. percutaneous ethanol injection for small hepatocellular carcinoma in cirrhosis: meta-analysis of randomized controlled trials. Am J Gastroenterol 2009; 104(2):514–24.
128. Llovet JM, Bruix J. Novel advancements in the management of hepatocellular carcinoma in 2008. J Hepatol 2008;48:S20–37.
129. Brunello F, Veltri A, Carucci P, et al. Radiofrequency ablation versus ethanol injection for early hepatocellular carcinoma: a randomized controlled trial. Scand J Gastroenterol 2008;43(6):727–35.
130. Shiina S, Teratani T, Obi S, et al. A randomized controlled trial of radiofrequency ablation with ethanol injection for small hepatocellular carcinoma. Gastroenterology 2005;129(1):122–30.
131. Lin S, Lin C, Lin C, et al. Randomised controlled trial comparing percutaneous radiofrequency thermal ablation, percutaneous ethanol injection, and percutaneous acetic acid injection to treat hepatocellular carcinoma of 3 cm or less. Gut 2005;54(8):1151–6.
132. Shibata T, Iimuro Y, Yamamoto Y, et al. Small hepatocellular carcinoma: comparison of radio-frequency ablation and percutaneous microwave coagulation therapy. Radiology 2002;223(2):331–7.

133. Yu NC, Lu D, Raman SS, et al. Hepatocellular carcinoma: microwave ablation with multiple straight and loop antenna clusters–pilot comparison with pathologic findings. Radiology 2006;239(1):269.

134. Brown DB, Gould JE, Gervais DA, et al. Transcatheter therapy for hepatic malignancy: standardization of terminology and reporting criteria. J Vasc Interv Radiol 2009;20(7):S425–34.

135. A comparison of lipiodol chemoembolization and conservative treatment for unresectable hepatocellular carcinoma. Groupe d'Etude et de Traitement du Carcinome Hépatocellulaire. N Engl J Med 1995;332(19):1256–61.

136. Riaz A, Memon K, Miller FH, et al. Role of the EASL, RECIST, and WHO response guidelines alone or in combination for hepatocellular carcinoma: radiologic-pathologic correlation. J Hepatol 2011;54(4):695–704.

137. Lencioni R, Llovet JM. Modified RECIST (mRECIST) assessment for hepatocellular carcinoma. Semin Liver Dis 2010;30:052–60 © Thieme Medical Publishers.

138. Bonekamp S, Jolepalem P, Lazo M, et al. Hepatocellular carcinoma: response to TACE assessed with semiautomated volumetric and functional analysis of diffusion-weighted and contrast-enhanced MR imaging data. Radiology 2011; 260(3):752–61.

139. Marelli L, Stigliano R, Triantos C, et al. Transarterial therapy for hepatocellular carcinoma: which technique is more effective? A systematic review of cohort and randomized studies. Cardiovasc Intervent Radiol 2007;30(1):6–25.

140. Llovet JM, Bruix J. Systematic review of randomized trials for unresectable hepatocellular carcinoma: chemoembolization improves survival. Hepatology 2003;37(2):429–42.

141. van Malenstein H, Maleux G, Vandecaveye V, et al. A randomized phase II study of drug-eluting beads versus transarterial chemoembolization for unresectable hepatocellular carcinoma. Onkologie 2011;34(7):368–76.

142. Lewis AL, Gonzalez M, Lloyd AW, et al. DC bead: in vitro characterization of a drug-delivery device for transarterial chemoembolization. J Vasc Interv Radiol 2006;17(2):335–42.

143. Lewis AL, Gonzalez MV, Leppard SW, et al. Doxorubicin eluting beads– 1: effects of drug loading on bead characteristics and drug distribution. J Mater Sci Mater Med 2007;18(9):1691–9.

144. Poon RT, Tso WK, Pang RW, et al. A phase I/II trial of chemoembolization for hepatocellular carcinoma using a novel intra-arterial drug-eluting bead. Clin Gastroenterol Hepatol 2007;5(9):1100–8.

145. Lammer J, Malagari K, Vogl T, et al. Prospective randomized study of doxorubicin-eluting-bead embolization in the treatment of hepatocellular carcinoma: results of the PRECISION V study. Cardiovasc Intervent Radiol 2010; 33(1):41–52.

146. Vogl TJ, Lammer J, Lencioni R, et al. Liver, gastrointestinal, and cardiac toxicity in intermediate hepatocellular carcinoma treated with PRECISION TACE with drug-eluting beads: results from the PRECISION V randomized trial. Am J Roentgenol 2011;197(4):W562–70.

147. Sangro B, Iñarrairaegui M, Bilbao JI. Radioembolization for hepatocellular carcinoma. J Hepatol 2012;56(2):464–73.

148. Kim YH, Kim DY. Yttrium-90 radioembolization for hepatocellular carcinoma: what we know and what we need to know. Oncology 2013;84(Suppl 1):34–9.

149. Mazzaferro V, Sposito C, Bhoori S, et al. Yttrium-90 radioembolization for intermediate-advanced hepatocellular carcinoma: a phase 2 study. Hepatology 2013;57(5):1826–37.

150. Salem R, Mazzaferro V, Sangro B. Yttrium 90 radioembolization for the treatment of hepatocellular carcinoma: biological lessons, current challenges and clinical perspectives. Hepatology 2013. [Epub ahead of print].
151. Seinstra BA, Defreyne L, Lambert B, et al. Transarterial RAdioembolization versus ChemoEmbolization for the treatment of hepatocellular carcinoma (TRACE): study protocol for a randomized controlled trial. Trials 2012;13(1):144.
152. Leung TW, Johnson PJ. Systemic therapy for hepatocellular carcinoma. Semin Oncol 2001;28:514–20 Elsevier.
153. Yeo W, Mok TS, Zee B, et al. A randomized phase III study of doxorubicin versus cisplatin/interferon α-2b/doxorubicin/fluorouracil (PIAF) combination chemotherapy for unresectable hepatocellular carcinoma. J Natl Cancer Inst 2005; 97(20):1532–8.
154. Louafi S, Boige V, Ducreux M, et al. Gemcitabine plus oxaliplatin (GEMOX) in patients with advanced hepatocellular carcinoma (HCC). Cancer 2007;109(7): 1384–90.
155. Cheng AL, Kang YK, Chen Z, et al. Efficacy and safety of sorafenib in patients in the Asia-Pacific region with advanced hepatocellular carcinoma: a phase III randomised, double-blind, placebo-controlled trial. Lancet Oncol 2009;10(1): 25–34.
156. Furuse J, Ishii H, Nakachi K, et al. Phase I study of sorafenib in Japanese patients with hepatocellular carcinoma. Cancer Sci 2008;99(1):159–65.
157. Lencioni R, Kudo M, Ye SL, et al. First interim analysis of the GIDEON (Global Investigation of therapeutic DEcisions in hepatocellular carcinoma and Of its treatment with sorafeNib) non-interventional study. Int J Clin Pract 2012;66(7): 675–83.
158. Johnson PJ, Qin S, Park JW, et al. Brivanib versus Sorafenib as first-line therapy in patients with unresectable, advanced hepatocellular carcinoma: results from the randomized phase III BRISK-FL Study. J Clin Oncol 2013;31:3517–24.
159. Cheng A, Kang Y, Lin D, et al. Phase III trial of sunitinib (Su) versus sorafenib (So) in advanced hepatocellular carcinoma (HCC). J Clin Oncol 2011; 29(Suppl 15):4000.
160. Santoro A, Simonelli M, Rodriguez-Lope C, et al. A phase-1b study of tivantinib (ARQ 197) in adult patients with hepatocellular carcinoma and cirrhosis. Br J Cancer 2013;108(1):21–4.
161. Buijs M, Reyes DK, Pawlik TM, et al. Phase 2 trial of concurrent bevacizumab and transhepatic arterial chemoembolization in patients with unresectable hepatocellular carcinoma. Cancer 2012;119:1042–9.

Staging of Biliary Tract and Primary Liver Tumors

Junichi Shindoh, MD, PhD, Jean-Nicolas Vauthey, MD*

KEYWORDS

- Staging • Hepatocellular carcinoma • Intrahepatic cholangiocarcinoma
- Bile duct cancer • Gallbladder cancer

KEY POINTS

- Tumor staging is important for stratifying patients according to prognosis and selecting adequate treatment options.
- A variety of staging systems are available for hepatobiliary malignancies. However, each staging system has its own strengths and weaknesses, and no perfect staging system exists.
- Patients with hepatobiliary malignancies often have decreased hepatic function from underlying liver disease.
- Tumor staging should be interpreted with care according to the status of patients, while understanding of the nature of each staging system.

INTRODUCTION

For patients with hepatobiliary malignancies, various therapeutic options are currently available, including surgical resection, ablation, transarterial chemoembolization (TACE), systemic therapy, and radiotherapy. To optimize the selection of these therapeutic options, adequate stratification of patients according to their prognosis is practically important. Among the hepatobiliary malignancies, hepatocellular carcinoma (HCC) is the most studied malignancy, and various staging systems have been proposed from both clinical and pathologic standpoints, such as the Cancer of the Liver Italian Program (CLIP) score, Barcelona Clinic Liver Cancer (BCLC) staging system, Liver Cancer Study Group of Japan (LCSGJ) staging system, or American Joint Committee on Cancer/International Union Against Cancer (AJCC/UICC) staging system. However, these staging systems have their relative strengths and weaknesses. In addition, for biliary tract cancers, several controversies remain regarding prognostic

Conflicts of Interest and Source of Funding: This research was supported in part by the National Institutes of Health through MD Anderson's Cancer Center Support Grant, CA016672. The authors report no conflicts of interest relevant to this article.
Department of Surgical Oncology, The University of Texas MD Anderson Cancer Center, 1515 Holcombe Boulevard, Unit 1484, Houston, TX 77030, USA
* Corresponding author.
E-mail address: jvauthey@mdanderson.org

Surg Oncol Clin N Am 23 (2014) 313–322
http://dx.doi.org/10.1016/j.soc.2013.11.003
1055-3207/14/$ – see front matter © 2014 Elsevier Inc. All rights reserved.

implications of tumor location or definition of regional lymph nodes. This article reviews currently used staging systems for hepatobiliary malignancies, and highlights their clinical relevance and controversies.

STAGING OF PRIMARY LIVER CANCER
HCC

CLIP score
The CLIP score was developed using data on 435 Italian patients with HCC treated with a range of surgical and nonsurgical therapies (**Table 1**),[1] and several subsequent validation studies confirmed the clinical relevance of this prognostic score.[2–4] The CLIP score includes more tumor-specific factors and offers better prognostic stratification than the conventional Okuda Staging System, which included tumor morphology, presence of ascites, serum albumin level, and serum bilirubin level as parameters for prognostic scoring.[5] However, the limitation of this staging system is its poor discriminatory power of prognosis in early and advanced stages of HCC. The parameter of tumor morphology includes a wide range of tumor sizes. Furthermore, vascular invasion, which is a potent prognostic factor for HCC, is not considered unless a portal vein tumor thrombus is present. Therefore, the clinical use of the CLIP score is limited, especially in the selection of therapeutic options.

BCLC staging system
The BCLC staging system (**Fig. 1**)[6] is one of the popular staging systems, especially in European countries. This system includes liver function, tumor characteristics, and performance status when addressing disease progression, and offers adequate therapeutic options based on the treatment algorithm. Although its usefulness was validated in several studies,[7–9] one of the major drawbacks of this staging system is that it is based on a single institutional experience. Furthermore, mixture of staging system and treatment algorithm may cause several problems in actual clinical settings. First, the surgical management is rather conservative in this system, and patients with lesions greater than 5 cm are not candidates for surgery. Because treatment for HCC has been changing over time and some patients actually benefit from multidisciplinary and/or sequential approach (eg, resection after TACE plus portal vein embolization, or orthotopic liver transplantation after TACE), simplified therapeutic recommendations for each tumor stage do not fit with actual clinical practice. Second, although the BCLC staging system considers both underlying liver disease and cancer progression, this system is rather a treatment algorithm than a pure cancer staging system, and accordingly, simple comparison with other staging systems is difficult.

Table 1
CLIP score

Variable	Points		
	0	1	2
Child-Pugh grade	A	B	C
Tumor morphology	Solitary and ≤50%	Multifocal and ≤50%	Massive or >50%
Serum α-fetoprotein	<400 ng/mL	≥400 ng/mL	
Portal vein thrombosis	Absent	Present	

From The Cancer of the Liver Italian Program (CLIP) investigators. A new prognostic system for hepatocellular carcinoma: a retrospective study of 435 patients: the Cancer of the Liver Italian Program (CLIP) investigators. Hepatology 1998;28:751–5; with permission.

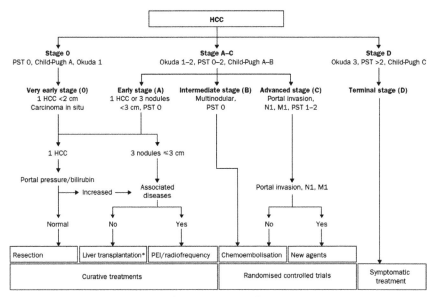

Fig. 1. BCLC staging system. PST, performance status. (*From* Llovet JM, Burroughs A, Bruix J. Hepatocellular carcinoma. Lancet 2003;362(9399):1907–17; with permission.)

LCSGJ staging system

The LCSGJ 4th edition staging system was developed by a working group of the International Hepato-Pancreato-Biliary Association using data on 21,711 Japanese patients who underwent liver resection for HCC.[10] T factor is determined based on how many of the following factors are present: tumor size ($\leq$2 cm or >2 cm), tumor number (solitary or multiple), and macrovascular invasion (present or absent). The stage is determined according to the T factor and presence of regional node metastasis (N) or distant metastasis (M) (**Table 2**). The strength of this staging system is that it is based on a large cohort from a Japanese nationwide survey by the LCSGJ. However, the limitations are that this staging system places equal weight on each of

Table 2 LCSGJ staging system			
T	T1		None of following factors
	T2		One of following factor
	T3		Two of following factors
	T4		Three of following factors or tumor rupture/direct invasion
			• Size >2 cm
			• Multiple tumor
			• Macrovascular invasion
Stage I			T1N0M0
Stage II			T2N0M0
Stage III			T3N0M0
Stage IVA			T4N0M0 or T1–3N1M0
Stage IVB			Any T/N, M1

From Makuuchi M, Belghiti J, Belli G, et al. IHPBA concordant classification of primary liver cancer: working group report. J Hepatobiliary Pancreat Surg 2003;10:26–30; with permission.

3 tumor-specific factors, and only macroscopic evidence of vascular invasion is accounted for in determining T factor.

AJCC/UICC staging system

The AJCC/UICC 7th edition TNM staging system[11] is a modification of the simplified TNM staging system based on a study from the International Cooperative Study Group on Hepatocellular Carcinoma that included data on 591 surgical patients from the United States, Japan, and France (**Table 3**).[12] The strength of this staging system was the use of centralized pathologic review, and its clinical relevance has been validated in various subsequent studies in patients treated with liver resection.[13–19] Validation was also performed using patients who underwent transplant in a multicenter study.[20] Because liver explantation enables complete removal of liver invaded by cancer, full staging of HCC is feasible depending on the progression of the initial cancer.

However, the limitation of the current edition of the AJCC/UICC staging system is that solitary HCC is not stratified with respect to size. Recent studies have reported excellent long-term outcomes in patients with solitary HCC up to 2 cm.[21–26] The size cutoff of 2 cm has been adopted in the LCSGJ and BCLC staging systems. Although the presence of microvascular invasion has been reported to be a strong prognostic factor in HCC,[10,27–29] its significance in small HCC has not yet been clarified.

A recent study from the International Cooperative Study Group on Hepatocellular Carcinoma reported that microvascular invasion does not affect patient prognosis in small HCCs up to 2 cm, and showed the potential for the reclassification of the current version of the AJCC/UICC staging system (**Fig. 2**, **Table 4**). This result is practically important because various curative therapeutic options can be selected for small tumors up to 2 cm, and also suggests that resection for the purpose of pathologic evaluation might not be necessary in patient selection for liver transplantation.[30,31]

INTRAHEPATIC CHOLANGIOCARCINOMA

Intrahepatic cholangiocarcinoma is an uncommon disease accounting for 5% to 30% of all primary liver malignancies.[32] Historically, the staging system for

Table 3			
AJCC/UICC 7th edition staging system			
T	T1		Solitary with no vascular invasion
	T2		Solitary with vascular invasion or multifocal ≤5 cm
	T3a		Multifocal >5 cm
	T3b		Involvement of a major branch of the portal vein or hepatic artery
	T4		Invasion of adjacent organs or rupture of HCC
Stage I			T1N0M0
Stage II			T2N0M0
Stage IIIA			T3aN0M0
Stage IIIB			T3bN0M0
Stage IIIC			T4N0M0
Stage IVA			Any TN1M0
Stage IVB			Any T/N, M1

From Edge SB, Byrd DR, Compton CC, et al, editors. AJCC cancer staging manual. 7th edition. New York: Springer; 2010; with permission.

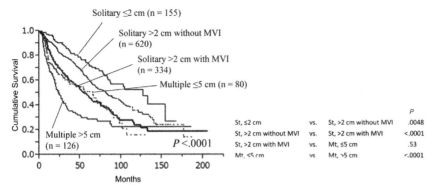

Fig. 2. Reclassification of AJCC/UICC staging system for solitary HCC. Mt, multiple tumors; MVI, microvascular invasion; St, solitary tumor. (*Adapted from* Shindoh J, Andreou A, Aloia TA, et al. Microvascular invasion does not predict long-term survival in hepatocellular carcinoma up to 2 cm: reappraisal of the staging system for solitary tumors. Ann Surg Oncol 2013;20(4):1223–9; with permission.)

intrahepatic cholangiocarcinoma has been identical to that of HCC. However, the current version of the AJCC/UICC staging system provides unique staging for this entity (**Table 5**) based on evidence from a study involving 598 patients from the Surveillance, Epidemiology, and End Results (SEER) database,[33] which was later validated in studies using international multicenter data.[34,35] Tumor size had no independent effect on survival, and multiple tumors and vascular invasion had similar prognostic influence.

STAGING OF BILIARY TRACT CANCER
Extrahepatic Bile Duct Cancer

For extrahepatic biliary tract cancers, different staging systems are used according to the location of the tumor (**Fig. 3**, **Table 6**). Because complete surgical resection is the

Table 4 Current AJCC/UICC staging system (7th edition) and new classification				
	AJCC Current (7th edition)	OS, Months, Median (Range)	New Classification	OS, Months, Median (Range)
T1	Solitary HCC without MVI	84.7 (76.1–100.4)	T1a Solitary HCC ≤2 cm	126.9 (83.8–NE)
			T1b Solitary HCC >2 cm without MVI	81.4 (69.0–97.2)
T2	Solitary HCC with MVI	60.6 (50.4–75.8)	T2 Solitary HCC >2 cm with MVI	55.0 (44.2–65.6)
	Multiple HCC ≤5 cm	55.9 (48.6–72.0)	Multiple HCC ≤5 cm	55.9 (48.6–72.0)
T3a	Multiple HCC >5 cm	27.7 (22.5–38.7)	T3a Multiple HCC >5 cm	27.2 (22.5–38.7)
T3b	Major vascular invasion	28.0 (15.4–43.3)	T3b Major vascular invasion	28.0 (15.4–43.3)

Abbreviations: MVI, microvascular invasion; NE, not estimated; OS, overall survival.
Adapted from Shindoh J, Andreou A, Aloia TA, et al. Microvascular invasion does not predict long-term survival in hepatocellular carcinoma up to 2 cm: reappraisal of the staging system for solitary tumors. Ann Surg Oncol 2013;20(4):1223–9; with permission.

Table 5
AJCC/UICC classification (7th edition) of intrahepatic cholangiocarcinoma

T	Tis	Carcinoma in situ
	T1	Solitary tumor without vascular invasion
	T2a	Solitary tumor with vascular invasion
	T2b	Multiple tumors, with or without vascular invasion
	T3	Tumor perforating the visceral peritoneum or involving the local extrahepatic structures by direct invasion
	T4	Tumor with periductal invasion

Stage 0	TisN0M0
Stage I	T1N0M0
Stage II	T2N0M0
Stage III	T3N0M0
Stage IVA	T4N0M0, Any T, N1M0
Stage IVB	Any T/N, M1

From Edge SB, Byrd DR, Compton CC, et al, editors. AJCC cancer staging manual. 7th edition. New York: Springer; 2010; with permission.

single most effective treatment for patients diagnosed with extrahepatic biliary tract cancer, preoperative evaluation of tumor progression is clinically important. However, most factors determining T stages are histopathologic parameters, and would not change the surgical management for the extrahepatic bile duct cancers. Accordingly, the staging system is less useful for the selection of treatment, unless remarkable vascular involvement, invasion to adjacent organs, or nodal/distant metastases is present on preoperative imaging studies. Furthermore, because bile duct cancer extends both laterally and longitudinally, the current staging system is difficult to apply in patients with wide cancer spread along the biliary tract.

In clinical settings, the distribution of cancer is most important for determining the surgical procedure, especially in patients with hilar cholangiocarcinoma. The Bismuth-Corlette classification[36] is a simple and useful classification offering adequate surgical management (**Fig. 4**). For types I, II, and IIIa hilar cholangiocarcinoma, an extended right hepatectomy is usually performed, whereas for type IIIb hilar cholangiocarcinoma, a left or extended left hepatectomy is needed.

Gallbladder Cancer

Gallbladder cancer is a relatively uncommon malignancy, and most cases are detected incidentally in cholecystectomies for cholelithiasis or cholecystitis. Unlike

Proximal Bile Duct and Gallbladder			
	N0 and M0	N1 and M0	N2 or M1
Tis	0		
T1	I		
T2	II	IIID	
T3	IIIA		IVB
T4	IVA		

Distal Bile Duct and Ampulla of Vater			
	N0 and M0	N1 and M0	M1
Tis	0		
T1	IA		
T2	IB	IIB	
T3	IIA		IV
T4	III		

Fig. 3. Staging for extrahepatic biliary cancers. M0, no distant metastasis; M1, presence of distant metastasis; N0, no regional lymph node metastasis; N1, regional lymph node metastasis (including nodes along the cystic duct, common bile duct, hepatic artery, and portal vein); N2, metastasis to periaortic, pericaval, superior mesenteric artery, and/or celiac artery lymph node. (*Data from* Edge SB, Byrd DR, Compton CC, et al, editors. AJCC cancer staging manual. vol. XV. 7th edition. Springer; 2010. p. 649.)

Table 6	
AJCC/UICC 7th classification for extrahepatic biliary cancer	
Hilar and Proximal Cholangiocarcinoma	
Tis	Carcinoma in situ
T1	Tumor confined to the bile duct, with extension up to the muscle layer or fibrous tissue
T2a	Tumor invades beyond the wall of the bile duct to surrounding adipose tissue
T2b	Tumor invades adjacent hepatic parenchyma
T3	Tumor invades unilateral branches of the portal vein or hepatic artery
T4	Tumor invades main portal vein or its branches bilaterally; or the common hepatic artery; or the second-order biliary radicals bilaterally; or unilateral second-order biliary radicals with contralateral portal vein or hepatic artery involvement
Gallbladder cancer	
Tis	Carcinoma in situ
T1	The tumor has grown into the lamina propria or the muscle layer (muscularis)
T2	The tumor has grown into perimuscular fibrous tissue
T3	The tumor has grown through the serosa and/or it has grown from the gallbladder directly into the liver and/or one nearby structure such as the stomach, duodenum, colon, pancreas, or bile ducts outside the liver
T4	The tumor has grown into one of the main blood vessels leading into the liver or it has grown into 2 or more organs outside of the liver
Distal cholangiocarcinoma	
Tis	Carcinoma in situ
T1	Tumor confined to the bile duct histologically
T2	Tumor invades beyond the wall of the bile duct
T3	Tumor invades the gallbladder, pancreas, duodenum, or other adjacent organs without involvement of the celiac axis, or the superior mesenteric artery
T4	Tumor involves the celiac axis, or the superior mesenteric artery
Ampulla of Vater	
Tis	Carcinoma in situ
T1	Tumor limited to ampulla of Vater or sphincter of Oddi
T2	Tumor invades duodenal wall
T3	Tumor invades pancreas
T4	Tumor invades peripancreatic soft tissues or other adjacent organs or structures other than pancreas

From Edge SB, Byrd DR, Compton CC, et al, editors. AJCC cancer staging manual. 7th edition. New York: Springer; 2010; with permission.

in the remainder of the gastrointestinal tract, the gallbladder lacks muscularis mucosa, and the presence of Rokitansky-Aschoff sinus–forming microscopic diverticula in the gallbladder wall would facilitate early tumor progression deep into the gallbladder wall. T stage is based on the depth of the tumor invasion in gallbladder cancer (see **Table 6**). Because the depth of invasion is associated with increased incidence of liver metastasis and nodal metastasis, T stage is a useful guide for concomitant or additional resection of the gallbladder bed and regional lymph nodes.[37] However, the limitation of the current staging system is that it does not differentiate clinical presentation according to tumor location (ie, serosal vs hepatic side).

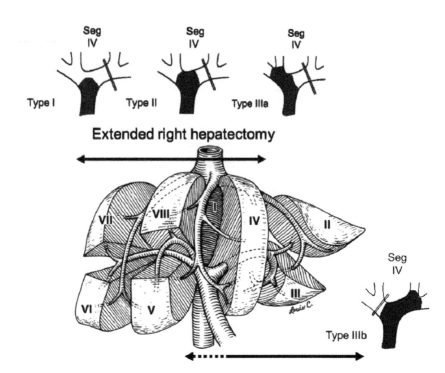

Fig. 4. Extent of hepatic resection according to Bismuth-Corlette classification of hilar chol-angiocarcinoma. (*Adapted from* Parikh AA, Abdalla EK, Vauthey JN. Operative considerations in resection of hilar cholangiocarcinoma. HPB 2005;7:254–8; with permission.)

SUMMARY

In the field of hepatobiliary malignancies, a variety of staging systems have been introduced in an effort to stratify patients based on prognosis and facilitate the selection of appropriate treatment strategies. However, each staging system has strengths and limitations, and no perfect staging system exists for these disease entities because of the variability in nature of the population used for the development of a staging system. In addition, because the hepatic function of the underlying liver is also a potent prognostic factor in hepatobiliary malignancies, interpretation of tumor staging and selection of treatment should be performed with care based on the comprehensive assessment of patient status.

REFERENCES

1. The Cancer of the Liver Italian Program (CLIP) investigators. A new prognostic system for hepatocellular carcinoma: a retrospective study of 435 patients: the Cancer of the Liver Italian Program (CLIP) investigators. Hepatology 1998;28:751–5.
2. The Cancer of the Liver Italian Program (CLIP) investigators. Prospective validation of the CLIP score: a new prognostic system for patients with cirrhosis and hepatocellular carcinoma. The Cancer of the Liver Italian Program (CLIP) Investigators. Hepatology 2000;31:840–5.

3. Levy I, Sherman M. Staging of hepatocellular carcinoma: assessment of the CLIP, Okuda, and Child-Pugh staging systems in a cohort of 257 patients in Toronto. Gut 2002;50:881–5.

4. Ueno S, Tanabe G, Sako K, et al. Discrimination value of the new western prognostic system (CLIP score) for hepatocellular carcinoma in 662 Japanese patients. Cancer of the Liver Italian Program. Hepatology 2001;34:529–34.

5. Okuda K, Ohtsuki T, Obata H, et al. Natural history of hepatocellular carcinoma and prognosis in relation to treatment. Study of 850 patients. Cancer 1985;56: 918–28.

6. Llovet JM, Bru C, Bruix J. Prognosis of hepatocellular carcinoma: the BCLC staging classification. Semin Liver Dis 1999;19:329–38.

7. Cillo U, Vitale A, Grigoletto F, et al. Prospective validation of the Barcelona Clinic Liver Cancer staging system. J Hepatol 2006;44:723–31.

8. Guglielmi A, Ruzzenente A, Pachera S, et al. Comparison of seven staging systems in cirrhotic patients with hepatocellular carcinoma in a cohort of patients who underwent radiofrequency ablation with complete response. Am J Gastroenterol 2008;103:597–604.

9. Marrero JA, Fontana RJ, Barrat A, et al. Prognosis of hepatocellular carcinoma: comparison of 7 staging systems in an American cohort. Hepatology 2005;41:707–16.

10. Makuuchi M, Belghiti J, Belli G, et al. IHPBA concordant classification of primary liver cancer: working group report. J Hepatobiliary Pancreat Surg 2003;10:26–30.

11. Edge S, Byrd D, Campton C, et al. AJCC cancer staging manual. 7th edition. New York: Springer; 2010.

12. Vauthey JN, Lauwers GY, Esnaola NF, et al. Simplified staging for hepatocellular carcinoma. J Clin Oncol 2002;20:1527–36.

13. Cheng CH, Lee CF, Wu TH, et al. Evaluation of the new AJCC staging system for resectable hepatocellular carcinoma. World J Surg Oncol 2011;9:114.

14. Kee KM, Wang JH, Lee CM, et al. Validation of clinical AJCC/UICC TNM staging system for hepatocellular carcinoma: analysis of 5,613 cases from a medical center in southern Taiwan. Int J Cancer 2007;120:2650–5.

15. Lei HJ, Chau GY, Lui WY, et al. Prognostic value and clinical relevance of the 6th Edition 2002 American Joint Committee on Cancer staging system in patients with resectable hepatocellular carcinoma. J Am Coll Surg 2006;203:426–35.

16. Poon RT, Fan ST. Evaluation of the new AJCC/UICC staging system for hepatocellular carcinoma after hepatic resection in Chinese patients. Surg Oncol Clin N Am 2003;12:35–50, viii.

17. Ramacciato G, Mercantini P, Cautero N, et al. Prognostic evaluation of the new American Joint Committee on Cancer/International Union Against Cancer staging system for hepatocellular carcinoma: analysis of 112 cirrhotic patients resected for hepatocellular carcinoma. Ann Surg Oncol 2005;12:289–97.

18. Varotti G, Ramacciato G, Ercolani G, et al. Comparison between the fifth and sixth editions of the AJCC/UICC TNM staging systems for hepatocellular carcinoma: multicentric study on 393 cirrhotic resected patients. Eur J Surg Oncol 2005; 31:760–7.

19. Wu CC, Cheng SB, Ho WM, et al. Liver resection for hepatocellular carcinoma in patients with cirrhosis. Br J Surg 2005;92:348–55.

20. Vauthey JN, Ribero D, Abdalla EK, et al. Outcomes of liver transplantation in 490 patients with hepatocellular carcinoma: validation of a uniform staging after surgical treatment. J Am Coll Surg 2007;204:1016–27.

21. Arii S, Yamaoka Y, Futagawa S, et al. Results of surgical and nonsurgical treatment for small-sized hepatocellular carcinomas: a retrospective and nationwide

survey in Japan. The Liver Cancer Study Group of Japan. Hepatology 2000;32: 1224–9.

22. Inoue K, Takayama T, Higaki T, et al. Clinical significance of early hepatocellular carcinoma. Liver Transpl 2004;10:S16–9.

23. Livraghi T, Meloni F, Di Stasi M, et al. Sustained complete response and complications rates after radiofrequency ablation of very early hepatocellular carcinoma in cirrhosis: is resection still the treatment of choice? Hepatology 2008;47:82–9.

24. Takayama T, Makuuchi M, Hirohashi S, et al. Early hepatocellular carcinoma as an entity with a high rate of surgical cure. Hepatology 1998;28:1241–6.

25. Todo S, Furukawa H. Living donor liver transplantation for adult patients with hepatocellular carcinoma: experience in Japan. Ann Surg 2004;240:451–9 [discussion: 59–61].

26. Yamashita Y, Tsuijita E, Takeishi K, et al. Predictors for microinvasion of small hepatocellular carcinoma </= 2 cm. Ann Surg Oncol 2012;19:2027–34.

27. Jonas S, Bechstein WO, Steinmuller T, et al. Vascular invasion and histopathologic grading determine outcome after liver transplantation for hepatocellular carcinoma in cirrhosis. Hepatology 2001;33:1080–6.

28. Liver Cancer Study Group of Japan. Primary liver cancer in Japan. Clinicopathologic features and results of surgical treatment. Ann Surg 1990;211:277–87.

29. Mazzaferro V, Regalia E, Doci R, et al. Liver transplantation for the treatment of small hepatocellular carcinomas in patients with cirrhosis. N Engl J Med 1996;334:693–9.

30. Belghiti J, Cortes A, Abdalla EK, et al. Resection prior to liver transplantation for hepatocellular carcinoma. Ann Surg 2003;238:885–92.

31. Sala M, Fuster J, Llovet JM, et al. High pathological risk of recurrence after surgical resection for hepatocellular carcinoma: an indication for salvage liver transplantation. Liver Transpl 2004;10:1294–300.

32. Kaczynski J, Hansson G, Wallerstedt S. Incidence, etiologic aspects and clinicopathologic features in intrahepatic cholangiocellular carcinoma—a study of 51 cases from a low-endemicity area. Acta Oncol 1998;37:77–83.

33. Nathan H, Aloia TA, Vauthey JN, et al. A proposed staging system for intrahepatic cholangiocarcinoma. Ann Surg Oncol 2009;16:14–22.

34. de Jong MC, Nathan H, Sotiropoulos GC, et al. Intrahepatic cholangiocarcinoma: an international multi-institutional analysis of prognostic factors and lymph node assessment. J Clin Oncol 2011;29:3140–5.

35. Farges O, Fuks D, Le Treut YP, et al. AJCC 7th edition of TNM staging accurately discriminates outcomes of patients with resectable intrahepatic cholangiocarcinoma: by the AFC-IHCC-2009 study group. Cancer 2011;117:2170–7.

36. Bismuth H, Corlette MB. Intrahepatic cholangioenteric anastomosis in carcinoma of the hilus of the liver. Surg Gynecol Obstet 1975;140:170–8.

37. Kokudo N, Makuuchi M, Natori T, et al. Strategies for surgical treatment of gallbladder carcinoma based on information available before resection. Arch Surg 2003;138:741–50.

Transarterial Therapies for Primary Liver Tumors

Adam D. Talenfeld, MD, Akhilesh K. Sista, MD,
David C. Madoff, MD*

KEYWORDS

- Transarterial • Chemoembolization • Radioembolization • Hepatocellular carcinoma
- Cholangiocarcinoma

KEY POINTS

- Choosing the appropriate transarterial modality to aggressively treat malignancy while preserving function and lower portal pressures is central to patient selection for transarterial therapy.
- Current transarterial techniques have been proved safe and effective in advanced hepatocellular carcinoma and Child B cirrhosis. The posttreatment prognosis for Child A patients continues to improve.
- Many modern transarterial therapies cause minimal postembolization syndrome and are therefore routinely provided as outpatient procedures.
- Meticulous imaging follow-up and retreatment of new or recurrent lesions is imperative for ensuring maximum survival after any transarterial therapy.
- Current transarterial treatment options are safer and more effective than treatments of a decade ago. New techniques will continue this trend via patient-specific therapies in the future.

INTRODUCTION

Transarterial therapy for hepatocellular carcinoma (HCC) was first described in the medical literature in the late 1970s.[1–3] In the 1980s, several reports discussed the feasibility of combining embolic and chemotherapeutic agents.[4–6] In 2002, 2 separate randomized controlled trials (RCTs) each showed longer survival by patients with HCC receiving transcatheter arterial chemoembolization (TACE) compared with those receiving best supportive care (BSC).[7,8] Since these two RCTs, novel transarterial techniques have continued to be developed, and the management of patients with primary liver cancer has also continued to evolve.

The authors have nothing to disclose.
Division of Interventional Radiology, Department of Radiology, New York-Presbyterian Hospital/Weill Cornell Medical Center, 525 East 68th Street, New York, NY 10065, USA
* Corresponding author. Division of Interventional Radiology, Department of Radiology, New York-Presbyterian Hospital/Weill Cornell Medical Center, 525 East 68th Street, P-518, New York, NY 10065.
E-mail address: dcm9006@med.cornell.edu

Surg Oncol Clin N Am 23 (2014) 323–351
http://dx.doi.org/10.1016/j.soc.2013.11.002
1055-3207/14/$ – see front matter © 2014 Elsevier Inc. All rights reserved.

surgonc.theclinics.com

The treatment of patients with HCC has become standardized as a result of several international guidelines.[9–12] **Fig. 1** describes a widely used algorithm that serves as the dominant general guideline for whether a patient undergoes transplantation, surgical resection, ablation, transarterial treatment, or systemic therapy. Because it is still a minority of patients with primary liver cancer who can be cured with resection or transplantation, percutaneous and transarterial interventional techniques remain essential in the management of patients with HCC and intrahepatic cholangiocarcinoma (ICC). Percutaneous techniques are addressed elsewhere in this issue by Clary and colleagues. This article describes current transarterial therapies in the management of primary liver cancers.

TRANSARTERIAL THERAPEUTIC OPTIONS

Table 1 lists the 5 main categories of transarterial therapy used in current practice. Transarterial therapies are usually performed under moderate sedation with independent radiology nursing supervision for most patients, including pulse oximetry, cardiac monitoring, and blood pressure monitoring. When warranted by a patient's comorbidities, procedures may be performed with light sedation or under deep sedation with anesthesiology assistance.

The wide availability of advanced cross-sectional imaging now frequently allows the interventionalist to forego aortic angiography, thus reducing x-ray exposure and contrast dose at the time of intervention. Focused sonographic examination in the interventional radiology suite often allows confirmation of hepatopetal portal flow, in many cases obviating routine superior mesenteric artery angiography.

Although conventional TACE (cTACE) has typically required inpatient admission for management of postprocedural pain, fever, and nausea, known as postembolization syndrome, many newer transarterial techniques cause less postembolization syndrome and are routinely performed as outpatient procedures.

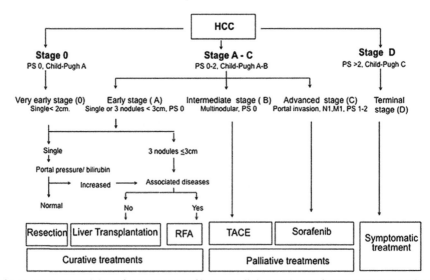

Fig. 1. Current guidelines for treatment of hepatocellular carcinoma by Breast Cancer Linkage Consortium (BCLC) stage. RFA, radiofrequency ablation. (*From* Bruix J, Sherman M, American Association for the Study of Liver Diseases. Management of hepatocellular carcinoma: an update. Hepatology 2011;53(3):1020–2; with permission.)

Table 1
Transarterial techniques

Transarterial Technique	Mechanism of Action	Advantages	Disadvantages
TACI	Intrahepatic chemotherapy, often suspended in oily contrast, without use of any other embolic	Absence of permanent embolic improves vessel patency for future transarterial treatment Low cost	Widely varying technique
cTACE, also called oily or Lipiodol TACE	Intrahepatic chemotherapy held in tumors by oily contrast, tumor ischemia by oil and additional temporary or permanent embolic material	Proved superior to supportive care by RCT Low cost	Widely varying technique Postembolization syndrome may require inpatient treatment
TAE also called bland embolization	Ischemic necrosis at the arteriolar level, typically with small (eg, 40–120 μm), permanent embolic material	Theoretically better side effect profile than cTACE Simplest transarterial technique, with potential for simple standardization Low cost	Less durable than DEB-TACE Potential for pulmonary emboli from small-particle treatment of large tumors near diaphragm Postembolization syndrome may require inpatient treatment
DEB-TACE	Intrahepatic chemotherapy slowly eluted by embolic microspheres	Less systemic chemotherapy leakage from liver than cTACE, with resultant lower systemic toxicity Can be less embolic than TAE or cTACE, with resultant lower ischemic toxicity to liver More standardized treatment technique than TACI or cTACE	Greater potency of individual microspheres requires possible prophylactic coiling of cystic or hepaticoenteric collateral arteries Postembolization syndrome may require inpatient treatment Greater cost than cTACE
Y90 radioembolization (TARE/SIRT)	Arterially directed intratumoral brachytherapy	Some data to support superior HCC downstaging vs TACE; role in PVT Radiation segmentectomy and lobectomy modifications of TARE may allow greater safety and effectiveness Fewer treatment sessions required than with other transarterial techniques Minimally embolic treatment allows safe lobar therapy despite PVT Less severe postembolization syndrome allows routine outpatient treatment	Each treatment requires coordination between interventional radiology; radiation safety; nuclear medicine; and, frequently, radiation oncology Meticulous angiographic technique required to avoid nontarget embolization Greatest per-treatment session cost of all transarterial techniques Small particle size may cause greater biliary toxicity than other transarterial techniques

Abbreviations: cTACE, conventional transarterial chemoembolization; DEB, drug-eluting bead; PVT, portal vein thrombosis; SIRT, selective internal radiotherapy; TACI, transarterial chemoinfusion; TAE, transarterial embolization; TARE, transarterial radioembolization.

cTACE

cTACE, the most widely practiced transarterial therapy, consists of filling the arterial supply of the target tumor or tumors with a mix of chemotherapy and embolic material. cTACE uses sterile iodinated poppy seed oil (Lipiodol Ultra-Fluide, Guerbet, Villepinte, France; previously also available as the Ethiodol brand) to create a viscous, highly radiopaque emulsion with a chemotherapeutic agent or agents that is infused into the tumoral arterial supply. This emulsion is typically either mixed with or followed by infusion of additional embolic material.

A variety of chemotherapeutic and embolic agents are currently in use in transarterial therapy for primary hepatic malignancy. Doxorubicin is currently the most commonly used chemotherapeutic in single-agent TACE in North America. Triple-agent TACE commonly uses a mix of cisplatin, doxorubicin (Adriamycin), and mitomycin C (CDM-TACE or CAM-TACE).

Spherical embolic material has generally replaced older, nonspherical embolic agents because of the availability of more tightly calibrated sizes and greater predictability of flow dynamics. Both temporary (eg, calibrated Gelfoam and starch microspheres) and permanent (eg, trisacryl gelatin [TAG] and spherical polyvinyl alcohol [PVA]) embolic agents are used, ranging in size from 40 to more than 1000 µm in diameter.

Transarterial Embolization

Although cTACE traditionally uses 100-µm to 500-µm diameter embolic, transarterial embolization without chemotherapy, also called bland embolization, as currently practiced more often makes use of smaller 50-µm PVA or 40-µm to 120-µm TAG microspheres in an effort to occlude the arteriolar tumoral blood supply while preserving patency of larger feeding arteries, allowing subsequent additional transarterial treatment. The primary procedural end point of both transarterial embolization (TAE) and TACE is the same: angiographic evidence of embolization (ie, stasis or near stasis) of arterial supply to the target tumors. However, the mechanisms of action differ, with bland embolization causing ischemia, whereas cTACE also relies on the chemotherapeutic effect for tumor necrosis. **Fig. 2** shows a case of HCC treated with the modern small-particle TAE technique.

Drug-eluting Bead TACE

First reported in the treatment of metastatic colorectal cancer in 2006 and for HCC in 2007,[13,14] drug-eluting bead (DEB) TACE is a modification of TACE in which a permanent embolic microsphere is soaked in a single chemotherapeutic agent in advance of the treatment session and then, once embolized transarterially, slowly elutes the agent within the tumor over a period of several days. Two products are currently available in the United States: LC Beads (Biocompatibles, BTG International Inc, West Conshohocken, PA) are PVA hydrogel microspheres, and QuadraSpheres (Merit Medical, South Jordan, UT) are hydrophilic microspheres consisting of sodium acrylate alcohol. For administration under fluoroscopic guidance, the chemotherapy-soaked microspheres are suspended in saline and aqueous iodinated contrast, usually without Lipiodol or any other additional embolic material.

Transarterial Chemoinfusion

Transarterial chemoinfusion (TACI), as the term is applied in the treatment of primary liver cancers, is typically defined as transarterial delivery of chemotherapy suspended in Lipiodol but without any other embolic material. Some investigators restrict the term TACI to exclude even Lipiodol. Others consider superselective TACE using a

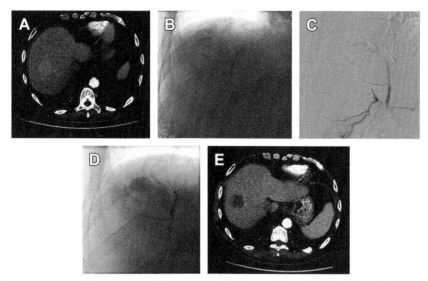

Fig. 2. A 60-year-old patient with hepatitis B infection and 4-cm HCC, on transplant list. (*A*) Pretreatment arterial phase computed tomography (CT) shows a 4-cm enhancing mass. (*B*) Preembolization angiography shows multiple feeding vessels off the segment 7 artery. (*C*) Post-TAE digital subtraction angiography (DSA) shows stasis in subsegmental tumor feeders and forward flow in nontargeted branches. (*D*) Fluoroscopy image after TAE shows dense tumor stain (static contrast in tumor and feeding vessels). (*E*) Arterial phase contrast CT 12 months after TAE shows 25% decrease in size and absence of enhancement (complete European Association for the Study of the Liver [EASL]/ Modified Response Evaluation Criteria In Solid Tumors [mRECIST] response).

temporary embolic (eg, Gelfoam) to be TACI; however, these are in the minority. TACI, as it is commonly defined, is currently less commonly used in North America than TACE and TAE.

Transarterial Radioembolization

Transarterial radioembolization (TARE), also known as selective internal radiotherapy (SIRT) or radiomicrobrachytherapy (RMB), was originally described in 1986 as transarterial infusion of ^{131}I-labeled Lipiodol for inoperable HCC.[15] Perhaps because of the greater regulatory requirements of open-source radiation therapy, development of TARE for liver cancer has been a more gradually evolving process. The first case series of yttrium-90 (Y90) TARE in humans was published in 1992 using resin microspheres in patients with metastatic colorectal cancer.[16] Glass and resin radiomicrobrachytherapy devices are now commercially available in North America with which to perform TARE. The TheraSphere (glass microspheres) device was approved by the US Food and Drug Administration (FDA) in 2000 as a humanitarian use device for patients with unresectable HCC. SIR-Spheres (resin microspheres) were granted premarket FDA approval in 2002 for treatment of metastatic colorectal carcinoma in the liver.

TheraSphere Y90 microspheres (BTG International Inc, West Conshohocken, PA) are nonbiodegradable glass microspheres with Y90 as an integral constituent. TheraSphere range from 20 to 30 μm in diameter and have a specific gravity of 3.6 g/dL and a specific activity of 2500 Bq/sphere. A 3-GBq vial contains 1.2×10^{6} microspheres (TheraSphere package insert). Specific doses are infused by ordering a predetermined-dose vial and coordinating the day and time of administration with published decay curves. Oversight by an institutional review board is required to administer TheraSphere.

SIR-Spheres (Sirtex Medical, Lane Cove, Australia) are resin microspheres onto which Y90 is bound. They range from 20 to 60 μm in diameter and have a specific gravity of 1.6 g/dL and a specific activity of 50 Bq/sphere. A 3-GBq vial contains 40×10^6 to 80×10^6 microspheres (SIR-Spheres package insert). SIR-Spheres arrive in a standard-dose vial on the day of treatment. The receiving institution's radiopharmacist decants an appropriate volume of spheres to achieve the prescribed activity for treatment. Use of SIR-Spheres for HCC and ICC is off-label.

Characteristics of Y90 that facilitate its use in transarterial radioembolization are common to both devices. Y90 is a pure beta particle emitter that decays to stable zirconium-90 (Zr-90) with a half-life of 64.1 days. The average energy of beta emission is 0.9367 MeV, with mean and maximum soft tissue penetrations of 2.5 and 10 mm, respectively. TARE takes advantage of the tendency of many tumors to recruit more arterial supply than benign hepatocytes, even some tumors that appear hypovascular on contrast computed tomography (CT) or magnetic resonance imaging (MRI). There is therefore shunting of hepatic arterial flow toward tumors and preferential deposition of radiomicrospheres within the tumors and away from benign liver tissue.

LANDMARK CLINICAL OUTCOMES, KEY CURRENT DATA, AND COMPARISONS OF MODERN TRANSARTERIAL TECHNIQUES

Although the literature on transarterial therapies for ICC continues to grow, the majority of research into transarterial therapy for primary liver cancer has focused on HCC. Text in this section will focus on HCC therapies. A summary of recent trials investigating transarterial therapies for ICC is listed in **Table 2**.

cTACE

Since the 2 seminal RCTs were published in 2002,[7,8] the most current large series reporting median overall survival (OS) for patients with HCC treated with cTACE are prospective and retrospective studies of 172 and 209 patients published in 2006 and 2008, respectively.[17,18] These 2 studies reported rates of median OS after cTACE of 19 and 20 months.

These larger series included heterogeneous patient populations that reflected modern practice; however, a more recent retrospective series of 67 patients treated with cTACE for early and very early malignancy (Barcelona Clinic for Liver Cancer [BCLC] stage A and 0) was published in 2012, reporting much longer survival. One-year, 2-year, and 3-year OS rates in this contemporary cTACE series were 90.9%, 86.1%, and 80.5%, respectively.[19]

Other developments in cTACE during the decade since its broad acceptance in clinical practice include:

- TACE in portal thrombus: a single-center registry series of 32 patients with Child A or B cirrhosis and main, left, and/or right portal vein occlusion was published showing safety of cTACE in this population and increases in survival compared with historical BSC controls. The investigators therefore suggested that portal vein thrombosis need not be an absolute contraindication to cTACE.[20] A subsequent retrospective case-control study of 125 patients with main portal tumor thrombus receiving either cTACE or BSC found significantly greater survival in the cTACE group.[21]

- Downstaging to transplant: a prospective study published in 2008 compared 129 patients with HCC listed for liver transplant with tumors meeting Milan criteria and 48 patients with hepatomas originally beyond Milan but within the Bologna Criteria with Downstage (BCDS).[22] Patients in the BCDS arm received either cTACE, radiofrequency ablation (RFA), percutaneous ethanol injection (PEI), laparoscopic resection, or a combination thereof. Subjects whose tumors showed a 3-month sustained successful downstaging to within Milan criteria were then listed. With a median follow-up of 2.5 years after transplant, there were no significant differences in disease-free survival or actuarial intention-to-treat survival between the groups.
- TACE alone for downstaging: a case series published in 2008 found that 22% of 76 patients with American Joint Commission for Cancer (AJCC) stage III or IV HCC could be successfully downstaged using cTACE to within Milan criteria by Response Evaluation Criteria In Solid Tumors (RECIST) imaging assessment of viable tumor. With a median follow-up of 20 months, patients who were transplanted after downstaging by cTACE had overall and disease-free survival of 94% and 88%, respectively, similar to AJCC stage II (Milan) historical controls.[23]
- Neoadjuvant TACE for resection: a prospective cohort study was conducted by Luo and colleagues[24] of 168 patients with large (>5 cm) or multinodular but resectable HCC who underwent either cTACE or resection as initial therapy. Those responding to cTACE by RECIST criteria who subsequently had their tumors resected had significantly longer 1-year, 3-year, and 5-year OS than those receiving primary resection (92%, 67%, and 50% vs 71%, 35%, and 24%). Patients who did not qualify for or refused resection went on to receive PEI. Median OS was similar between the TACE plus PEI group and the primary resection group. There were significantly fewer complications in the TACE group than in the primary resection group.

cTACE Versus Surgical Resection

A case-control study of 185 BCLC A patients with Child A cirrhosis receiving either cTACE or partial hepatectomy found no difference in 1-year, 3-year, and 5-year OS rates between the treatment groups: 91%, 66%, and 52% after cTACE versus 93%, 71%, and 57% after resection ($P = .239$). The 1-year, 3-year, and 5-year recurrence-free survival rates after cTACE and resection were 68%, 28%, and 17%, and 78%, 55%, and 35%, respectively ($P<.0001$).[25] This difference between OS and recurrence-free survival highlights the importance of imaging surveillance and retreatment as necessary after transarterial therapy.

TAE

The only RCT of TAE versus BSC for HCC, conducted in 1998, performed proximal embolization using Gelfoam and steel coils and did not find a difference in survival between the treatment groups.[26] Despite the technique of TAE having changed significantly since that time, there has not been another RCT. The largest study conducted to date is a single-center case series published in 2008 of 322 patients mostly in Okuda stage 1 and 2 that found a median OS of 21 months. The same study found 1-year, 2-year, and 3-year OS rates of 66%, 46%, and 33% for the series, and 84%, 66%, and 51% when patients with portal vein invasion or extrahepatic disease were excluded.[27] **Fig. 3** shows the average sizes of microspheres used for the different transarterial modalities.

Table 2
Summary of recent key trials of transarterial therapies for ICC

Primary Author, Year	Study Type	Type(s) of Treatment	Number of Subjects	Mean or Median# of Treatment Sessions	Noncirrhotic or CP A	ECOG 0 (%)	ECOG 1 (%)	ECOG 2+ (%)	Prior Chemotherapy (%)	Prior External Beam Radiotherapy (%)	Prior Thermal Ablation (%)	Prior Surgical Resection (%)	Single Tumor (%)	Peripheral/No Ductal Invasion (%)	Unilobar Disease (%)	Extrahepatic (%)	PVT/Vascular Invasion (%)	Hypervascular Tumor (%)	Approx % Liver Replaced by Tumor (<25%, <50%, <75%)	Treatment Response Imaging Criteria at 3 mo or First After Treatment	Objective Response (%), SD (%), PD (%)	Median OS (mo)
Aliberti et al,[92] 2008	CC	Doxorubicin DEB-TACE vs systemic fluorouracil	11/9	2.6	—	—	—	—	b	b	b	b	—	—	—	—	—	—	—	RECIST	91, 0, 0	13/7
Gusani et al,[93] 2008	CS	cTACE: gemcitabine, cisplatin, oxaliplatin or gem-cis combo; all with TAG microspheres	42	3.5	—	—	—	—	—	—	—	—	—	12	—	45	—	—	—	RECIST	0, 57, 43	9.1
Ibrahim et al,[94] 2008	CS	Glass microspheres TARE	24	2	—	42	50	8	29	—	—	4c	46	71	33	33	38	—	83, 13, 4	World Health Organization; EASL	27, 68, 5; 86, —, —d	14.9e
Kim et al,[36] 2008	CS	Cisplatin TACI (n = 13) or cisplatin, Lipiocol and Gelfoam cTACE (n = 36)	49	3	82	—	—	—	4f	33f	—	—	29	90	—	51	—	73	—	RECIST	55, 31, 14	10
Poggi et al,[95] 2009	CC	Systemic gem-ox vs systemic gem-ox + oxaliplatin DEB-TACE	11/9	3.3	91/100	—	—	0	—	—	—	0/22c	—	—	—	0	—	—	—	RECIST	0/44, 73/56, 27/0	20/30e

Study		Treatment	No.		60	28	12	72	8	40	60	20	48	0			Criteria		
Saxena et al,[96] 2010	CS	Resin microspheres TARE	25	—	—	—	—	—	—	—	—	—	—	0	—	40, 60, 0	RECIST	26, 48, 22	9.3[e]
Kiefer et al,[97] 2011	CS	cTACE: cisplatin, doxorubicin and mitomycin C with PVA spheres	62	2.7	89	10	1	29	3	5	11	—	—	—	—	—	RECIST	11, 64, 24	15[9]
Park et al,[98] 2011	CC	cTACE: cisplatin, Lipiodol and Gelfoam vs BSC	72/83	2.5	65/54	32/41	3/5	0/0	0/0	0/0	0/0	43/53	49/51	54/60	18[b]/12[h]	—	RECIST	23/NA, 67/NA, 11/NA	12.2/3.3
Shen et al,[37] 2011	CC	Fluorouracil or carboplatin, epirubicin and hydroxycam-ptothecin TACl ± Lipiodol cTACE vs systemic therapy or BSC only	53/72	—	60/61	—	—	—	—	100, 4[f] 100, 4[c]	63/68 92/83	—	6/10	—	—	—	—	—	12/5
Hoffman et al,[99] 2012	CS	Resin microspheres TARE	33	1	52	21	27	82	3	6	36	30	36	24	0	76/24/0	RECIST	36, 52, 15	22
Kuhlmann et al,[100] 2012	CC	Irinotecan DEB-TACE vs cTACE: mitomycin C + Gelfoam vs systemic oxaliplatin + gemcitabine	26/10/31 1.6/1.4/NA		100/100/100	62/70/65	35/30/32	4/0/3	19/200	4/10/3	—	4/0/23	—	42/40/90	—	—	RECIST	3/12.5/26, 42/12.5/45, 50/75/29	11.7/5.7/11.0[i]
Rafi et al,[101] 2013	PCS	Resin microspheres TARE	19	1.6	5	74	21	100	0	0	0	32	58	58	—	—	RECIST	11, 68, 21	11.5

(continued on next page)

Table 2
(continued)

Primary Author, Year	Study Type	Type(s) of Treatment	Number of Subjects	Mean or Median[a] of Treatment Sessions	Noncirrhotic or CP A	ECOG 0 (%)	ECOG 1 (%)	ECOG 2+ (%)	Prior Chemotherapy (%)	Prior External Beam Radiotherapy (%)	Prior Thermal Ablation (%)	Prior Surgical Resection (%)	Single Tumor (%)	Peripheral/No Ductal Invasion (%)	Unilobar Disease (%)	Extrahepatic (%)	PVT/Vascular Invasion (%)	Hypervascular Tumor (%)	Approx % Liver Replaced by Tumor (<25%, <50%, <75%)	Treatment Response Imaging Criteria at 3 mo or First After Treatment	Objective Response (%), SD (%), PD (%)	Median OS (mo)
Vogl et al,[102] 2012	CS	cTACE: mito C, gem, mito-gem, or mito-cis gem-cis, + Lipiodol and starch spheres	115	7.1	46	—	—	—	—	—	—	—	30	—	23	0	0	54	—	RECIST	9, 57, 33	13
Hyder et al,[103] 2013	CS	cTACE (gem-cis, cis-dox-mito, gem, cis, or other); doxorubicin, cisplatin or other DEB-TACE; TAE; Y90	198	—	—	59	36	4	28	—	2	12	48	12	—	20	80	—	—	mRECIST; EASL	25, 62, 13; 34, 48, 18	13.2

Data from different treatment arms are separated by forward slashes "/."

Abbreviations: CC, case control; cis, cisplatin; cis-dox-mito, cisplatin plus doxorubicin plus mitomycin C; CP, Child-Pugh classification of severity of cirrhosis; CS, case series; DEB, drug-eluting bead; dox, doxorubicin; EASL, European Association for the Study of the Liver criteria for measuring enhancing tumor; ECOG PS, Eastern Cooperative Oncology Group Performance Status 0–4; gem, gemcitabine; gem-cis, gemcitabine plus cisplatin; mito C, mitomycin C; mito-cis, mitomycin C plus cisplatin; mito-gem, mitomycin C plus gemcitabine; MR, minor response (WHO criteria only); mRECIST, modified RECIST criteria for measuring enhancing tumor; MWA, microwave ablation; OS, overall survival; PCS, prospectively gathered case series; PD, progression of disease; PR, partial response; PVA, polyvinyl alcohol microspheres; RECIST, Response Evaluation Criteria in Solid Tumors (National Cancer Institute); RFA, radiofrequency ablation; SD, stable disease; TAG, trisacryl gelatin microspheres; WHO, World Health Organization; ±, Gelfoam or permanent embolic.

[a] Study combined patients with ICC and hepatic metastases from pancreatic carcinoma.
[b] All patients had prior chemotherapy and/or surgery; specific quantities not specified.
[c] After transarterial therapy.
[d] SD and PD not reported.
[e] Resections after transarterial therapy not censored from survival data.
[f] Concurrent with transarterial therapy.
[g] Study combined patients with ICC and intrahepatic adenocarcinoma of unknown primary.
[h] All patients by this finding deemed to have recurrence after resection.
[i] Fifty-five percent of patients receiving systemic therapy had extrahepatic cholangiocarcinoma or gallbladder carcinoma.

Adapted from Talenfeld AD, Holzwanger DJ, Madoff DC. Transarterial and percutaneous therapies for unresectable intrahepatic cholangiocarcinoma. In: Herman J, Pawlik T, Thomas CR Jr, editors. Biliary tract and gallbladder cancer: a multidisciplinary approach. 2nd edition. New York: Springer; 2014; with permission.

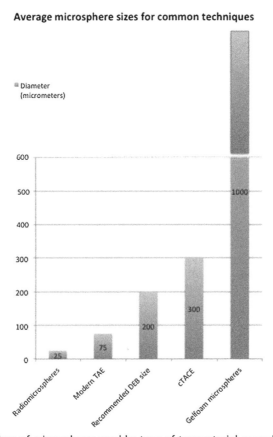

Fig. 3. Average sizes of microspheres used by type of transarterial procedure.

cTACE Versus TAE

To date, there has been no adequately powered prospective trial showing improved survival for ICC or HCC by adding transarterial chemotherapy to embolization (TACE vs TAE).[28] One of the 2 randomized, controlled trials to show superiority of cTACE compared with BSC contained a subgroup treated with TAE that experienced survival similar to those treated with cTACE.[8] The trial was stopped when superiority of TACE to BSC was shown, before demonstration of statistical significance in the smaller bland-embolization subgroup. With publication of these RCTs, cTACE became the standard of care for unresectable HCC; however, multiple meta-analyses of cTACE and TAE for HCC have failed to show superiority of cTACE compared with bland embolization.[29,30]

cTACE Versus TACI

There is limited evidence that chemoembolization is superior to transarterial chemoinfusion without embolization (TACI) for HCC.[31,32] One recent randomized study of 161 patients treated with TACE or TACI found no survival difference between the treatment groups.[33] Another recent propensity score–matched prospective cohort study of 11,030 patients found significantly longer survival of patients treated with TACE compared with those receiving TACI.[34] Multiple studies have also recently suggested superior efficacy of TACE compared with TACI in the treatment of ICC.[35–37] A retrospective study has found that a treatment program of either TACI or a combination of TACI and Gelfoam cTACE can be effective in downstaging patients to within Milan criteria.[38]

Doxorubicin Versus Cisplatin and Single Versus Multiple Chemotherapy cTACE

There is little information favoring use of one chemotherapeutic agent or group of agents over another in cTACE. One of the 2 RCTs to first show improved survival of TACE compared with BSC performed doxorubicin single-agent cTACE, whereas the other used cisplatin as its single transarterial chemotherapy.[7,8] Since then, several dedicated studies have been performed.

- Retrospective series of 133 and, recently, 202 patients showed significantly longer OS at 5 and 3 years with cisplatin cTACE versus doxorubicin or epirubicin cTACE, respectively.[39,40]
- A randomized, controlled trial of 415 patients receiving either epirubicin or doxorubicin failed to show a difference in survival, as did a smaller recent RCT of epirubicin versus CAM-TACE in 51 patients.[41,42]
- A recent retrospective study of 122 patients found a significantly greater imaging response to treatment and lower rate of disease progression in those treated with CAM-TACE than those treated with doxorubicin single-agent TACE.[43]

DEB-TACE

A recent single-institution registry-based study of doxorubicin DEB-TACE in 104 Child A, Eastern Cooperative Oncology Group (ECOG) performance status 1 patients with early and intermediate stage (BCLC A and B) HCC found a median OS of 48 months, which was more than twice as long as generally cited for cTACE.[44] A recent retrospective study of 45 Child A and B patients with BCLC A and B stage HCC noted a median 5-year survival of 62%.[45]

A retrospective study of 61 patients with hepatoma treated with either 100-µm to 300-µm or 300-µm to 500-µm doxorubicin-eluting microspheres found significantly lower rates of postembolization syndrome and fatigue in patients receiving the smaller DEBs (8% and 36%) than in those receiving the larger DEBs (40% and 70%). The investigators also noted a trend toward more complete imaging response to treatment in the smaller DEBs group.[46]

DEB-TACE Versus cTACE

In 2010, the first RCT of single-agent doxorubicin cTACE versus doxorubicin DEB-TACE found in a study population of 212 subjects that DEBs were associated with fewer side effects and decreased hepatic and systemic toxicity, thereby extending the indication of TACE to Child B and ECOG 1 patients.[47] There were fewer severe adverse events and a similar number of total adverse events (AEs). Although there were no significant differences in survival between treatment groups by study end at 6 months median follow-up, there was greater imaging evidence of response to treatment and longer time to progression (TTP) in Child B patients receiving DEB-TACE than those in the cTACE group. The investigators acknowledged that longer follow-up was likely required to show a survival advantage of one treatment arm rather than the other.

DEB-TACE Versus TAE

A recent RCT of 87 patients with HCC comparing DEB-TACE with 100-µm to 300-µm and/or 300-µm to 500-µm doxorubicin-loaded PVA microspheres versus bland PVA microspheres of the same size documented nearly half the rate of local recurrence at 12 months and a longer TTP in those treated with DEB-TACE versus TAE.[48] The investigators acknowledged that trials comparing DEB-TACE with smaller particle bland embolization are necessary in light of modern TAE techniques.

A small study of transplant patients' explanted native livers after having received neoadjuvant TAE (n = 8) or DEB-TACE (n = 8) found complete histologic necrosis in 77% of hepatomas treated with DEB-TACE versus only 27% of those treated with TAE.[49]

TARE

In the largest published series of Y90 TARE to date, 291 patients with unresectable HCC were treated with glass radiomicrospheres. Median OS in Child A subjects was 17 months, whereas Child B subjects experienced a median OS of 8 months.[50] Based on subgroup analysis, the investigators recommended TARE for Child A patients with portal vein thrombosis. A prior series of 108 patients found a median OS of 20 months for early Okuda stage patients and approximately 11 months for intermediate stage patients.[51]

TARE Versus cTACE

As shown by several comparative studies performed to date, TARE and cTACE seem in general to have similar safety and efficacy. Some studies suggest relative strengths of one technique rather than the other.

- The first study directly comparing cTACE and Y90 TARE, published in 2009, retrospectively compared 86 patients with T3 (intermediate stage) HCC treated with either CAM-cTACE or glass microsphere TARE. Significantly more patients were successfully downstaged to T2 in the TARE group (58%) versus the cTACE group (31%). Event-free survival was also significantly longer in the TARE cohort (18 months) than in the TACE group (7 months).[52]
- Two retrospective studies comparing cTACE and glass or resin microsphere Y90 TARE were published the next year and 1 recently published retrospectively matched cohort study of single-center registry data all found similar toxicity and survival outcomes between the two treatment groups.[53–55]
- A retrospective study published in 2011 found less abdominal pain and longer TTP in 123 patients treated with glass microsphere TARE (13 months) than in 122 patients treated with CAM-cTACE (8 months). These investigators found similar survival between the cohorts; however, a post-hoc analysis by the investigators suggested that a sample size of more than 1000 subjects would be necessary to show a significant survival difference between TACE and TARE.[56]

Combined Transarterial and Percutaneous Therapies

Several recent studies have shown successful local control of solitary medium-sized hepatomas by combination transarterial and percutaneous therapy, extending the range of potentially curative nonsurgical treatment to larger tumors than previously possible.

Combined TACE and RFA Versus RFA Alone

Three separate studies have shown superiority of TACE-RFA compared with RFA alone.

- In 2010, a small RCT of 37 patients with solitary 3-cm to 5-cm diameter hepatomas randomized to RFA or cTACE plus RFA found significantly lower local tumor progression at 3 years in patients treated with both RFA and TACE (6%) than in those treated with RFA alone (39%).[57]

- In 2010, a retrospective series of 117 patients receiving either TACE plus RFA (n = 62) or surgical resection (n = 55) found no difference in 1-year, 3-year, and 5-year median OS between groups: 100%, 95%, and 65% in the TACE-RFA group and 92%, 83%, and 77% in the resection group.[58]
- In 2011, a retrospective series (n = 123) of RFA with or without subsegmental cTACE for solitary HCCs 3 to 5 cm in diameter revealed markedly better tumor control with combined therapy than with RFA alone (60% vs 24% at 3 years' follow-up).[59]

COMBINED TAE AND RFA VERSUS RESECTION

Similar to the study by Luo and colleagues[24] using TACE and PEI, a recent case-control series of 73 Okuda stage 1 patients with solitary HCC lesions up to 7 cm in diameter receiving either resection (n = 40) or TAE followed by RFA (n = 33) revealed that, with median follow-up of 11 years, there was no difference in survival between the treatment groups. Median OS was 66 months in the resection group versus 58 months in the TAE-RFA group (P = .39). There was also no difference in rates of intrahepatic (P = .35) or metastatic (P = .48) progression. Surgical patients sustained more complications (P = .004), longer hospitalizations (P<.001), and were more likely to require hospital readmission within 30 days of discharge (P = .03).[60]

Fig. 4 shows a 3-cm hepatoma abutting the stomach and body wall that was treated with a combination of doxorubicin DEB-TACE and percutaneous microwave ablation.

TACE PLUS PORTAL VEIN EMBOLIZATION

TACE combined with portal vein embolization (PVE) is another strategy used largely to improve resectability of liver tumors.[61,62] This approach works by occluding both the arterial tumor blood supply and the portal blood supply to the tumor-bearing liver to be resected. This technique has been used to improve the safety and rate of resection in patients with cirrhotic livers but also has been used to treat large HCCs in patients not considered to be candidates for resection based on their underlying liver disease.

Data for the combined approach solely for liver tumor treatment are limited and largely anecdotal. However, 2 retrospective studies evaluating the strategy for resection have been published in recent years. A case-control series published in 2006 of 18 patients receiving TACE before PVE and 18 patients receiving only PVE found that patients receiving the combined procedure had significantly greater rates of future liver remnant hypertrophy (67% vs 28%), higher likelihood of complete histologic tumor necrosis (83% vs 6%), and increased recurrence-free survival at 5 years (37% vs 19%).[61]

Supporting these earlier findings, another case-control series of 71 patients receiving cTACE-PVE and 64 patients receiving PVE alone was published in 2011 and showed that TACE-PVE was associated with lower risk of liver failure (4% vs 12%), better 5-year OS (72% vs 38%), and greater recurrence-free survival (61% vs 38%) than PVE alone.[62]

Combined cTACE and Sorafenib

Phase II and III trials of TACE with sorafenib have shown mixed results. Larger phase III trials are ongoing.

- Several phase II trials of sorafenib with cTACE for HCC have suggested that this combination therapy is safe and possibly effective.[63,64]
- A midsized, double-blinded, randomized controlled trial was performed in 2012 in which 80 patients with Child A cirrhosis and BCLC stage B (intermediate)

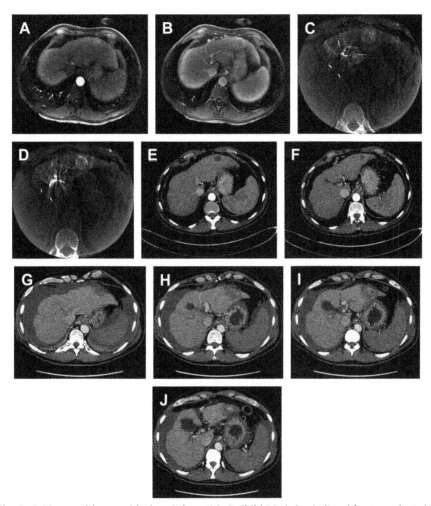

Fig. 4. A 66-year-old man with chronic hepatitis C, Child B9 cirrhosis, listed for transplant. (*A*) A 3-cm mildly arterially enhancing HCC abutting the anterior capsule of segment 2 and abdominal wall. (*B*) Portal phase magnetic resonance image showing the lesion's posterior-inferior aspect abutting posterior liver capsule and the stomach. Note recanalized umbilical vein. (*C, D*) C-arm CT angiogram images obtained with microcatheter in the common trunk of segments 2 to 3 confirms appropriate positioning for DEB-TACE. A dominant feeding vessel is present, although there was additional supply to the tumor from both segmental branches. (*E, F*) CT 2 months after DEB-TACE demonstrated nodular recurrence inferiorly. (*G–J*) Immediate post–percutaneous microwave ablation arterial phase contrast CT images show zone of ablation surrounding site of previously embolized tumor and spanning lateral segments. Note artificial ascites infused throughout the ablation to separate the lateral liver from the body wall, stomach, and colon.

HCC from chronic hepatitis C infection received cTACE with Lipiodol, mitomycin C, doxorubicin, and Gelfoam and were randomly assigned to either sorafenib 400 mg twice a day or placebo beginning at postprocedure day 30. cTACE was repeated up to 4 times at 4-week to 6-week intervals as needed for imaging evidence of viable tumor.[65] Nine patients in the sorafenib arm were excluded because of intolerance of sorafenib toxicities. Nine patients in the placebo arm were excluded because of refusal or failure to adhere to the study protocol. Median TTP in the sorafenib arm was 9.2 months, compared with 4.9 months in the placebo arm ($P<.001$). Metachronous, multicentric HCC progression was significantly less frequent in the sorafenib arm ($P<.05$).

- A large multi-institution RCT of 458 subjects randomized to cTACE and sorafenib versus cTACE and placebo reported no significant difference in TTP between study arms. cTACE was performed with a Lipiodol, epirubicin, doxorubicin, cisplatin, mitomycin, and Gelfoam cocktail. Patients were not randomized until after an imaging response to treatment was documented, sometimes after multiple TACE sessions. The investigators acknowledged that, because patients were not randomized for a median of 9.3 weeks, this delay in beginning sorafenib could have confounded results.[66]
- A double-blinded, controlled, randomized multicenter phase III trial of 204 patients with HCC treated with TACE and randomized to sorafenib or placebo completed enrollment in 2013.[67]

NOVEL TRANSARTERIAL THERAPIES AND FUTURE DIRECTIONS

A new family of anticancer drugs is being assessed for clinical trials of transarterial administration. 3-Bromopyruvate and ethylbromopyruvate are potent inhibitors of glycolysis, with preferential efficacy in tumor cells, and they lack the aerobic metabolic pathways found in normal hepatocytes and other differentiated, benign cells. Animal studies of these novel metabolic anticancer agents are promising, and clinical studies are pending.[68–70]

Several recent studies have shown that imaging criteria based on diameter of any residual tumor enhancement rather than diameter of the entire (enhancing and non-enhancing) tumor better predict survival after transarterial therapy for HCC.[71–73] More accurate imaging biomarkers will fill a long-standing need for more accurate restaging in research and clinical practice.

Phase III Trials in Progress Seek to Further Delineate the Role of TARE with Respect to Systemic and Other Transarterial Therapies

- Transarterial Radioembolization versus Chemoembolization for Treatment of Hepatocellular Carcinoma (TRACE): phase III RCT of TARE versus DEB-TACE for unresectable HCC is currently enrolling patients, with a target of 140 randomizations.
- A Phase III Clinical Trial of Intra-arterial TheraSphere in the Treatment of Patients with Unresectable Hepatocellular Carcinoma (STOP-HCC) is enrolling patients on standard-of-care sorafenib randomized to include or not include TARE.

Modifications of Standard TARE Have Been Described That Portend a Shift Toward a Goal of Transarterial Tumor Ablation

- The concept of radiation lobectomy was first described as a case report in 2009, in which a supratherapeutic second right lobar TARE procedure was performed to treat multifocal metastatic colorectal cancer that had progressed after a prior resin microsphere Y90 TARE treatment using 1.43 GBq of activity. The patient was not a candidate for surgical hepatectomy.[74] Having estimated an adequate volume of future liver remnant in the metastasis-free left lobe, the investigators administered the second treatment with the plan of ablating the right lobe using a supratherapeutic 2.0-GBq aliquot of spheres. At the time of publication, the patient was 20 months after treatment and without intrahepatic recurrence.

- A series of 101 patients with inoperable unilobar right liver HCC or ICC tumors was subsequently described who were treated with lobar glass microsphere TARE at standard doses.[75] Of these 101 treated patients, 20 patients experienced 52% median decrease in right lobar volume and 40% median increase in left lobar volume. There were no grade 3 or greater bilirubin toxicities. Tumor response in these 20 patients ranged from 55% to 70% by size criteria, and 5-year survival in the radiation lobectomy subgroup was 46%. **Fig. 5** shows a case of inoperable mixed HCC-ICC treated with TARE who had complete imaging response to treatment and findings of radiation lobectomy 1 year later.
- Radiation segmentectomy was described in 2011, in which, by administering lobar doses of transarterial brachytherapy to individual segments, zones of complete tumor ablation might be created encapsulating the visible tumor and creating the transarterial equivalent of a negative margin.[76] Highly tumoricidal therapy administered segmentally can spare the rest of the liver any exposure, preserving function. This initial study showed equal effectiveness with superior safety profile compared with conventional TARE.
- Boosted-SIRT was described in 2013 as a new model for TARE dosimetry based on MAA (macro-aggregated albumin) single-photon emission CT (SPECT) imaging rather than traditional liver and tumor volumetry. By incorporating a physiologic assessment of tumor and benign hepatic parenchyma radiotracer uptake, this model may allow both greater treatment effectiveness and equal or lesser toxicity than conventional dosimetry.[77]

PATIENT AND TECHNIQUE SELECTION, COMPLICATIONS, AND CONCERNS
Patient Selection

Box 1 lists historical, current, and developing indications for transarterial therapy for HCC. Indications for treatment of ICC are similar. As indicated by the table and described in detail earlier, both the scope of indications for treatment and the number of specific transarterial treatment options have continued to grow over time.

Technique Selection

Beyond the American Association for the Study of Liver Diseases guidelines shown in **Fig. 1** directing the selection of patients for whom transarterial therapy is recommended, determining the specific transarterial treatment to offer a patient is more complex. Liver function, severity of portal hypertension and hepatic vascular anatomy, extrahepatic comorbidities and functional status, as well as tumor size, vascularity, and distribution each play a role in the recommendation about how, where, and with what to provide intra-arterial treatments.

In general, embolic treatments to more than one lobe are staged to decrease the risk of liver failure and portal hypertensive complications.[78] More highly embolic treatments tend to be administered on a segmental or subsegmental level, whereas less embolic treatments are preferred when lobar therapy is required by widely distributed tumor. Transarterial lidocaine may be administered immediately before embolization and has been shown to decrease the pain that is the hallmark of postembolization syndrome.[79]

Box 2 lists contraindications to transarterial treatment of primary liver cancers. Most contraindications arise from moderate- to poorly-compensated cirrhosis. Because all transarterial techniques come at some cost to liver function, the goal of patient selection for transarterial therapy is to separate out those patients whose benign hepatic disease renders them poor candidates for treatment of their hepatic malignancy.

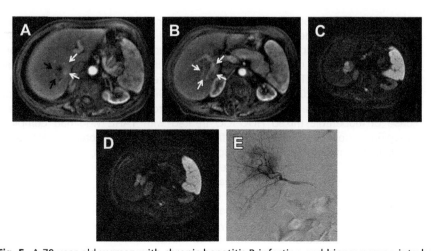

Fig. 5. A 79-year-old woman with chronic hepatitis B infection and biopsy-proven intrahepatic mixed hepatocellular cholangiocarcinoma (HCC-ICC) with progression of disease on systemic chemotherapy. (*A*) Axial arterial phase postcontrast magnetic resonance image shows a mixed cystic (*black arrows*) and solid (*white arrows*) lesion on the margin of segments 6 and 7 corresponding with the biopsy-proven lesion. (*B*) More inferiorly, the lesion is more solid (*white arrows*) and surrounds the posterior right portal vein. (*C*) Pre-TARE diffusion weighted image (DWI) shows markedly restricted diffusion in cystic component of mixed HCC-ICC and moderate to markedly restricted diffusion in the more medial, solid portion of the lesion. (*D*) Pre-TARE DWI just inferior to image C shows restricted diffusion corresponding with the HCC-ICC lesion on either side of the posterior right portal vein branch. (*E*) Microcatheter angiography performed via the right hepatic artery shows heterogeneous tumor blush corresponding with the known partly cystic segment 6/7 tumor. (*F*) Axial fused single-photon emission computed tomography CT images from Bremsstrahlung scan immediately after transarterial radioembolization with a delivered activity of 18.6 mCi (0.69 GBq) of ^{90}Y-resin microspheres infused via the right hepatic artery: white and yellow represent areas of greatest deposition of microspheres, almost all within the target HCC-ICC; gray represents least deposition of microspheres; and light blue is blooming artifact from activity within the right liver. (*G*, *H*) Arterial phase axial images through the superior and inferior aspects of the lesion 1 year after TARE show near-complete resolution of enhancement (EASL/mRECIST complete response). (*I*, *J*) Superior and inferior DWI 1 year after TARE show a small focus of restricted diffusion corresponding with the residual cystic component of the lesion. No restricted diffusion is shown corresponding with any residual solid tumor. Findings in *G–J* are compatible with RECIST partial response and mRECIST/EASL complete response. The patient was alive and asymptomatic at the time of this publication, 12 months after TARE treatment.

Complications and Concerns

The overall severe complication rate for transarterial therapy is 4% to 7%, with a 30-day mortality of ~1%.[80] Postembolization syndrome, consisting of nausea, abdominal pain, and fever, occurs in most patients receiving lobar TACE and is not considered a complication but the expected side effect of acute arterial ischemia and inflammation. Older techniques, such as lobar cTACE, are associated with more severe postembolization syndrome than newer, less embolic transarterial modalities and more selective infusions.[81]

Table 3 is adapted from the Society of Interventional Radiology Standard of Practice Committee's quality improvement guidelines for transarterial therapy, and

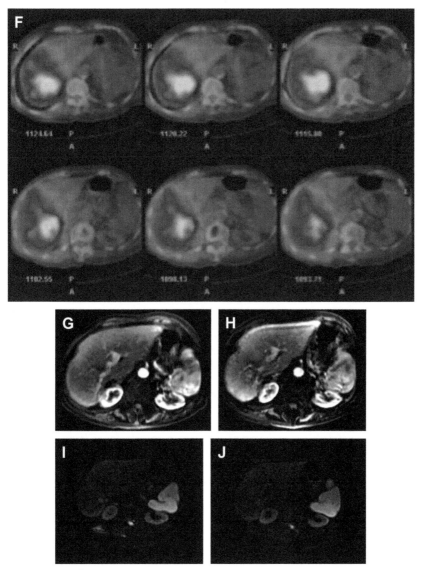

Fig. 5. (*continued*)

lists the most frequently reported major complications associated with cTACE.[82] These complications are generally representative of the risk profile of transarterial therapies. Some modality-specific concerns are discussed later.

TAE

Investigators expert in TAE advocate using 40-μm to 120-μm TAG microspheres and segmental or subsegmental infusion to maximize tumor necrosis, minimize hepatic toxicity, and maintain vessel patency for possible future treatments.[27,81] A review of more than 850 bland embolizations performed with 40-μm to 120-μm TAG

> **Box 1**
> **Indications for transarterial therapy for hepatocellular carcinoma**
>
> Original
>   Unresectable, intermediate stage HCC (BCLC B), Child-Pugh class A
> Newer
>   Child class B
>   Advanced stage HCC (BCLC C)
>   Bridge to transplantation
>   Downstaging for transplantation
>   Neoadjuvant for surgical resection
>   Combined with percutaneous ablation for AJCC T3 tumors
> Future/developing
>   Combined with systemic therapy
>   Combined with PVE
>   With curative intent

microspheres at a quaternary care center revealed 3 periprocedural patient deaths caused by proven or suspected pulmonary microsphere emboli. The investigators cautioned against the use of small microspheres for the treatment of tumors 10 cm or larger.[83]

Proponents of TAE cite the lack of systemic toxicity that bland embolization offers. Although use of Lipiodol in cTACE is intended to lock the chemotherapy within hepatic tumors, pharmacokinetic studies have shown that chemotherapeutic agents are poorly retained within the liver during cTACE, with systemic doses from cTACE being similar to those seen with traditional intravenous chemotherapy infusion.[84] Those favoring bland embolization also argue that it results in less pruning of the hepatic arterial circulation compared with cTACE because of the lack of chemotherapeutic toxicity on the endothelium.[81]

DEB-TACE

Because of the increased per-volume potency of drug-eluting microspheres compared with the components of cTACE, an expert panel recently recommended intraprocedural use of C-arm CT to identify origins of the cystic artery and hepaticoenteric collaterals and coil embolize these arteries if they cannot be avoided during treatment.[85]

Despite the greater potential toxicity compared with the bland spheres used in TAE and cTACE, a recent case series of 237 patients treated with doxorubicin DEB-TACE found a 30-day mortality of 1.2% and a National Cancer Institute Common Terminology Criteria for Adverse Events (CTCAE, version 3.0) grade 4 adverse event rate of 5.5% (irreversible liver failure and cholecystitis).[86] Most AEs were grades 1 and 2. There was a 0.5% rate of grade 3 AEs in the form of pleural effusion. These rates compare favorably with the recently published professional society guidelines for TACE.[82] A recent series of 121 patients with BCLC stage C (advanced HCC) disease treated with doxorubicin DEB-TACE found no grade 4 or 5 AEs and a rate of 1% of

---

Box 2
Contraindications to transarterial therapies

- Decompensated cirrhosis
  - Impaired hepatic metabolic function
    - Hypoalbuminemia (<2.5 mg/dL)[a]
    - Poorly controlled encephalopathy[a]
    - Hyperbilirubinemia (>2–4 mg/dL)[a]
  - Complications of portal hypertension
    - Child-Pugh class C
    - Severe ascites
- Acute illness
  - Acute hepatitis/transaminitis
  - Active gastrointestinal bleeding
- Systemic comorbidity
  - ECOG PS greater than 2
  - Renal insufficiency (Cr >2.0 mg/dL)[a]
  - Neutropenia[b]
  - Cardiomyopathy[b]
- Tumor factors
  - Greater than 75% tumor burden in liver[a]
  - Portal vein thrombus[a]
  - Extrahepatic malignancy[a]
- Vascular/anatomic factors
  - Inability to protect extrahepatic organs from DEB or Y90 microspheres
  - Severe arterial disease precluding catheterization
  - Uncorrectable hepatopulmonary shunting
  - Compromised sphincter of Oddi[a]

[a] Relative contraindication; many groups advocate treating superselectively up to a bilirubin of 4 mg/dL and with reduced contrast for patients with creatinine levels up to 2.0 mg/dL. Large tumor burden requires staged treatment. Portal vein thrombus requires minimally embolic technique. Compromised sphincter of Oddi requires a prophylactic antibiotic course and counseling regarding risk of abscess. To justify treatment, hepatic malignancy should be the expected cause of a patient's greatest future morbidity or mortality.
[b] Potentially exacerbated by doxorubicin administration, not applicable to TAE and TARE.

---

grade 3 AEs, suggesting that DEB-TACE may be safe and effective for patients with all but end-stage disease.[87]

TARE

In contrast with conventional external beam radiation, which necessarily passes through benign tissue en route to tumor and can therefore only deliver 30 to 35 Gy of radiation before causing radiation-induced liver disease, histologic studies have confirmed the expected accumulation of radioembolic microspheres in tumoral arterioles at a

Table 3
Reported complication rates from transarterial chemoembolization

Complication	Rate (%)
Liver failure	2.3
Abscess with functional sphincter of Oddi	1–2
Postembolization syndrome requiring extended stay or readmission	4.6
Abscess with biliary-enteric anastomosis/biliary stent/sphincterotomy with premedication	0–15
Surgical cholecystitis	<1
Biloma requiring percutaneous drainage	<1
Pulmonary arterial oil embolus	<1
Gastrointestinal hemorrhage/ulceration	<1
Iatrogenic dissection preventing treatment	<1
Death within 30 d	2–4

Adapted from Brown DB, Nikolic B, Covey AM, et al. Quality improvement guidelines for transhepatic arterial chemoembolization, embolization, and chemotherapeutic infusion for hepatic malignancy. J Vasc Interv Radiol 2012;23(3):287–94; with permission.

concentration greater than 50 times that in adjacent normal liver.[88,89] As a result, intraarterial Y90 TARE can be used to deliver up to 150 Gy per infused volume of liver safely.[90] Because the radiomicrospheres are merely a carrier for microvascular brachytherapy and are not designed to induce ischemia, the procedure is usually well tolerated, with little to none of the postembolization syndrome seen with TAE or TACE.

Gastrointestinal ulcer formation from nontarget embolization occurs in less than 2% of cases. Radiation pneumonitis is more common with higher lung shunt fractions and repeat sessions. Hepatotoxicity is the most common adverse event, complicating approximately 15% of radioembolic procedures.[91]

SUMMARY

In the decade since being proved to improve survival, transarterial therapies have gained worldwide acceptance as standard of care for inoperable primary liver cancer. Multiple recent studies suggest a doubling of median OS after conventional TACE, TAE, and DEB-TACE compared with standards from 10 years ago, with OS at 3 years in Child A, BCLC B patients frequently approaching or exceeding 50%.

DEB-TACE, beyond being applied with ever-greater effectiveness in Child A, BCLC B patients, is increasingly being used safely and effectively in Child B and BCLC C patients. TAE, with or without intrahepatic chemotherapy, has been applied in combination with percutaneous ablation to effectively control tumors up to 5 cm in diameter. Superselective embolizations and lobar radioembolizations allow patients routinely to be treated in an ambulatory setting.

In the coming years, newer transarterial therapies such as radiation segmentectomy, boosted-TARE, TACE-PVE, and transarterial infusion of cancer-specific metabolic inhibitors promise to continue improving survival and quality of life, even for patients with advanced disease. Transarterial therapy with curative intent may become possible as a consequence of one or more of these developments.

REFERENCES

1. Tadavarthy SM, Knight L, Ovitt TW, et al. Therapeutic transcatheter arterial embolization. Radiology 1974;112:13–6.
2. Yamada R, Nakatsuka H, Nakamura K, et al. Hepatic artery embolization in 32 patients with unresectable hepatoma. Osaka City Med J 1980;26:81–96.
3. Wheeler PG, Melia W, Dubbins P, et al. Non-operative arterial embolization in primary liver tumors. BMJ 1979;2:242–4.
4. Patt YZ, Chuang VP, Wallace S, et al. Hepatic arterial chemotherapy and occlusion for palliation of primary hepatocellular and unknown primary neoplasms in the liver. Cancer 1983;51(8):1359–63.
5. Sasaki Y, Imaoka S, Kasugai, et al. A new approach to chemoembolization therapy for hepatoma using ethiodized oil, cisplatin, and gelatin sponge. Cancer 1987;60:1194–203.
6. Hirai K, Kawazoe Y, Yamashita K, et al. Arterial chemotherapy and transcatheter arterial embolization therapy for non-resectable hepatocellular carcinoma. Cancer Chemother Pharmacol 1989;23(Suppl):S37–41.
7. Lo CM, Ngan H, Tso WK, et al. Randomized controlled trial of transarterial Lipiodol chemoembolization for unresectable hepatocellular carcinoma. Hepatology 2002;35:1164–71.
8. Llovet JM, Real MI, Montana X, et al. Arterial embolization or chemoembolization versus symptomatic treatment in patients with unresectable hepatocellular carcinoma: a randomized controlled trial. Lancet 2002;359:1734–9.
9. Bruix J, Sherman M, Llovet JM, et al. Clinical management of hepatocellular carcinoma. Conclusions of the Barcelona-2000 EASL conference. J Hepatol 2001;35(3):421–30.
10. Bruix J, Sherman M, Practice Guidelines Committee, American Association for the Study of Liver Disease. Management of hepatocellular carcinoma. Hepatology 2005;42(5):1208–36.
11. Bruix J, Sherman M. American Association for the Study of Liver Diseases. Management of hepatocellular carcinoma: an update. Hepatology 2011;53(3):1020–2.
12. Llovet JM, Bru C, Bruix J. Prognosis of hepatocellular carcinoma: the BCLC staging classification. Semin Liver Dis 1999;19(3):329–38.
13. Aliberti C, Tilli M, Benea G, et al. Transarterial chemoembolization (TACE) of liver metastases from colorectal cancer using irinotecan-eluting beads: preliminary results. Anticancer Res 2006;26:3793–6.
14. Poon RT, Tso WK, Pang RW, et al. A phase I/II trial of chemoembolization for hepatocellular carcinoma using a novel intra-arterial DEB. Clin Gastroenterol Hepatol 2007;5(9):1100–8.
15. Park CH, Suh JH, Yoo HS, et al. Evaluation of intrahepatic I-131 ethiodol on a patient with hepatocellular carcinoma. Therapeutic feasibility study. Clin Nucl Med 1986;11(7):514–7.
16. Gray BN, Anderson JE, Burton MA, et al. Regression of liver metastases following treatment with yttrium-Y90 microspheres. Aust N Z J Surg 1992;62(2):105–10.
17. Georgiades CS, Liapi E, Frangakis C, et al. Prognostic accuracy of 12 liver staging systems in patients with unresectable hepatocellular carcinoma treated with transarterial chemoembolization. J Vasc Interv Radiol 2006;17:1619–24.
18. Brown DB, Chapman WC, Cook RD, et al. Chemoembolization of hepatocellular carcinoma: patient status at presentation and outcome over 15 years at a single center. AJR Am J Roentgenol 2008;190:608–15.

19. Bargellini I, Sacco R, Bozzi E, et al. Transarterial chemoembolization in very early and early-stage hepatocellular carcinoma patients excluded from curative treatment: a prospective cohort study. Eur J Radiol 2012;81:1173–8.

20. Georgiades CS, Hong K, D'Angelo M, et al. Safety and efficacy of transarterial chemoembolization in patients with unresectable hepatocellular carcinoma and portal vein thrombosis. J Vasc Interv Radiol 2005;16:1653–9.

21. Chung GE, Lee JH, Kim HY, et al. Transarterial chemoembolization can be safely performed in patients with hepatocellular carcinoma invading the main portal vein and may improve overall survival. Radiology 2011;258:627–34.

22. Ravaioli M, Grazi GL, Piscaglia F, et al. Liver transplantation for hepatocellular carcinoma: results of down-staging in patients initially outside the Milan selection criteria. Am J Transplant 2008;8:2547–57.

23. Chapman WC, Majella Doyle MB, Stuart JE, et al. Outcomes of neoadjuvant transarterial chemoembolization to downstage hepatocellular carcinoma before liver transplantation. Ann Surg 2008;248:617–25.

24. Luo J, Peng ZW, Guo RP, et al. Hepatic resection versus transarterial Lipiodol chemoembolization as the initial treatment for large, multiple, and resectable hepatocellular carcinomas: a prospective nonrandomized analysis. Radiology 2011;259:286–95.

25. Hsu KF, Chu CH, Chan DC, et al. Superselective transarterial chemoembolization vs. hepatic resection for resectable early-stage hepatocellular carcinoma in patients with Child-Pugh class A liver function. Eur J Radiol 2012;81:466–71.

26. Bruix J, Llovet JM, Castells A, et al. Transarterial embolization versus symptomatic treatment in patients with advanced hepatocellular carcinoma: results of a randomized, controlled trial in a single institution. Hepatology 1998;27(6):1578–83.

27. Maluccio MA, Covey AM, Porat LB, et al. Transcatheter arterial embolization with only particles for the treatment of unresectable hepatocellular carcinoma. J Vasc Interv Radiol 2008;19(6):862–9.

28. Brown DB, Cardella JF, Sacks D, et al. Quality improvement guidelines for transhepatic arterial chemoembolization, embolization and chemotherapeutic infusion for hepatic malignancy. J Vasc Interv Radiol 2009;20:S219–26.

29. Camma C, Schepis F, Orlando A, et al. Transarterial chemoembolization for unresectable hepatocellular carcinoma: meta-analysis of randomized controlled trials. Radiology 2002;224(1):47–54.

30. Marelli L, Stigliano R, Triantos C, et al. Transarterial therapy for hepatocellular carcinoma: which technique is more effective? A systematic review of cohort and randomized studies. Cardiovasc Intervent Radiol 2007;30(1):6–25.

31. Maeda S, Fujiyama S, Tanaka M, et al. Survival and local recurrence rates of hepatocellular carcinoma patients treated by transarterial chemolipiodolization with and without embolization. Hepatol Res 2002;23:202–10.

32. Ikeda M, Maeda S, Shibata J, et al. Transcatheter arterial chemotherapy with and without embolization in patients with hepatocellular carcinoma. Oncology 2004;66(1):24–31.

33. Okusaka T, Kasugai H, Shioyama Y, et al. Transarterial chemotherapy alone versus transarterial chemoembolization for hepatocellular carcinoma: a randomized phase III trial. J Hepatol 2009;51(6):1030–6.

34. Takayasu K, Shigeki A, Iwao I, et al. Overall survival after transarterial Lipiodol infusion chemotherapy with or without embolization for unresectable hepatocellular carcinoma: a propensity score analysis. AJR Am J Roentgenol 2010;194:830–7.

35. Vogl TJ, Schwarz W, Eichler K, et al. Hepatic intraarterial chemotherapy with gemcitabine in patients with unresectable cholangiocarcinomas and liver metastases of pancreatic cancer: a clinical study on maximum tolerable dose and treatment efficacy. J Cancer Res Clin Oncol 2006;132:745–55.
36. Kim JH, Yoon HK, Sung KB, et al. Transcatheter arterial chemoembolization or chemoinfusion for unresectable intrahepatic cholangiocarcinoma: clinical efficacy and factors influencing outcomes. Cancer 2008;113:1614–22.
37. Shen WF, Zhong W, Liu Q, et al. Adjuvant transcatheter arterial chemoemboliza-tion for intrahepatic cholangiocarcinoma after curative surgery: retrospective control study. World J Surg 2011;35:2083–91.
38. De Luna W, Sze DY, Ahmed A, et al. Transarterial chemoinfusion for hepatocel-lular carcinoma as downstaging therapy and a bridge toward liver transplanta-tion. Am J Transplant 2009;9:1158–68.
39. Kamada K, Nakanishi T, Kitamoto M, et al. Long-term prognosis of patients undergoing transcatheter arterial chemoembolization for unresectable hepato-cellular carcinoma: comparison of cisplatin Lipiodol suspension and doxoru-bicin hydrochloride emulsion. J Vasc Interv Radiol 2001;12:847–54.
40. Yodono H, Matsuo K, Shinohara A, et al. A retrospective comparative study of epirubicin-Lipiodol emulsion and cisplatin Lipiodol suspension for use with transcatheter arterial chemoembolization for treatment of hepatocellular carci-noma. Anticancer Drugs 2011;22:277–82.
41. Kawai S, Tani M, Okamura J, et al. Prospective and randomized trial of Lipiodol transcatheter arterial chemoembolization for treatment of hepatocellular carci-noma: comparison of epirubicin and doxorubicin (second cooperative study). The Cooperative Study Group for Liver Cancer Treatment of Japan. Semin Onol 1997;24:S6–38 S36–45.
42. Sahara S, Kawai N, Sato M, et al. Prospective evaluation of transcatheter arterial chemoembolization (TACE) with multiple anticancer drugs (epirubicin, cisplatin, mitomycin c, 5-fluorouracil) compared with TACE with epirubicin for treatment of hepatocellular carcinoma. Cardiovasc Intervent Radiol 2012;35(6):1363–71.
43. Petruzzi NJ, Frangos AJ, Fenkel JM, et al. Single-center comparison of three chemoembolization regimens for hepatocellular carcinoma. J Vasc Interv Radiol 2013;24(2):266–73.
44. Burrel M, Reig M, Forner A, et al. Survival of patients with hepatocellular carci-noma treated by transarterial chemoembolisation (TACE) using drug eluting beads. Implications for clinical practice and trial design. J Hepatol 2012; 56(6):1330–5.
45. Malagari K, Pomoni M, Sotirchos VS, et al. Long term recurrence analysis post drug eluting bead (DEB) chemoembolization for hepatocellular carcinoma (HCC). Hepatogastroenterology 2013;60(126):1413–9.
46. Padia SA, Shivaram G, Bastawrous S, et al. Safety and efficacy of DEB chemo-embolization for hepatocellular carcinoma: comparison of small-versus medium-size particles. J Vasc Interv Radiol 2013;24:301–6.
47. Lammer J, Malagari K, Vogl T, et al. Prospective randomized study of doxorubicin-eluting-bead embolization in the treatment of hepatocellular carci-noma: results of the PRECISION V study. Cardiovasc Intervent Radiol 2010; 33:41–52.
48. Malagari K, Pomoni M, Kelekis A, et al. Prospective randomized comparison of chemoembolization with doxorubicin-eluting beads and bland embolization with BeadBlock for hepatocellular carcinoma. Cardiovasc Intervent Radiol 2010; 33(3):541–51.

49. Nicolini A, Martinetti L, Crespi S, et al. Transarterial chemoembolization with epirubicin-eluting beads versus transarterial embolization before liver transplantation for hepatocellular carcinoma. J Vasc Interv Radiol 2010;21:327–32.

50. Salem R, Lewandowski RJ, Mulcahy MF, et al. Radioembolization for hepatocellular carcinoma using yttrium-Y90 microspheres: a comprehensive report of long-term outcomes. Gastroenterology 2010;138:52–64.

51. Geschwind JF, Salem R, Carr BI, et al. Yttrium-90 microspheres for the treatment of hepatocellular carcinoma. Gastroenterology 2004;127:S107–10.

52. Lewandowski RJ, Kulik LM, Riaz A, et al. A comparative analysis of transarterial downstaging for hepatocellular carcinoma: chemoembolization versus radioembolization. Am J Transplant 2009;9:1920–8.

53. Kooby DA, Egnatashvili V, Srinivasan S, et al. Comparison of yttrium-Y90 radioembolization and transcatheter arterial chemoembolization for the treatment of unresectable hepatocellular carcinoma. J Vasc Interv Radiol 2010;21:224–30.

54. Carr BI, Kondragunta V, Buch SC, et al. Therapeutic equivalence in survival for hepatic arterial chemoembolization and yttrium Y90 microsphere treatments in unresectable hepatocellular carcinoma: a two-cohort study. Cancer 2010;116:1305–14.

55. Moreno-Luna LE, Yang JD, Sanchez W, et al. Efficacy and safety of transarterial radioembolization versus chemoembolization in patients with hepatocellular carcinoma. Cardiovasc Intervent Radiol 2013;36(3):714–23.

56. Salem R, Lewandowski RJ, Kulik L, et al. Radioembolization results in longer time-to-progression and reduced toxicity compared with chemoembolization in patients with hepatocellular carcinoma. Gastroenterology 2011;140:497–507.e2.

57. Morimoto M, Numata K, Kondou M, et al. Midterm outcomes in patients with intermediate-sized hepatocellular carcinoma: a randomized controlled trial for determining the efficacy of radiofrequency ablation combined with transcatheter arterial chemoembolization. Cancer 2010;116(23):5452–60.

58. Kagawa T, Koizumi J, Kojima SI, et al. Transcatheter arterial chemoembolization plus radiofrequency ablation therapy for early stage hepatocellular carcinoma. Cancer 2010;116:3638–44.

59. Kim JH, Won HJ, Shin YM, et al. Medium-Sized (3.1–5.0 cm) hepatocellular carcinoma: transarterial chemoembolization plus radiofrequency ablation versus radiofrequency ablation alone. Ann Surg Oncol 2011;18:1624–9.

60. Elnekave E, Erinjeri JP, Brown KT, et al. Long-term outcomes comparing surgery to embolization-ablation for treatment of solitary HCC <7 cm. Ann Surg Oncol 2013;20:2881–6.

61. Ogata S, Belghiti J, Farges O, et al. Sequential arterial and portal vein embolizations before right hepatectomy in patients with cirrhosis and hepatocellular carcinoma. Br J Surg 2006;93(9):1091–8.

62. Yoo H, Kim JH, Ko GY, et al. Sequential transcatheter arterial chemoembolization and portal vein embolization versus portal vein embolization only before major hepatectomy for patients with hepatocellular carcinoma. Ann Surg Oncol 2011;18(5):1251–7.

63. Pawlik TM, Reyes DK, Cosgrove D, et al. Phase II Trial of sorafenib combined with concurrent transarterial chemoembolization with DEBs for hepatocellular carcinoma. J Clin Oncol 2011;29(30):3960–7.

64. Park JW, Koh YH, Kim HB, et al. Phase II study of concurrent transarterial chemoembolization and sorafenib in patients with unresectable hepatocellular carcinoma. J Hepatol 2012;56:1336–42.

65. Sansonno D, Lauletta G, Russi S, et al. Transarterial chemoembolization plus sorafenib: a sequential theme for HCV-related intermediate stage hepatocellular carcinoma: a randomized clinical trial. Oncologist 2012;17:359–66.
66. Kudo M, Imanaka K, Chida N, et al. Phase III study of sorafenib after transarterial chemoembolisation in Japanese and Korean patients with unresectable hepatocellular carcinoma. Eur J Cancer 2011;47:2117–27.
67. Hoffman K, Glimm H, Radeleff B, et al. Prospective, randomized, double-blind, multi-center, phase III clinical study on transarterial chemoembolization (TACE) combined with sorafenib versus TACE plus placebo in patients with hepatocellular cancer before liver transplantation – HeiLivCa. BMC Cancer 2008;8:349–56.
68. Choi YH. Novel intraarterial therapy for liver cancer using ethylbromopyruvate dissolved in an iodized oil. Acad Radiol 2011;18:471–8.
69. Liapi E, Geschwind JF. Interventional oncology: new options for interstitial treatments and intravascular approaches. Targeting tumor metabolism via a locoregional approach: a new therapy against liver cancer. J Hepatobiliary Pancreat Sci 2010;17:405–6.
70. Vali M, Liapi E, Kowalski J, et al. Intraarterial therapy with a new potent inhibitor of tumor metabolism (3-bromopyruvate): identification of therapeutic dose and method of injection in an animal model of liver cancer. J Vasc Interv Radiol 2007;18:95–102.
71. Memon K, Kulik L, Lewandowski RJ, et al. Radiographic response to locoregional therapy in hepatocellular carcinoma predicts patient survival times. Gastroenterology 2011;141:526–35.
72. Gillmore R, Stuart S, Kirkwood A, et al. EASL and mRECIST responses are independent prognostic factors for survival in hepatocellular carcinoma patients treated with transarterial embolisation. J Hepatol 2011;55:1309–16.
73. Shim JH, Lee HC, Kim SO, et al. Which response criteria best help predict survival of patients with hepatocellular carcinoma following chemoembolization? A validation study of old and new models. Radiology 2012;262(2):708–18.
74. Siddiqi NH, Devlin PM. Radiation Lobectomy – A minimally invasive treatment model for liver cancer: case report. J Vasc Interv Radiol 2009;20:664–9.
75. Gaba R, Lewandowski RJ, Kulik LM, et al. Radiation lobectomy: preliminary findings of hepatic volumetric response to lobar yttrium-Y90 radioembolization. Ann Surg Oncol 2009;16(6):1587–96.
76. Riaz A, Gates VL, Atassi B, et al. Radiation segmentectomy: a novel approach to increase safety and efficacy of radioembolization. Int J Radiat Oncol Biol Phys 2011;79:163–71.
77. Garin E, Lenoir L, Edeline J, et al. Boosted selective internal radiation therapy with Y90-loaded glass microspheres (B-SIRT) for hepatocellular carcinoma patients: a new personalized promising concept. Eur J Nucl Med Mol Imaging 2013;40:1057–68.
78. Brown KT, Koh BY, Brody LA, et al. Particle embolization of hepatic neuroendocrine metastases for control of pain and hormonal symptoms. J Vasc Interv Radiol 1999;10:309–403.
79. Lee SH, Hahn ST, Park SH. Intraarterial lidocaine administration for the relief of pain resulting from transarterial chemoembolization of hepatocellular carcinoma: its effectiveness and optimal timing of administration. Cardiovasc Intervent Radiol 2001;24:368–71.
80. Liapi E, Geschwind JF. Transcatheter arterial chemoembolization for liver cancer: is it time to distinguish conventional from drug-eluting chemoembolization? Cardiovasc Intervent Radiol 2011;34:37–49.

81. Erinjeri JP, Salhab HM, Covey AM. Arterial patency after repeated hepatic artery bland particle embolization. J Vasc Interv Radiol 2010;21(4):522–6.

82. Brown DB, Nikolic B, Covey AM, et al. Quality improvement guidelines for transhepatic arterial chemoembolization, embolization, and chemotherapeutic infusion for hepatic malignancy. J Vasc Interv Radiol 2012;23(3):287–94.

83. Brown KT. Fatal pulmonary complications after arterial embolization with 40–120 micron tris-acryl gelatin microspheres. J Vasc Interv Radiol 2004;15:197–200.

84. Varela M, Real MI, Burrel M, et al. Chemoembolization of hepatocellular carcinoma with drug eluting beads: efficacy and doxorubicin pharmacokinetics. J Hepatol 2007;46:474–81.

85. Lencioni R, de Baere T, Burrel M, et al. Transcatheter treatment of hepatocellular carcinoma with doxorubicin-loaded DC bead (DEBDOX): technical recommendations. Cardiovasc Intervent Radiol 2012;35:980–5.

86. Malagari K, Pomoni M, Spyridopoulos TN, et al. Safety profile of sequential transcatheter chemoembolization with DC Bead: results of 237 hepatocellular carcinoma (HCC) patients. Cardiovasc Intervent Radiol 2011;34(4):774–85.

87. Prajapati HJ, Dhanasekaran R, El-Rayes BF, et al. Safety and efficacy of doxorubicin DEB transarterial chemoembolization in patients with advanced hepatocellular carcinoma. J Vasc Interv Radiol 2013;24(3):307–15.

88. Ingold JA, Reed GB, Kaplan HS, et al. Radiation hepatitis. Am J Roentgenol Radium Ther Nucl Med 1965;93:200–8.

89. Campbell AM, Bailey IH, Burton MA. Analysis of the distribution of intra-arterial microspheres in human liver following hepatic yttrium-90 microsphere therapy. Phys Med Biol 2000;45(4):1023–33.

90. Kennedy AS, Nutting C, Coldwell D, et al. Pathologic response and microdosimetry of (90)Y microspheres in man: review of four explanted whole livers. Int J Radiat Oncol Biol Phys 2004;60:1552–63.

91. Sangro B, D'Avola D, Inarrairaegui M, et al. Transarterial therapies for hepatocellular carcinoma. Expert Opin Pharmacother 2011;12(7):1057–73.

92. Aliberti C, Benea G, Tilli M, et al. Chemoembolization (TACE) of unresectable intrahepatic cholangiocarcinoma with slow-release doxorubicin-eluting beads: preliminary results. Cardiovasc Intervent Radiol 2008;31:883–8.

93. Gusani NJ, Balaa FK, Steel JL, et al. Treatment of unresectable cholangiocarcinoma with gemcitabine-based transcatheter arterial chemoembolization (TACE): a single-institution experience. J Gastrointest Surg 2008;12(1):129–37.

94. Ibrahim SM, Mulcahy MF, Lewandowsky RJ, et al. Treatment of unresectable cholangiocarcinoma using yttrium-90 microspheres: results from a pilot study. Cancer 2008;113:2119–28.

95. Poggi G, Amatu B, Quaretti P, et al. OEM-TACE: A new therapeutic approach in unresectable intrahepatic cholangiocarcinoma. Cardiovasc Interv Radiology 2009;32(6):1187–92.

96. Saxena A, Bester L, Chua TC, et al. Yttrium-90 radiotherapy for unresectable intrahepatic cholangiocarcinoma: a preliminary assessment of this novel treatment option. Ann Surg Oncol 2010;17:484–91.

97. Kiefer MV, Albert M, McNally M, et al. Chemoembolization of intrahepatic cholangiocarcinoma with cisplatin, doxorubicin, mitomycin C, Ethiodol and polyvinyl alcohol: a 2-center study. Cancer 2011;117:1498–505.

98. Park SY, Kim JH, Yoon HJ, et al. Transarterial chemoembolization versus supportive therapy in the palliative treatment of unresectable intrahepatic cholangiocarcinoma. Clin Radiol 2011;66:322–8.

99. Hoffman RT, Paprottka PM, Schon A, et al. Transarterial hepatic yttrium-90 radio-embolization in patients with unresectable intrahepatic cholangiocarcinoma: factors associated with prolonged survival. Cardiovasc interv radiol 2012;35: 105–16.
100. Kuhlmann JB, Euringer W, Spangenberg HC, et al. Treatment of unresectable cholangiocarcinoma: conventional transarterial chemoembolization compared with drug eluting bead-transarterial chemoembolization and systemic chemotherapy. Eur J Gastroenterol Hepatol 2012;4:437–43.
101. Rafi S, Piduru SM, El-Rayes B, et al. Yttrium-90 radioembolization for unresectable standard-chemorefractory intrahepatic cholangiocarcinoma: survival, efficacy and safety study. Cardiovasc interv radiol 2013;36:440–8.
102. Vogl TJ, Naguib NN, Nour-Eldin NE, et al. Transarterial chemoembolization in the treatment of patients with unresectable cholangiocarcinoma: Results and prognostic factors governing treatment success. Int J Cancer 2012;131(3):733–40.
103. Hyder O, Marsh JW, Salem R, et al. Intra-arterial therapy for advanced intrahepatic cholangiocarcinoma: a multi-institutional analysis. Ann Surg Oncol 2013; 20:3779–86.

An Emerging Role for Radiation Therapy in the Treatment of Hepatocellular Carcinoma and Intrahepatic Cholangiocarcinoma

Jennifer Y. Wo, MD[a],*, Laura A. Dawson, MD[b],
Andrew X. Zhu, MD, PhD[c], Theodore S. Hong, MD[a]

KEYWORDS

- Hepatobiliary cancers • Radiation therapy • Stereotactic body radiation therapy

KEY POINTS

- Because of recent technologic advancements in radiation treatment planning, hepatobiliary imaging techniques, breathing motion reduction strategies, and image guidance, radiation therapy is re-emerging as a potentially effective treatment of locally advanced, unresectable hepatocellular carcinoma (HCC).
- Outcomes from early experiences of prospective studies evaluating liver stereotactic body radiation therapy (SBRT) for treatment of HCC seem promising, with improved survivals compared with historical controls.
- Liver directed radiation therapy, including three-dimensional conformal radiotherapy, SBRT, and charged-particle radiotherapy, may be a safe, alternative treatment options for patients with locally advanced HCC who are unsuitable for other local therapies and a potential bridging therapy for patients awaiting transplantation.
- Despite increasing conformal therapy, decline in baseline liver function is a potential treatment-related complication. As a result, large, multi-institutional, prospective, phase 3 studies are needed to definitively establish the benefit of radiation therapy. To this end, RTOG 1112 (Radiation Therapy Oncology Group 1112), a phase 3, randomized cooperative group trial study of sorafenib versus SBRT followed by sorafenib in locally advanced HCC, is open to accrual.

The authors have nothing to disclose.
[a] Department of Radiation Oncology, Massachusetts General Hospital, 100 Blossom Street, Cox 3, Boston, MA 02114, USA; [b] Department of Radiation Oncology, Princess Margaret Cancer Centre, 610 University Avenue, Toronto, ON M5G 2M9, Canada; [c] Department of Medical Oncology, Massachusetts General Hospital, 55 Fruit Street, Boston, MA 02114, USA
* Corresponding author.
E-mail address: jwo@partners.org

Surg Oncol Clin N Am 23 (2014) 353–368
http://dx.doi.org/10.1016/j.soc.2013.10.007
1055-3207/14/$ – see front matter © 2014 Elsevier Inc. All rights reserved.

HEPATOCELLULAR CARCINOMA

Most patients with hepatocellular carcinoma (HCC) present with locally advanced, unresectable disease, as a result of tumor extension or invasion of major vasculature. For patients not suitable for transplantation, resection, or ablation, locoregional therapies, including transarterial chemoembolization (TACE) and radiation therapy, and systemic therapies may be available. TACE does not completely eradicate HCC, but has been shown to be an effective palliative strategy with improved survival compared with best supportive care,[1,2] particularly in patients with multifocal involvement. However, for large HCC (>10 cm) or HCC with portal vein thrombus, TACE is less effective. The SHARP (Sorafenib Hepatocellular Carcinoma Assessment Randomized Protocol) study established sorafenib, a multikinase inhibitor, as an effective systemic agent when compared with placebo among patients unsuitable for TACE, with Child-Pugh class A, with an improvement in median overall survival from 7.9 to 10.7 months.[3]

In contrast, historically, the role of radiation therapy has been limited in the treatment of HCC. However, with recent technological advancements in radiation treatment planning, imaging techniques, breathing motion reduction strategies, and image guidance, there has been increasing interest in evaluating conformal liver directed radiation therapy. Early published data have yielded promising results, with high rates of local control and acceptable rates of radiation-related toxicity; however, despite increasingly conformal therapy, decline in liver function as a treatment-related toxicity can occur and must be carefully monitored.[4,5] Worldwide, focal radiation treatment delivery to the liver has been gaining traction, as shown by the rapidly increasing body of literature over the last 10 years.[6] Because of the prevalence of HCC in Asia, most of the published series have emerged out of Korea, Japan, and recently, China. This review surveys the recently published data evaluating radiation therapy as a potential treatment of hepatobiliary primary tumors. Although the potential role of radiation therapy in the treatment of liver metastases has also been recently established, this review does not directly address this topic and focuses only on treatment of primary liver tumors.

Radiation-Induced Liver Toxicity

Radiation oncologists have been traditionally hesitant to irradiate the liver because of concerns of radiation-induced liver disease (RILD). Classic RILD is defined as the triad of anicteric hepatosplenomegaly, ascites, and increased alkaline phosphatase levels ($\geq$2 times upper limits of normal), which typically develops 2 weeks to 3 months after completion of therapy. Patients may also develop nonclassic RILD, which manifests as increased transaminase levels (typically $\geq$5 times upper limits of normal) or a decline in liver function test (defined by increase in Child-Pugh score of $\geq$2) in the absence of classic RILD. Centrilobular congestion and hyperemia with surrounding hepatocyte atrophy are the pathologic hallmarks of RILD. Although classic RILD can occur in patients with intact pretreatment hepatic function, nonclassic RILD is most frequently appreciated in patients with poor baseline liver function in the setting of HCC. In addition, evaluation of RILD is confounded by the natural progression of a patient's underlying hepatic dysfunction over time. In addition, radiation has been associated with reactivation of hepatitis B, which can further lead to worsening of hepatic function abnormalities. Currently treatment of RILD is mainly supportive, with administration of diuretics for fluid imbalance as needed.

Ingold and colleagues[7] published the first report of dose-limiting toxicities with whole-liver irradiation, in which there was a 44% risk of RILD in patients treated with 35 Gy or more. Subsequently, in the 1980s, the Radiation Therapy Oncology Group (RTOG) launched several prospective studies evaluating the toxicity and efficacy of liver directed irradiation. RTOG 84-05 launched a dose escalation study of whole-liver irradiation for patients with liver metastases from 27 Gy to a planned 36 Gy in 1.5-Gy fractions administered twice daily. Approximately 10% of patients treated to 33 Gy developed RILD compared with 0% of patients treated with 27 to 30 Gy. Based on the results of this study, 33 Gy in fractions of 1.5 Gy to the whole liver was deemed unsafe.[8] Because of the toxicity observed in early studies and inability to conform radiation to include only the involved portions of the liver, interest in continued pursuit of liver directed radiation therapy waned.

Partial Liver Tolerance and Re-emergence of Fractionated Conformal Radiotherapy

HCC has traditionally been considered a radioresistant tumor; however, this likely reflects hesitation of treating the liver with ablative doses because of concerns of excessive toxicity. Significant recent developments in imaging modalities and more refined imaging protocols have improved tumor detection and tumor delineation, thereby allowing for more focused radiation therapy to the areas of tumor involvement and greater sparing of uninvolved liver parenchyma. Given these advancements, based on the rationale of the viability of patients after partial hepatectomy, and the liver functioning as a parallel organ, radiation oncologists postulated that it should be feasible to deliver tumoricidal doses to the intrahepatic tumors if an adequate amount of normal liver tissue could be spared. Accomplishing this goal necessitated both conformal radiation therapy (CRT) delivery and development of a normal tissue complication model for the normal liver tissue to be spared. Optimal treatment strategy was predicated on understanding of the volume effect of partial liver irradiation in order to maximize tumor control probabilities without significantly increasing normal tissue complication probabilities (NTCP). To achieve this goal, through a series of prospective studies of fractionated conformal radiation, the University of Michigan developed an NTCP model that quantitatively described the relationship between dose and volumes irradiated and the probability of developing classic RILD.[9] In this model, radiation dose is individualized based on the volume of normal liver that can be spared without exceeding a 5% to 20% risk for RILD.

Successive clinical trials from the University of Michigan established the ability to treat unresectable liver tumors with conformal hyperfractionated radiation therapy with concurrent hepatic arterial fluorodeoxyuridine with excellent outcomes.[10–12] In the phase 2 study from the University of Michigan, among 128 patients enrolled with liver tumors, including 46 patients with intrahepatic cholangiocarcinoma (ICC), 47 patients with colorectal metastases, and 35 patients with HCC, the investigators reported an impressive median survival of 15.8 months and 3-year survival of 17%. Compared with historical controls stratified by disease type, patients in this study had significantly improved overall survival, with median survival in HCC, ICC, and metastatic colorectal cancer reaching 15.2, 13.3, and 17.2 months, respectively. On multivariate analysis, tumor dose was a significant predictor for improved survival. Patients receiving doses of 75 Gy or greater had significantly higher overall survival compared with patients receiving lower doses (23.9 months vs 14.9 months, $P<.01$). In addition, the investigators noted a predominantly local pattern of failure for patients with hepatobiliary tumors, suggesting that dose intensification may further improve on outcomes. The association between tumor dose and improved survival suggested the importance of dose response. Based on these promising results, there was renewed interest in reassessing the potential for liver directed irradiation, particularly with intensification of local therapy for unresectable hepatobiliary tumors.[11]

Subsequently, the French RTG1 multicenter prospective phase 2 study[13] sought to assess the feasibility, safety, and efficacy of high-dose three-dimensional (3D) CRT (66 Gy in 2-Gy fractions) for cirrhotic patients with HCC (1 ≤5 cm or 3 ≤3 cm). Sustained local control was reported in 78% of 25 assessable patients. Grade 4 toxicities were reported only in patients with Child-Pugh class B, all of whom had grade 3 abnormalities before initiation of treatment. In addition to these prospective studies, numerous retrospective series have emerged from Asia. Seong and colleagues[14] have published the largest retrospective series to date, of 398 patients with HCC treated at 10 institutions in Korea. These investigators reported 1-year overall survival of 45%, with no grade 3 or higher toxicity. This study similarly confirmed the prognostic significance of radiation dose, with improved 2-year survival reported among patients treated with a biological effective dose of 53.1 Gy or greater.

Thus, over the last decade, there has been an increasing body of literature establishing the use of CRT in treatment of HCC. Although most studies are small and retrospective, reported local control and survival outcomes have been promising. Incorporation of 3D-CRT planning has permitted delivery of higher doses of radiation to localized intrahepatic malignancies.

Stereotactic Body Radiation Therapy

Stereotactic body radiation therapy (SBRT) is a radiation technique that delivers high doses of precisely targeted radiation therapy in a few fractions to a tumor and minimizes radiation dose to adjacent normal tissue structures (**Fig. 1**). Because of improved precision of treatment delivery and improved immobilization over the last 5 years, liver directed SBRT has emerged as a promising treatment of primary liver tumors. Despite its relatively recent adoption into clinical practice, liver SBRT was first described in the early 1990s by Blomgren and colleagues,[15] who reported an objective response rate of 70%. More recently, Tse and colleagues[4] published a phase 1 experience of SBRT for unresectable HCC and ICC. In this study, all patients were required to have Child-Pugh A liver function with more than 800 cm³ of uninvolved liver. Radiation dose was dependent on the volume of liver irradiated, and the estimated risk of liver toxicity based on a normal tissue complication model with radiation dose was

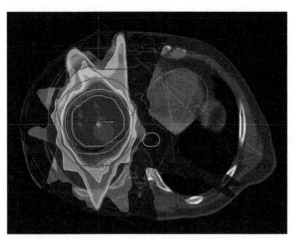

Fig. 1. Representative slice from a liver SBRT plan for a patient with unresectable HCC. Note the ability of the beams to conform to the involved liver with relative sparing of the esophagus and heart.

escalated in 3 predefined toxicity strata of 5%, 10%, and 20%. In total, 31 patients with HCC and 10 patients with ICC were enrolled and completed the prescribed 6-fraction SBRT treatment. With a median tumor size of 173 mL (range, 9–1913 mL) and median dose of 36 Gy (range, 24–54 Gy), no RILD or treatment-related grade 4/5 toxicity was seen within 3 months of completion of SBRT. Based on the favorable tolerance of this regimen, a maximum tolerated dose was not achieved. Seven patients (17%) developed a decline in liver function from Child-Pugh class A to B within 3 months of completion of treatment, although progression of underlying cirrhosis may have contributed to some of the decline in liver function. Overall, the median survival for all patients was 13.4 months, with a 1-year survival rate of 51% and 1-year in-field local control rate of 65%. The promising results from this phase 1 study laid a foundation for future studies.

Expanding on this phase 1 experience, Bujold and colleagues[5] recently published their expanded phase 1/2 experience of 102 patients with locally advanced HCC unsuitable for standard locoregional therapies. All patients were Child-Pugh class A, with at least 700 mL of uninvolved liver. The primary end point of the study was local control at 1 year. Generally, doses of 30 to 54 Gy in 6 fractions were prescribed and administered every other day over 2 weeks. Dose was determined according to a radiobiological model of normal tissue complications based on the effective irradiated liver volumes. In addition, the initial trial design had no limitations on number of lesions or size limits; trial 2 subsequently stipulated no more than 5 discrete liver tumors, with a maximal diameter of 15 cm. Tumor vascular thrombus (TVT) was present in 55%. Despite the advanced stage of patients enrolled, the investigators reported an impressive 1-year local control rate of 87%. When evaluating best responses, 11% of patients had a complete response (CR), 43% of patients had a partial response (PR), and 44% of patients had stable disease (SD). With a median follow-up of 31.4 months, the median time to local recurrence had not yet been reached. Median overall survival was reported at 17 months. Absence of tumor vein thrombus and treatment on trial 2, likely because of improved patient selection and possible improvements in treatment targeting and delivery, were associated with improved overall survival. A summary of recent SBRT studies for HCC is provided in **Table 1**.

Evaluation of treatment response for patients treated with SBRT for HCC can be challenging. To date, there have been few studies that have attempted to establish radiographic correlates of response. Since 2001, the European Association for the Study of the Liver (EASL) has suggested that tumor necrosis, defined as nonenhanced areas by spiral computed tomography (CT), should be considered the optimal method to assess tumor response.[21] Traditionally, prospective studies have evaluated tumor response by axial bidimensional RECIST (Response Evaluation Criteria In Solid Tumors) criteria; however, some studies suggest underestimation of HCC tumor response to SBRT when evaluated by RECIST criteria.[22] A recent study from Indiana University evaluated radiologic response in 26 patients with HCC treated with SBRT at Indiana University enrolled in a phase 1 or 2 trial. Eligibility criteria included solitary tumors of 6 cm or smaller or up to 3 lesions with sum diameters of 6 cm or less, and well-compensated cirrhosis. Patients received 3 to 5 fractions of SBRT, and the median SBRT dose was 42 Gy (range, 24–48 Gy). On posttreatment scans, abnormal enhancement on arterial and venous phases of images of peritumoral liver was seen in all cases by 6 months, consistent with radiation-induced inflammation. After a median follow-up of 13 months, per RECIST criteria, 4 patients had a CR, 15 had a PR, and 7 achieved SD at 12 months. The mean tumor dimension decreased by 35%, 37%, 48%, and 55%, respectively, at 3 months, 6 months, 9 months, and 12 months compared with pretreatment size. In contrast, by EASL criteria, the

Table 1
Summary of SBRT literature for treatment of primary liver tumors

Author, Year	Study Design	Number of Patients	Tumor Size	Portal Vein Thrombus (%)	Dose (Gy)	Number of Fractions	1-Y Overall Survival (%)	Grade ≥3 Toxicity (%)
Bujold et al,[5] 2013	Phase 1/2	102	Trial 1: no limits Trial 2: maximum dimension 15 cm	55	24–54	6	55	36
Andolino et al,[16] 2011	Retrospective	60	1–6.5 cm	NA	24–48	3–5	67 at 2 y	37
Cardenes et al,[17] 2010	Phase 1	17	≤6 cm	18	36–48	3–4	75	18
Kwon et al,[18] 2010	Retrospective	42	≤100 mL	0	30–39	3	93	2
Seo et al,[19] 2010	Retrospective	38	<10 cm	NA	33–57	3–4	69	0
Tse et al,[4] 2008	Phase 1	31	9–1913 mL	0	37.5	4	75	29
Méndez Romero et al,[20] 2006	Phase 1/2	8	NA	25	25–30	3–5	75	12.5

Abbreviation: NA, not applicable.

mean percent necrosis was 59%, 69%, 81%, and 92%, respectively, at 3 months, 6 months, 9 months, and 12 months. Because the percentage necrosis was greater than percentage size reduction at each time point, the investigators suggested that nonenhancement on imaging may be a more useful early indicator than size reduction in evaluating HCC response to SBRT in the first 6 to 12 months, supporting EASL criteria.[23] It is hoped that future studies will further elucidate optimal radiographic correlates to assess tumor response to liver directed radiation therapy.

Portal Vein Thrombosis

Patients with advanced HCC with portal vein thrombosis (PVTT) represent a subset of patients with particularly poor prognosis, with a median survival of only 2 to 4 months if left untreated.[24] Many of the standard treatment modalities, including resection, percutaneous ethanol injection, and radiofrequency ablation (RFA), are contraindicated, particularly if PVTT is located in the main trunk or any of the main portal vein branches. TACE confers limited treatment efficacy and can be associated with a risk of liver insufficiency as a result of treatment-related ischemia. Radiation therapy has been increasingly explored as a potential treatment option with the goal of recanalization of the portal vein, either alone, or in combination with TACE. In 1989, Takagi and colleagues[25] first reported an impressive response rate of 29% among 7 patients with HCC and PVTT treated with radiation therapy. Since that time, numerous single-institutional series have been published, which have reported improved outcomes compared with historical controls, suggesting a potential benefit to treatment with radiation therapy for this patient subset (**Table 2**).

Although response of PVTT dissolution can be slow, recanalization of the PVTT has been reported.[32] The Tsukuba group have looked at the efficacy of radiotherapy (RT) for patients with HCC in the setting of PVTT, with impressive local progression-free survival of 21 months, and 2-year and 5-year progression-free survival of 46% and 20%, respectively.[30] In another series from Southern China, 41 patients with HCC with associated PVTT or thrombus of the inferior vena cava were treated to a median dose of 36 Gy in 6 fractions targeting the tumor thrombus. A total of 36% achieved a CR, 39% achieved PR, 17% achieved SD, and 7% showed progressive disease. Xi and colleagues[26] reported a median survival of 13 months and a 1-year overall survival of 50.3%. More recently, as discussed earlier, the University of Toronto phase 1/2 prospective trial included 56 (55%) patients with TVT. Consistent with other studies, PVTT was the strongest adverse prognostic factor, with a median survival of 10.6 months versus 21.5 months for HCC with and without PVTT, respectively.[5] After adjusting for other known prognostic factors, TVT was associated with significantly increased mortality, with a hazard ratio of 2.47 (95% CI, 1.25–4.88; $P = .01$). Based on these data, for patients with HCC who present with PVTT, radiation therapy may be an effective therapy either alone or in combination with TACE.

Charged-Particle RT

Because of the relatively low radiation tolerance to normal liver tissue, particle beam RT, including proton beam RT and carbon ion beam therapy, have been explored as a means to further minimize radiation exposure to normal liver tissue. Theoretically, particle beam RT may offer distinct biological and physical advantages. Because of favorable depth dose characteristics with the Bragg peak, charged particles allow for precise dose application, with maximal sparing of normal tissue (**Fig. 2**). The role of charged-particle RT for primary hepatobiliary tumors is undefined. In addition, whether or not charged-particle RT is more effective or better tolerated than photon SBRT remains to be seen, particularly given its prohibitive cost.

Table 2
Summary of SBRT literature for treatment of primary liver tumors with tumor vein thrombus

Author, Year	Study Design	Number of Patients	RT Dose	Fractionation Schema	Median Survival (mo)	Rate of Grade 3 or Higher Toxicity (%)
Bujold et al,[5] 2013	Prospective	56	24–54 Gy	6 fractions	44% (1-y OS)	36[a]
Xi et al,[26] 2013	Retrospective	41	30–48 Gy	6 fractions	13	2.4
Rim et al,[27] 2012	Retrospective	45	38–65 Gy	1.8–2.5 Gy/fraction	11.2	2
Yoon et al,[28] 2012	Retrospective	412	21–60 Gy (with TACE)	2–5 Gy/fraction	10.6	10
Chuma et al,[29] 2011	Retrospective	20	30–48 Gy	7–16 fractions	12	15
Sugahara et al,[30] 2009	Retrospective	35	55 GyE–77 GyE (protons)	2.2–5.5 GyE/fraction	22	8.6
Huang et al,[31] 2009	Retrospective	326	60 Gy	2–3 Gy/fraction	4	0

[a] Grade 3+ toxicity reported for all patients.

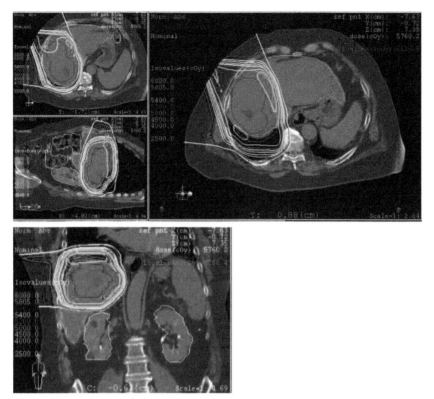

Fig. 2. Representative slice from a proton radiation treatment plan for a patient with unresectable HCC treated to a planned total of 58 Gy in 15 fractions.

With respect to proton RT, numerous single-institutional series have been published evaluating its efficacy and toxicity for treatment of HCC. The largest experience of proton beam RT for treatment of HCC comes from the University of Tsukuba, who reviewed outcomes of 318 patients treated between 2001 and 2007. Three radiation dose schemes were used, depending on tumor location. Most patients treated on the study were Child-Pugh class A. A total dose of 77.5 GyE in 35 fractions was used for tumors within 2 cm of digestive organs, 72.6 GyE in 22 fractions was used for tumors within 2 cm of the porta hepatis, and 66 GyE in 10 fractions was delivered to peripheral tumors more than 2 cm from the digestive tract and porta hepatis. With a median follow-up of 19 months, 3-year and 5-year overall survival was 64.7% and 44.6%, respectively. Baseline hepatic function, tumor classification, performance status, and size of planning tumor volume were all independently associated with overall survival. Treatment-related toxicity was minimal, with no treatment-related deaths and only 5 patients developing grade 3 toxicity (4 skin toxicity, 1 gastrointestinal toxicity). Approximately 20% of patients went on to receive at least 1 or more additional courses of proton RT, with 5-year overall survival of 51%.[33]

More recently, Bush and colleagues[34] published a phase 2 prospective trial of 76 patients treated at Loma Linda University with proton RT for HCC. Fifty-four percent of patients were outside the Milan criteria, 24% with Child-Pugh class C, and 16% had MELD (Model for End-Stage Liver Disease) score greater than 15; therefore, patients in this study represented relatively advanced stage HCC, with many patients with decompensated liver disease. All patients received 63 Gy delivered in 4.2-Gy daily fractions for 15 fractions over a 3-week period. A median progression-free survival time of 36 months was reported, with significantly improved progression-free survival for patients within the Milan criteria. Twenty percent of patients developed local treatment failure, which occurred at an average onset of 18 months (range, 2–60 months). As in other series, distant intrahepatic failure was the predominant pattern of failure. Similar to the Tsukuba experience, treatment was extremely well tolerated, with no grade 3 toxicity. Five patients experienced gastrointestinal bleeding, which was medically managed effectively. Based on these studies, proton therapy has shown early evidence of favorable safety and encouraging antitumor activity for patients with unresectable HCC.

There has been limited prospective experience of carbon ion in the treatment of HCC. In 2004, Kato and colleagues[35] published promising results from the first prospective study of carbon ion RT for HCC. The dose escalation schema consisted of 15 fractions delivered with increasing total doses starting at 49.5 Gy (relative biological effectiveness [RBE]) up to 79.5 Gy (RBE). These investigators reported 1- year and 5-year local control rates of 92% and 81%, respectively. Based on their phase 1 study, the investigators suggested an overall dose of 72 Gy (RBE) to optimize local tumor control, with minimization of treatment-related toxicities.[35] More recently, the University of Heidelberg has reported their phase 1 clinical experience of 6 patients with 7 HCC lesions treated with hypofractionated RT (4 × 10 Gy). At time of publication, with a median follow-up of 11 months, they reported 100% local control, with 4 lesions showing a PR and the remaining 3 lesions remaining stable.[36]

Only 1 series has retrospectively compared the efficacy of proton beam and carbon ion RT. Komatsu and colleagues[37] published their large retrospective analysis of 343 consecutive patients treated with either proton RT (n = 242) or carbon ion therapy (n = 101) on 12 different prospective treatment protocols at the Hyogo Ion Beam Medical Center in Kobe, Japan. Among patients treated with proton RT, these investigators reported 5-year local control and overall survival rates of 90.2% and 38%, respectively. Among patients treated with carbon ion, the 5-year local control and survival rates were 93% and 36.3%. Late toxicities of grade 3 or higher were observed in 8 patients on proton RT and in 4 patients on carbon ion therapy, and 4 of 12 patients were diagnosed with RILD. When analyzed by radiation modalities, there was no difference in overall survival or local control between these 2 therapies. Although results were retrospective, proton and carbon ion therapies for HCC were comparable in terms of long-term outcomes. These promising studies suggest that charged ion RT is a potentially effective treatment strategy for treatment of primary liver tumors. However, future prospective clinical studies and cost-effective analyses are necessary to provide a more robust evaluation of efficacy, toxicity, and cost for photon, proton, and carbon ion RT.

BRIDGE TO TRANSPLANT

For patients with advanced HCC who are potential candidates for liver transplantation, local therapy, in the form of either RFA or TACE, have traditionally been considered potential bridging therapies to transplantation. Numerous recently published single-institutional reports have now suggested a role for CRT as a potential bridging therapy. Sandroussi and colleagues[38] recently published the University of Toronto experience of 10 patients listed for liver transplantation in whom either previous local therapies had failed or who were not believed to be suitable for standard local therapies because of poor liver function or suboptimal anatomy. With a median dose of

33 Gy administered in 1 to 6 fractions, no treated tumors progressed during or after treatment. In-field tumor control was achieved with all patients, 7 of 9 tumors showing 10% to 50% tumor regression. Of the 5 patients who went for liver transplantation, no complications were attributed to the liver radiation. Explant pathology, available for all 5 patients, was notable for tumor necrosis and fibrosis, ranging from 40% to 90%. With a median follow-up of 14 months, all transplanted patients remained cancer free.

Similarly, in the reported phase 2 proton experience from Loma Linda University, Bush and colleagues[34] discussed the outcome of 18 patients who underwent liver transplantation after treatment. With an average time from treatment to transplantation of 13 months, the 3-year survival was 70%. Pathologic examination of explanted livers showed 33% pathologic CR, with no residual gross or microscopic HCC. In addition, 39% of patients had residual microscopic disease, and 28% of patients had gross residual disease. Facciuto and colleagues[39] recently reported of 27 patients with HCC treated at Mount Sinai University with SBRT as a bridging therapy to liver transplant. Of the 17 patients who went on to liver transplantation, based on pathologic evaluation, 37% were responders, including 14% with CR, 23% with PR, and 63% with no response. A series from Baylor Medical Center reported similar rates of pathologic response, with a CR noted in 27% of explanted tumors. Microscopic and macroscopic residual was appreciated in 27% and 54% of tumors, respectively.[40] These series suggest that liver SBRT for HCC may be a safe and alternative treatment option in patients with HCC and cirrhosis awaiting transplantation.

COMBINATION THERAPY
Sorafenib and Radiation Therapy

Despite high rates of local control after SBRT, distant liver failure remains the predominant site of failure for patients with HCC. Sorafenib (Nexavar) is a small-molecule multikinase inhibitor that targets tumor-cell proliferation and tumor angiogenesis by inhibiting the Raf/MAPK/ERK signaling pathway and the receptor tyrosine kinase of vascular endothelial growth factor receptors 1, 2, and 3 and platelet-derived growth factor receptor β. The SHARP trial established sorafenib as an active systemic agent in the treatment of advanced HCC, conferring an improvement in median survival of 2.8 months compared with placebo.[3] Recent in vitro and in vivo studies suggest that low-dose sorafenib may act as a radiosensitizer in HCC cells via downregulation of STAT3 phosphorylation.[41] One retrospective review studied 23 patients with advanced HCC treated in Taiwan with radiation therapy and sunitinib (a tyrosine kinase inhibitor with a similar mechanism to sorafenib), given at least 1 week before and 2 weeks after radiation therapy. With a median radiation dose of 52.5 Gy in 15 fractions, the objective response rate was 74%. The 1-year survival rate was 70%, with maintenance sunitinib being the most significant prognostic factor for survival. Based on these results, the investigators concluded that conformal hypofractionated RT and sunitinib could be delivered safely in patients with HCC.[42] However, data from an early phase 1 study from the University of Toronto combining a 6-fraction SBRT with escalating doses of sorafenib before, during, and after RT suggested that higher doses of sorafenib (400 mg daily) when combined with radiation delivered to a higher effective liver volume (Veff 30%–60%), may yield significant grade 3+ toxicity. RTOG 1112 is an ongoing phase 3 study of sorafenib versus SBRT followed by sorafenib in HCC. In this study, sorafenib will be delivered after completion of radiation, rather than concurrently with radiation, to reduce the risk of treatment toxicity.

TACE and Radiation Therapy

Because PVTT is a major obstacle to performing TACE, there has been interest in combining RT and TACE. RT targeted to the PVTT may decrease intravascular tumor growth and maintain portal blood flow, allowing the maintenance of normal liver blood flow, further limiting intrahepatic tumor spread, and thereby potentially allowing for additional TACE.[43,44] Zhang and colleagues[45] performed a retrospective analysis evaluating the benefit of the addition of RT to percutaneous transhepatic portal vein stenting (PTPVS) and TACE among 45 patients with HCC complicated by main portal vein tumor thrombus. With an objective response rate of 35.6%, the investigators reported that the addition of radiation therapy was associated with significantly higher rates of stent patency rates and longer mean patency times. Radiation therapy after PTPVS-TACE was also associated with improved 1-year survival of 32% versus 6.9% (P<.01), suggesting that sequential therapy by PTPVS-TACE-3D-CRT is possibly an effective treatment modality for HCC complicated by main portal vein tumor thrombus.[45] Similarly, a recent series from Korea suggested the potential benefit of TACE and RT for stabilizing or improving PVTT in patients with advanced HCC. In this series, patients identified with PVTT underwent TACE followed by 3D-CRT 2 to 3 weeks after completion of TACE. For most patients, the gross target volume included the PVTT and a 2-cm to 3-cm margin into the contiguous HCC as determined by dynamic enhanced CT or magnetic resonance imaging. On follow-up scans performed 2 to 3 months after completion of radiation therapy, the objective response rate of PVTT was 39.6% and the progression-free rate of PVTT was 85.6%.[28] It is hoped that future studies including randomized clinical trials will further elucidate the relative benefit of each of these treatment modalities.

PRIMARY ICC

Because of extensive involvement of the primary tumor and predisposition for distant metastases, less than 30% of patients with ICC present with resectable disease. ICC is a rare, locally aggressive cancer, and surgical resection is the only known curative therapy. Most patients present with unresectable disease. Similarly to HCC, nonsurgical options for patients with unresectable or recurrent disease include chemotherapy, external-beam RT (EBRT), TACE, RFA, although the last 2 techniques are less well studied with ICC. Despite treatment with EBRT, patients frequently fail within the treatment field, suggesting the potential for a role for dose escalation.

Few published studies have solely addressed the efficacy of RT for treatment of primary ICC. More frequently, these tumors have been included in prospective studies that enroll all liver tumors, with a preponderance of HCC. As mentioned earlier, a phase 2 study of conformal hyperfractionated radiation therapy with concurrent hepatic arterial fluorodeoxyuridine from the University of Michigan[11] included 46 patients with ICC. Compared with historical controls, patients with ICC had significantly improved overall survival with median survival of 13.3 months.

Even more recently, the Mayo Clinic reported the outcomes of 10 patients with ICC treated with abdominal SBRT, although this study included primary unresectable and recurrent disease. Sites treated included liver (n = 10), abdominal lymph nodes (n = 1), and adrenal gland (n = 1). The median prescription dose was 55 Gy, administered in 3 or 5 consecutive daily fractions over 1 week. With a median follow-up of 14 months, local control was 100%, although 4 patients developed distant intrahepatic failure. Two patients experienced serious late toxicities: one required placement of a biliary stent for grade 3 biliary stenosis, and another developed grade 5 liver failure.[46] Therefore, based on initial promising data, SBRT seems to be a safe, effective, and noninvasive treatment option for carefully selected patients with unresectable ICC. The role of radiation therapy needs to be prospectively validated in large, multi-institutional studies.

FUTURE DIRECTION

Radiation therapy is re-emerging as a potentially effective treatment of locally advanced, unresectable HCC. Outcomes from early experiences of prospective studies seem promising, with improved survival compared with historical controls. Cure of early stage and unresectable HCC may be possible with high-quality radiation therapy. Many questions remain, including determination of the ideal radiation dose and fractionation schema, optimal patient selection criteria based on tumor size, tumor location, extent of vascular involvement, and baseline liver function, and the role of radiation therapy compared with other localized standard treatments, including RFA or TACE. Advancements in functional imaging may further aid with targeting the most resistant portions of the tumor by administering concomitant radiation boost to those regions and also permit relative sparing for uninvolved liver. Further investigation to identify strategies that may further minimize liver-related toxicity will be increasingly important as the role of radiation therapy to the liver expands.

Despite a renewed interest globally in radiation therapy in the treatment of locally advanced HCC, RT has not been incorporated into international HCC treatment consensus guidelines because of the lack of level I evidence. Large, multi-institutional, prospective, phase 3 studies are needed to definitively establish the benefit of radiation therapy. To this end, RTOG 1112, a phase 3, randomized cooperative group trial study of sorafenib versus SBRT followed by sorafenib in locally advanced HCC, is open to accrual. In addition, dedicated early phase trials should further investigate the role of liver directed radiation therapy for Child-Pugh class B patients.

Although promising, the data regarding the efficacy and tolerability of hypofractionated radiation therapy for the treatment of ICC are still in its nascent stages. Radiation therapy may provide meaningful local biliary tumor control; however, hypofractionated regimens may incur the risk of significant biliary toxicity. Future studies are necessary to further define the ideal patient selection criteria and optimal dose fractionation schema for patients with ICC.

REFERENCES

1. Llovet JM, Real MI, Montana X, et al. Arterial embolisation or chemoembolisation versus symptomatic treatment in patients with unresectable hepatocellular carcinoma: a randomised controlled trial. Lancet 2002;359(9319):1734–9.
2. Lo CM, Ngan H, Tso WK, et al. Randomized controlled trial of transarterial lipiodol chemoembolization for unresectable hepatocellular carcinoma. Hepatology 2002;35(5):1164–71.
3. Llovet JM, Ricci S, Mazzaferro V, et al. Sorafenib in advanced hepatocellular carcinoma. N Engl J Med 2008;359(4):378–90.
4. Tse RV, Hawkins M, Lockwood G, et al. Phase I study of individualized stereotactic body radiotherapy for hepatocellular carcinoma and intrahepatic cholangiocarcinoma. J Clin Oncol 2008;26(4):657–64.
5. Bujold A, Massey CA, Kim JJ, et al. Sequential phase I and II trials of stereotactic body radiotherapy for locally advanced hepatocellular carcinoma. J Clin Oncol 2013;31(13):1631–9.

6. Klein J, Dawson LA. Hepatocellular carcinoma radiation therapy: review of evidence and future opportunities. Int J Radiat Oncol Biol Phys 2013;87(1):22–32.
7. Ingold JA, Reed GB, Kaplan HS, et al. Radiation hepatitis. Am J Roentgenol Radium Ther Nucl Med 1965;93:200–8.
8. Russell AH, Clyde C, Wasserman TH, et al. Accelerated hyperfractionated hepatic irradiation in the management of patients with liver metastases: results of the RTOG dose escalating protocol. Int J Radiat Oncol Biol Phys 1993;27(1):117–23.
9. Dawson LA, Normolle D, Balter JM, et al. Analysis of radiation-induced liver disease using the Lyman NTCP model. Int J Radiat Oncol Biol Phys 2002;53(4): 810–21.
10. Lawrence TS, Tesser RJ, ten Haken RK. An application of dose volume histograms to the treatment of intrahepatic malignancies with radiation therapy. Int J Radiat Oncol Biol Phys 1990;19(4):1041–7.
11. Ben-Josef E, Normolle D, Ensminger WD, et al. Phase II trial of high-dose conformal radiation therapy with concurrent hepatic artery floxuridine for unresectable intrahepatic malignancies. J Clin Oncol 2005;23(34):8739–47.
12. Robertson JM, Lawrence TS, Dworzanin LM, et al. Treatment of primary hepatobiliary cancers with conformal radiation therapy and regional chemotherapy. J Clin Oncol 1993;11(7):1286–93.
13. Mornex F, Girard N, Beziat C, et al. Feasibility and efficacy of high-dose three-dimensional-conformal radiotherapy in cirrhotic patients with small-size hepatocellular carcinoma non-eligible for curative therapies–mature results of the French Phase II RTF-1 trial. Int J Radiat Oncol Biol Phys 2006;66(4):1152–8.
14. Seong J, Lee IJ, Shim SJ, et al. A multicenter retrospective cohort study of practice patterns and clinical outcome on radiotherapy for hepatocellular carcinoma in Korea. Liver Int 2009;29(2):147–52.
15. Blomgren H, Lax I, Naslund I, et al. Stereotactic high dose fraction radiation therapy of extracranial tumors using an accelerator. Clinical experience of the first thirty-one patients. Acta Oncol 1995;34(6):861–70.
16. Andolino DL, Johnson CS, Maluccio M, et al. Stereotactic body radiotherapy for primary hepatocellular carcinoma. Int J Radiat Oncol Biol Phys 2011;81(4): e447–53.
17. Cardenes HR, Price TR, Perkins SM, et al. Phase I feasibility trial of stereotactic body radiation therapy for primary hepatocellular carcinoma. Clin Transl Oncol 2010;12(3):218–25.
18. Kwon JH, Bae SH, Kim JY, et al. Long-term effect of stereotactic body radiation therapy for primary hepatocellular carcinoma ineligible for local ablation therapy or surgical resection. Stereotactic radiotherapy for liver cancer. BMC Cancer 2010;10:475.
19. Seo YS, Kim MS, Yoo SY, et al. Preliminary result of stereotactic body radiotherapy as a local salvage treatment for inoperable hepatocellular carcinoma. J Surg Oncol 2010;102(3):209–14.
20. Méndez Romero A, Wunderink W, Hussain SM, et al. Stereotactic body radiation therapy for primary and metastatic liver tumors: a single institution phase I–II study. Acta Oncol 2006;45(7):831–7.
21. Bruix J, Sherman M, Llovet JM, et al. Clinical management of hepatocellular carcinoma. Conclusions of the Barcelona-2000 EASL conference. European Association for the Study of the Liver. J Hepatol 2001;35(3):421–30.
22. Forner A, Ayuso C, Varela M, et al. Evaluation of tumor response after locoregional therapies in hepatocellular carcinoma: are response evaluation criteria in solid tumors reliable? Cancer 2009;115(3):616–23.

23. Price TR, Perkins SM, Sandrasegaran K, et al. Evaluation of response after stereotactic body radiotherapy for hepatocellular carcinoma. Cancer 2012; 118(12):3191–8.
24. Llovet JM, Bustamante J, Castells A, et al. Natural history of untreated nonsurgical hepatocellular carcinoma: rationale for the design and evaluation of therapeutic trials. Hepatology 1999;29(1):62–7.
25. Takagi H, Takayama H, Yamada S, et al. Radiation therapy of hepatocellular carcinoma. Nihon Shokakibyo Gakkai Zasshi 1989;86(2):237–45 [in Japanese].
26. Xi M, Zhang L, Zhao L, et al. Effectiveness of stereotactic body radiotherapy for hepatocellular carcinoma with portal vein and/or inferior vena cava tumor thrombosis. PLoS One 2013;8(5):e63864.
27. Rim CH, Yang DS, Park YJ, et al. Effectiveness of high-dose three-dimensional conformal radiotherapy in hepatocellular carcinoma with portal vein thrombosis. Jpn J Clin Oncol 2012;42(8):721–9.
28. Yoon SM, Lim YS, Won HJ, et al. Radiotherapy plus transarterial chemoembolization for hepatocellular carcinoma invading the portal vein: long-term patient outcomes. Int J Radiat Oncol Biol Phys 2012;82(5):2004–11.
29. Chuma M, Taguchi H, Yamamoto Y, et al. Efficacy of therapy for advanced hepatocellular carcinoma: intra-arterial 5-fluorouracil and subcutaneous interferon with image-guided radiation. J Gastroenterol Hepatol 2011;26(7):1123–32.
30. Sugahara S, Nakayama H, Fukuda K, et al. Proton-beam therapy for hepatocellular carcinoma associated with portal vein tumor thrombosis. Strahlenther Onkol 2009;185(12):782–8.
31. Huang YJ, Hsu HC, Wang CY, et al. The treatment responses in cases of radiation therapy to portal vein thrombosis in advanced hepatocellular carcinoma. Int J Radiat Oncol Biol Phys 2009;73(4):1155–63.
32. Lin CS, Jen YM, Chiu SY, et al. Treatment of portal vein tumor thrombosis of hepatoma patients with either stereotactic radiotherapy or three-dimensional conformal radiotherapy. Jpn J Clin Oncol 2006;36(4):212–7.
33. Nakayama H, Sugahara S, Tokita M, et al. Proton beam therapy for hepatocellular carcinoma: the University of Tsukuba experience. Cancer 2009;115(23): 5499–506.
34. Bush DA, Kayali Z, Grove R, et al. The safety and efficacy of high-dose proton beam radiotherapy for hepatocellular carcinoma: a phase 2 prospective trial. Cancer 2011;117(13):3053–9.
35. Kato H, Tsujii H, Miyamoto T, et al. Results of the first prospective study of carbon ion radiotherapy for hepatocellular carcinoma with liver cirrhosis. Int J Radiat Oncol Biol Phys 2004;59(5):1468–76.
36. Habermehl D, Debus J, Ganten T, et al. Hypofractionated carbon ion therapy delivered with scanned ion beams for patients with hepatocellular carcinoma–feasibility and clinical response. Radiat Oncol 2013;8:59.
37. Komatsu S, Fukumoto T, Demizu Y, et al. Clinical results and risk factors of proton and carbon ion therapy for hepatocellular carcinoma. Cancer 2011;117(21):4890–904.
38. Sandroussi C, Dawson LA, Lee M, et al. Radiotherapy as a bridge to liver transplantation for hepatocellular carcinoma. Transpl Int 2010;23(3):299–306.
39. Facciuto ME, Singh MK, Rochon C, et al. Stereotactic body radiation therapy in hepatocellular carcinoma and cirrhosis: evaluation of radiological and pathological response. J Surg Oncol 2012;105(7):692–8.
40. O'Connor JK, Trotter J, Davis GL, et al. Long-term outcomes of stereotactic body radiation therapy in the treatment of hepatocellular cancer as a bridge to transplantation. Liver Transpl 2012;18(8):949–54.

41. Huang CY, Lin CS, Tai WT, et al. Sorafenib enhances radiation-induced apoptosis in hepatocellular carcinoma by inhibiting STAT3. Int J Radiat Oncol Biol Phys 2013;86(3):456–62.

42. Chi KH, Liao CS, Chang CC, et al. Angiogenic blockade and radiotherapy in hepatocellular carcinoma. Int J Radiat Oncol Biol Phys 2010;78(1):188–93.

43. Yamada K, Izaki K, Sugimoto K, et al. Prospective trial of combined transcatheter arterial chemoembolization and three-dimensional conformal radiotherapy for portal vein tumor thrombus in patients with unresectable hepatocellular carcinoma. Int J Radiat Oncol Biol Phys 2003;57(1):113–9.

44. Zeng ZC, Fan J, Tang ZY, et al. A comparison of treatment combinations with and without radiotherapy for hepatocellular carcinoma with portal vein and/or inferior vena cava tumor thrombus. Int J Radiat Oncol Biol Phys 2005;61(2):432–43.

45. Zhang XB, Wang JH, Yan ZP, et al. Hepatocellular carcinoma with main portal vein tumor thrombus: treatment with 3-dimensional conformal radiotherapy after portal vein stenting and transarterial chemoembolization. Cancer 2009;115(6): 1245–52.

46. Barney BM, Olivier KR, Miller RC, et al. Clinical outcomes and toxicity using stereotactic body radiotherapy (SBRT) for advanced cholangiocarcinoma. Radiat Oncol 2012;7:67.

Systemic and Targeted Therapy for Biliary Tract Tumors and Primary Liver Tumors

Melanie Byrne Thomas, MD

KEYWORDS

- Bile duct cancer cholangiocarcinoma • Hepatocellular carcinoma
- Systemic therapy • Chemotherapy • Targeted therapies

KEY POINTS

- There are limited effective chemotherapy options that have shown clinical benefit for patients with metastatic bile duct and hepatocellular carcinoma.
- Cancers of the biliary tract and primary tumors of the liver are challenging malignancies to treat in the advanced disease setting. These tumors are known as being chemotherapy resistant, as is well documented in the numerous negative clinical trials that have been conducted using conventional cytotoxic chemotherapy agents.
- There is emerging understanding of the unique biology of hepatobiliary cancers that will lead to development of targeted anticancer therapies for hepatobiliary cancers.

INTRODUCTION

Most patients with cancer of the bile ducts and liver eventually develop advanced disease that is not treatable with surgery, radiation therapy, or other liver-directed treatment options. These patients seek systemic therapy hoping for prolonged survival and palliation of tumor-related symptoms such as pain, anorexia, ascites, and fatigue. A large number of clinical trials have been conducted over several decades to evaluate a variety of chemotherapy agents in both tumor types. However, few chemotherapy regimens have produced level-1 evidence of clinical benefit to patients.

THE CHALLENGES OF DEVELOPING AN EFFECTIVE SYSTEMIC THERAPY FOR ADVANCED BILIARY TRACT AND LIVER CANCERS

When evaluating systemic therapy for solid tumors, there are several factors that affect the design of clinical trials, selection of study end points, and the agents to be studied. The factors relevant to biliary tract cancer are summarized in this article.

Hollings Cancer Center, College of Medicine, Medical University of South Carolina, 86 Jonathan Lucas Street, Charleston, SC 29425, USA
E-mail address: thomasmb@musc.edu

Surg Oncol Clin N Am 23 (2014) 369–381
http://dx.doi.org/10.1016/j.soc.2013.11.004
1055-3207/14/$ – see front matter © 2014 Elsevier Inc. All rights reserved.

Clinical Behavior

As is the case in many solid tumors, but particularly in cholangiocarcinoma, a wide range of tumor behavior is observed. Many of these tumors display indolent clinical behavior, may remain stable for many months, and seem to grow slowly and progress over years rather than months. These indolent intrahepatic cholangiocarcinomas (ICCs) often do not cause tumor-related symptoms until the tumor burden is extensive. Other cholangiocarcinomas have a more aggressive phenotype, progress rapidly, and result in more tumor-related morbidity.[1]

Imaging Characteristics

Tumors of the bile ducts appear radiographically in 2 general forms: the mass-forming ICCs appear as low-attenuation masses with irregular peripheral enhancement, and may be accompanied by liver capsule retraction, satellite nodules, and peripheral intrahepatic ductal dilatation. The periductal infiltrating cholangiocarcinomas are characterized by growth along dilated or narrowed bile ducts without mass formation.[2] Both ICC and extrahepatic cholangiocarcinoma (EHCC) are highly desmoplastic tumors and tend to spread along bile duct walls and periductal tissue, which makes them challenging to image adequately with conventional imaging techniques in order to establish a baseline and assess radiographic tumor response.[3–8]

Tumor Biology

The putative cell of origin in ICC and EHCC, the cholangiocytes, are multifunctional proproliferative cells. Cholangiocytes produce stimulatory cytokines (including transforming growth factor, interleukin-6, platelet-derived growth factor, tumor necrosis factor) as part of both autocrine and paracrine modulatory pathways. They mediate inflammation in the liver, which is known to play a key role in the initiation and maintenance of carcinogenesis.[9,10] The liver-cholangiocyte microenvironment is thought to be procarcinogenic. Cholangiocytes are also able to detoxify foreign substances as a normal cellular function, and thus are inherently chemotherapy resistant.[11–13]

Patient Comorbid Conditions

Patients with malignancies of the bile ducts or hepatocytes commonly have underlying liver disease that contributes in varying degrees to the initiation and progression of these cancers, as well as to whether the patient is a reasonable candidate for palliative systemic therapy. Comorbid liver-related conditions include fibrosis, cirrhosis, portal hypertension, altered drug metabolism, coagulopathy, hypoalbuminemia, thrombocytopenia, and ascites.

Cirrhosis can have a profound impact on tolerance and efficacy of anticancer drug therapy. The liver is central to the metabolism of most foreign and endogenous substances in the body. Hepatic metabolism involves oxidative pathways, primarily via the cytochrome P (CYP) 450 enzyme system, and additional metabolic steps, which include conjugation to a glucuronide, a sulfate, or glutathione. In cirrhosis, the total liver cell mass is reduced and distortion of the microcirculation of the liver and collagen deposition lead to impaired sinusoidal transport and reduced extraction of protein-bound substances. Hepatic cirrhosis not only decreases drug metabolizing enzyme activity but also alters the absorption, plasma protein binding, distribution, and renal excretion of drugs. Intrahepatic vascular shunts that develop as a consequence of cirrhosis allow drugs to be routed around hepatocytes, thus decreasing their first-pass extraction. However, all routes of hepatic metabolism are not equally impaired.

As hepatic dysfunction progresses in cirrhotic patients, reduced synthesis of albumin occurs and leads to a decrease in the plasma protein binding of drugs. In the setting of hypoalbuminemia, for drugs that are more than 90% protein bound, the increase in the free drug fraction may have substantial clinical consequences. The CYP3A4 subfamily, the most common hepatic enzyme in adult humans, oxidizes more than 50% of currently used drugs. Several studies have shown significant decreases in the CYP3A protein levels in patients with cirrhosis, although contradictory data do exist. Therefore, it is difficult to predict the disposition of a drug in liver disease, and each agent must be studied individually to provide a rationale for adjusting doses.

SYSTEMIC THERAPY FOR BILIARY TRACT CANCERS: STATE OF THE CLINICAL SCIENCE

A large number of clinical trials of chemotherapy using single agents, doublets, and multidrug combinations have been published in recent years. Most trials were conducted to ascertain whether chemotherapy can provide clinical benefit to patients with advanced cancer of the biliary tract, in terms of palliation of tumor-related symptoms or increased survival. Most trials have been small, single-arm studies that commonly evaluate tumor response rate at the primary end point. For trials that follow the RECIST (Response Evaluation Criteria in Solid Tumors) 1.1 guidelines, tumor response is defined as complete response (disappearance of all target lesions) or partial response (at least a 30% decrease in the sum of diameters of target lesions, taking as reference the baseline sum diameters).[14] Tumor response is an indication of antitumor activity, but may not correlate with clinical benefit to patients with advanced disease. A few prospective chemotherapy clinical trials have included subgroup analyses to ascertain whether there are differences in clinical outcome based on ICC, EHCC, or gallbladder cancer. However, because of the many challenges in conducting prospective clinical trials in these patients, there have not yet been separate trials in ICC and EHCC, or trials that are stratified by tumor location that are adequately powered to identify differences in chemotherapy benefit. Selected studies are summarized in **Table 1**.

In April 2010, the Advanced Biliary Cancer (ABC)-02 trial was published, and this was the first phase III, randomized controlled trial in subjects with advanced biliary tract cancer. The ABC-02 trial compared doublet therapy consisting of gemcitabine and cisplatin with single-agent gemcitabine in 410 patients with locally advanced or metastatic biliary tract cancer. The combination of gemcitabine plus cisplatin showed improved progression-free survival (PFS) and overall survival (OS) compared with gemcitabine alone. In this trial, 59% (241 patients) had bile duct tumors, but the site of disease within the bile duct was not specified. After a median follow-up of 8.2 months, the combination group had significantly improved OS (11.7 vs 8.1 months).[15] This regimen is currently considered the standard-of-care, first-line therapy for patients with advanced cancer of the bile ducts and gallbladder. The results of the ABC-02 trial have prompted many investigators to conduct trials in the second-line setting, as well as of novel targeted anticancer agents based on existing understanding of the molecular carcinogenesis of biliary tract cancers.

ADVANCING TREATMENT OF BILIARY TRACT CANCER BY INCORPORATING TARGETED THERAPIES INTO CLINICAL TRIALS

There remains a significant unmet medical need to develop effective and safe systemic therapy regimens for patients with advanced cholangiocarcinoma. The 2 main areas of unmet clinical need are to extend the benefit of gemcitabine and cisplatin, potentially by adding one or more targeted agents to the combination, and to develop

Table 1
Selected cytotoxic chemotherapy regimens for biliary tract cancer

Regimen	Study Phase	Sample Size	Response Rate (%)	PFS TTP (mo)	Overall Survival (mo)
Gemcitabine plus cisplatin vs gemcitabine[15]	III	410	81[a]	8.0	11.7
			71	5.0	8.1
Gemcitabine[16]	II	24	13	—	7.2
Gemcitabine plus 5-fluorouracil[17]	II	42	1	—	9.7
Gemcitabine plus S-1[18]	II	35	34.3	TTP 5.9	11.6
Gemcitabine plus cisplatin[19]	II	43	28	—	8.4
Gemcitabine plus capecitabine[20]	II	45	31	—	14
GEMOX[21]	II	53	18.9	PFS 4.8	8.3
GEMOX plus cetuximab[22]	II	30	63	—	11.6
CAPEOX[23]	II	65	37 (GB, ECC)	—	12.8
			0 (ICC)		16.8
Capecitabine[24]	II	26	19	—	8.1
FOLFIRI[25]	II	30	10	PFS:	OS:
		17 ICC		3	5.9
		13 GB		5.9	9.75

Abbreviations: CAPEOX, oxaliplatin plus capecitabine; FOLFIRI, 5-fluorouracil plus leucovorin plus irinotecan; GB, gallbladder; GEMOX, gemcitabine plus oxaliplatin; PFS, progression-free survival; TTP, time to progression.
  [a] Tumor control rate = stable disease + partial response + complete response.

effective regimens for patients who have failed first-line chemotherapy. However, the numerous single-arm clinical trials in advanced biliary tract cancer conducted over the previous 2 decades have made little progress.[26,27] Some trials of single-agent targeted therapies, and combinations with cytotoxic agents, have been reported, as listed in **Table 2**.

The foremost task in biliary tract cancer research is to improve understanding of the key molecular carcinogenetic mechanisms, with a focus on identifying the oncogenic driver mechanisms or mutations. **Table 3** summarizes several of the potential therapeutic targets in biliary tract cancer that have been identified and, in some cases, evaluated in preclinical models. Given the high cost, the time required to complete, and low yield of empirical clinical trials, it is essential that a better understanding of the potential efficacy of new agents and combinations be obtained in the preclinical setting. In order to identify potential relevant molecular targets(s) or combinations of targets in ICC and/or EHCC, some concepts are particularly important:

- The results from measuring overexpression of a potential molecular target are highly variable depending on the quality of tumor specimen analyzed.
- Consistent overexpression of a receptor or a protein does not guarantee that it is a driver mechanism in the cancer or an actionable target for drug development.
- Screening of potential new agents and combinations in cholangiocarcinoma cell lines, of which there are few, is one step in assessing new therapeutics. However, cell lines have lost many characteristics of the original tumor and thus have significant limitations in predicting behavior of human tumors.

Table 2
Clinical trials of targeted therapies for biliary tract cancer

Regimen	Study Phase	Sample Size	Response Rate (%)	PFS TTP (mo)	Overall Survival (mo)
Bevacizumab plus erlotinib[28]	II	49	18.4	TTP 4.4	9.9
Sorafenib[29]	II	31	—	3	9
Sorafenib[30]	II	46	0	PFS 3	9
Lapatinib[31]	II	17	—	PFS 1.8	5.2
Selumetinib[32]	II	28	12	3.7	9.8
Erlotinib[33]	II	42	8	—	7.5
GEMOX plus Panitumumab[34]	II	46	33	PFS 8.3	10.0
GEMOX vs	RIII	133	29	PFS 4.2	9.5
GEMOX plus erlotinib[35]	First line	135	15.7	PFS 5.8	9.5
Sunitinib[36]	II, 2nd line	56	8.9	1.7	4.8
GEMOX plus bevacizumab[37]	II, 1st line	35	40	7	12.7

- Development of new anticancer drugs in cholangiocarcinoma must use appropriate preclinical models. The ideal models include the role of the tumor microenvironment.[40,43,73]
- Genetic and genomic profiling using powerful bioinformatics techniques holds the promise of identifying validated molecular targets in both populations and individuals that provide rationales for determining suitable targets for drugs in ICC and EHCC.
- Future clinical trials should stratify by tumor location, if targets differ by site, and enrich the trial patient population by the target of interest.

Several recent studies that used advanced molecular analytical approaches to ICC have provided insight into molecular classifications of these tumors than can inform the development of rationales for future clinical trials in this malignancy. Llovet and colleagues[68] identified 2 classes of cholangiocarcinoma through genomic identification of significant targets in cancer (GISTIC) analysis of specimens from 149 subjects. The categories, including a proliferative class and inflammatory class, had different gene signatures, activated oncogenic pathways, and clinical outcomes. This work represents important progress in developing therapeutic biomarkers in cholangiocarcinoma.

SYSTEMIC THERAPY FOR HEPATOCELLULAR CARCINOMA: CURRENT MANAGEMENT

Hepatocellular carcinoma (HCC) is a heterogeneous malignancy in terms of cause and molecular carcinogenesis. HCCs are clinically chemotherapy-resistant tumors, and this observation is supported by low response rates across a wide variety of chemotherapy agents. Cytotoxic chemotherapy agents have shown no clinical benefit to patients with HCC, and can be toxic in individuals with underlying liver dysfunction. Over the course of the previous decades, numerous clinical trials of a wide variety of chemotherapeutic and hormonal agents had shown little or no activity in this complex malignancy.

Table 3
Novel targeted agents with preclinical rationale for the treatment of biliary tract cancer

Pathway/Target	Rationale	Outcome
EGFR plus VEGF inhibition	Both EGFR and VEGF overexpression common in cholangiocarcinoma	Vandetanib, dual VEGF2/EGFR inhibitor significantly decreased in cell lines and xenografts[38,39]
PDGF	Myofibroblasts are abundant in cholangiocarcinoma microenvironment and display procarcinogenic crosstalk with cancer cells, mediated partly by PDGF-B[40–42]	Cytotoxic agent navitoclax induced apoptosis in CAF in a cholangiocarcinoma rat model[43]
EGFR	ERB1 and ERB2 overexpression are prominent in biliary tract.[44–48] Activating mutations rate very low[49]	Several preclinical studies suggest benefit of therapeutic efficacy with EGFR inhibitors[50]
COX	COX plays important role in biliary cancer cell signaling[51–54]	COX-2 inhibitor NS-398 showed dose-dependent growth inhibition in rat model of cholangiocarcinoma[55]
VEGF expression	VEGF expression linked to poor prognostic features and decreased survival[29,30,38,56–58]	Some suggestion of clinical benefit shown in single-arm clinical trials[29,30,37,58,59]
MEK ERK	MEK is critical element of Ras/Raf/MEK/ERK signal transduction pathway[60,61]	Evidence of gallbladder cancer cell line growth inhibition by MEK inhibitor UO126[62,63]
c-MET (hepatocyte growth factor)	Several studies show overexpression of c-MET overexpression in preclinical cholangiocarcinoma models[64–66]	NK4, which acts as an HGF antagonist and angiogenesis inhibitor, when transfected cholangiocarcinoma cell line clones, showed cell growth inhibition by arresting cell cycle progression[67]
Molecular subclasses including inflammatory and proliferative subclasses	This important work may provide biomarkers of therapeutic efficacy to design biomarker-driven clinical trials[68,69]	—
BRAF-activating mutations	Present in 7% of cholangiocarcinoma specimens[68–70]	—
Hedgehog signaling	Sonic hedgehog ligand highly expressed by human cholangiocarcinoma tissue specimens and cell lines[42,71,72]	In vitro inhibition of sonic hedgehog signaling decreased epithelial-mesenchymal transition and cholangiocarcinoma cell viability[71]

Abbreviations: CAF, cancer-associated fibroblasts; COX, cyclooxygenase; EGFR, epidermal growth factor receptor; ERB, eukaryotic ribosome biogenesis protein; ERK, extracellular signal regulated kinase; HGF, hepatocyte growth factor; MEK, mitogen-activated ERK; VEGF, vascular endothelial growth factor.

Table 4
Randomized prospective trials of cytotoxic chemotherapy in HCC

Regimen	Study Phase	Sample Size	RR	Survival (mo)
PIAF vs Adriamycin[74]	III	94/94	20.9 vs 10.5	8.6 vs 6.83
Nolatrexed vs Adriamycin[75]	III	444	1.4 vs 4.0	5.5 vs 8 ($P = .0068$)

Until recently there was no published evidence that systemic chemotherapy improves OS in any subset of patients with HCC. The most widely used agent has been Adriamycin as a single agent or in combination. A pivotal phase III trial of Adriamycin versus combination chemotherapy (platinum, interferon, Adriamycin, 5-fluorouracil [PIAF]) showed a statistically significant difference in response rate (RR) favoring PIAF, but no survival difference.[74] **Table 4** includes the results of the phase II PIAF versus Adriamycin study, as well as one of the few other large randomized trials completed in HCC. Given the disappointing results of the trial by Yeo and colleagues,[74] clinicians have become skeptical about the prospects for developing an effective systemic therapy for HCC.

Several molecular pathways seem to be commonly aberrant in HCCs, such as growth factor expression, angiogenesis, and cell cycle control. A placebo-controlled international phase III trial of sorafenib was conducted in patients with HCC with Child-Pugh A cirrhosis and showed superior survival in the sorafenib arm compared with placebo (10.7 months vs 7.9 months; $P = .00058$).[76] The approval of sorafenib in 2007 for the treatment of patients with HCC in both the United States and the

Table 5
Clinical trials of novel targeted therapies for HCC

Regimen	Study Phase	Sample Size	Response Rate (%)	PFS TTP (mo)	Overall Survival (mo)
Sorafenib vs placebo[76]	III	299 vs 303	<1	5.5	10.7 vs 7.9
Sorafenib vs placebo[77]	III	150 vs 76	2.2	2.8	6.5
Bevacizumab	II	43	14	—	NA
Bevacizumab[78]	II	46	13	6.9	12.4
Bevacizumab plus erlotinib[79]	II	40	25	9	15.65
Bevacizumab plus erlotinib[28]	II	49	18.4	4.4	9.9
Bevacizumab plus erlotinib[80]	II	59	24	7.2	13.7
Brivanib[81]	II	55	—	2.7	10
Erlotinib[82]	II	40	0	—	10.75
Erlotinib[33]	II	38	9	—	13
Lapatinib[31]	II	40	5	2.3	6.2
Lapatinib[83]	II	26	0	1.9	12
Selumetinib[32]	II	28	12	3.7	9.8
Erlotinib[33]	II	42	8	—	7.5
GEMOX plus Panitumumab[34]	II	46	33	PFS 8.3	10.0
GEMOX vs	RIII	133	29	PFS 4.2	9.5
GEMOX plus erlotinib[35]	First line	135	15.7	PFS 5.8	9.5
Sunitinib[36]	II, 2nd line	56	8.9	1.7	4.8
GEMOX plus bevacizumab[37]	II, 1st line	35	40	7	12.7

European Union represents a paradigm shift in the treatment of advanced HCC, and is a clinically meaningful therapeutic advancement in this challenging malignancy. A subsequent prospective controlled trial of sorafenib in Asian patients with the same design and eligibility criteria as the SHARP (Sorafenib HCC Assessment Randomized Protocol) trial, showed an improvement in OS with similar hazard ratio to that of the SHARP trial. However, the Asian study showed significantly lower absolute benefit (6.2 months median survival in the study arm vs 10.7 months in SHARP) and possibly overall lower tolerance of sorafenib. Understanding the reasons for such a differential effect is essential to inform the design of future trials in HCC and underscore the importance of identifying stratification factors in future clinical trials, such as hepatic function, ethnicity, disease cause, and tumor molecular profile.

Despite sorafenib not yielding radiographic tumor shrinkage, the traditional measure of antitumor activity, it does affect carcinogenic activity in HCC, based on prolongation of both time to tumor progression and OS. The demonstration of improved patient outcome of a targeted chemotherapeutic agent in this challenging malignancy has also generated renewed enthusiasm among clinicians, and an increase in clinical research efforts worldwide. Sorafenib also provides a platform on which to build future comparative, adjuvant, and combination clinical trials to further improve patient outcome. **Table 5** summarizes several of the many phase II and III clinical trials that have been conducted as follow-on studies to the pivotal SHARP study. The challenge going forward is to identify those agents that, in combination with sorafenib, have the greatest potential for improved efficacy while maintaining patient safety.

SUMMARY

Tumors of the biliary tract and HCC are important malignancies worldwide; they are complex tumors with heterogeneous carcinogenic mechanisms that are steadily increasing in incidence in the United States and other Western countries. Most patients diagnosed with both biliary tract cancer and HCC have advanced disease, and these patients represent the highest priority for development of effective therapies. Advanced HCC remains a significant unmet medical need for which available research resources should be prioritized. It is hoped that current and future clinical trials will identify additional effective systemic agents, combination systemic therapies, and combined modality options. As advancements in developing personalized therapy continue to evolve in other tumors, it will be essential for the HCC community to develop tissue, serum, and other validated biomarkers that can help identify those patients who will benefit most from emerging treatment options.

REFERENCES

1. Blechacz B, Komuta M, Roskams T, et al. Clinical diagnosis and staging of cholangiocarcinoma. Nat Rev Gastroenterol Hepatol 2011;8:512–22.
2. Chung YE, Kim MJ, Park YN, et al. Varying appearances of cholangiocarcinoma: radiologic-pathologic correlation. Radiographics 2009;29:683–700.
3. Inui K, Yoshino J, Miyoshi H. Differential diagnosis and treatment of biliary strictures. Clin Gastroenterol Hepatol 2009;7:S79–83.
4. Motosugi U, Ichikawa T, Nakajima H, et al. Cholangiolocellular carcinoma of the liver: imaging findings. J Comput Assist Tomogr 2009;33:682–8.
5. Kim SH, Lee WJ, Lim HK, et al. Sclerosing hepatic carcinoma: helical CT features. Abdom Imaging 2007;32:725–9.

6. Gu XJ, Wang BF, Liu R. Application of (18)F-fluorodeoxyglucose positron emission tomography/computed tomography in preoperative assessment of hilar cholangiocarcinoma. Zhonghua Yi Xue Za Zhi 2012;92:1409–12 [in Chinese].

7. Alvaro D, Bragazzi MC, Benedetti A, et al. Cholangiocarcinoma in Italy: a national survey on clinical characteristics, diagnostic modalities and treatment. Results from the "Cholangiocarcinoma" committee of the Italian Association for the Study of Liver disease. Dig Liver Dis 2011;43:60–5.

8. Lee SW, Kim HJ, Park JH, et al. Clinical usefulness of 18F-FDG PET-CT for patients with gallbladder cancer and cholangiocarcinoma. J Gastroenterol 2010; 45:560–6.

9. Wehbe H, Henson R, Meng F, et al. Interleukin-6 contributes to growth in cholangiocarcinoma cells by aberrant promoter methylation and gene expression. Cancer Res 2006;66:10517–24.

10. Fava G, Alpini G, Rychlicki C, et al. Leptin enhances cholangiocarcinoma cell growth. Cancer Res 2008;68:6752–61.

11. Marin JJ, Romero MR, Briz O. Molecular bases of liver cancer refractoriness to pharmacological treatment. Curr Med Chem 2010;17:709–40.

12. Namwat N, Amimanan P, Loilome W, et al. Characterization of 5-fluorouracil-resistant cholangiocarcinoma cell lines. Chemotherapy 2008;54:343–51.

13. Kongpetch S, Kukongviriyapan V, Prawan A, et al. Crucial role of heme oxygenase-1 on the sensitivity of cholangiocarcinoma cells to chemotherapeutic agents. PLoS One 2012;7:e34994.

14. Eisenhauer EA, Therasse P, Bogaerts J, et al. New Response Evaluation Criteria in Solid Tumours: revised RECIST guideline (version 1.1). Eur J Cancer 2009;45: 228–47.

15. Valle J, Wasan H, Palmer DH, et al. Cisplatin plus gemcitabine versus gemcitabine for biliary tract cancer. N Engl J Med 2010;362:1273–81.

16. Lin MH, Chen JS, Chen HH, et al. A phase II trial of gemcitabine in the treatment of advanced bile duct and periampullary carcinomas. Chemotherapy 2003;49: 154–8.

17. Alberts SR, Al-Khatib H, Mahoney MR, et al. Gemcitabine, 5-fluorouracil, and leucovorin in advanced biliary tract and gallbladder carcinoma: a North Central Cancer Treatment Group phase II trial. Cancer 2005;103:111–8.

18. Sasaki T, Isayama H, Nakai Y, et al. Multicenter phase II study of S-1 monotherapy as second-line chemotherapy for advanced biliary tract cancer refractory to gemcitabine. Invest New Drugs 2012;30:708–13.

19. Thongprasert S, Napapan S, Charoentum C, et al. Phase II study of gemcitabine and cisplatin as first-line chemotherapy in inoperable biliary tract carcinoma. Ann Oncol 2005;16:279–81.

20. Knox JJ, Hedley D, Oza A, et al. Combining gemcitabine and capecitabine in patients with advanced biliary cancer: a phase II trial. J Clin Oncol 2005;23: 2332–8.

21. Jang JS, Lim HY, Hwang IG, et al. Gemcitabine and oxaliplatin in patients with unresectable biliary cancer including gall bladder cancer: a Korean Cancer Study Group phase II trial. Cancer Chemother Pharmacol 2010;65:641–7.

22. Gruenberger B, Schueller J, Heubrandtner U, et al. Cetuximab, gemcitabine, and oxaliplatin in patients with unresectable advanced or metastatic biliary tract cancer: a phase 2 study. Lancet Oncol 2010;11:1142–8.

23. Nehls O, Oettle H, Hartmann JT, et al. Capecitabine plus oxaliplatin as first-line treatment in patients with advanced biliary system adenocarcinoma: a prospective multicentre phase II trial. Br J Cancer 2008;98:309–15.

24. Patt YZ, Hassan MM, Aguayo A, et al. Oral capecitabine for the treatment of hepatocellular carcinoma, cholangiocarcinoma, and gallbladder carcinoma. Cancer 2004;101:578–86.
25. Feisthammel J, Schoppmeyer K, Mossner J, et al. Irinotecan with 5-FU/FA in advanced biliary tract adenocarcinomas: a multicenter phase II trial. Am J Clin Oncol 2007;30:319–24.
26. Furuse J, Kasuga A, Takasu A, et al. Role of chemotherapy in treatments for biliary tract cancer. J Hepatobiliary Pancreat Sci 2012;19:337–41.
27. Eckmann KR, Patel DK, Landgraf A, et al. Chemotherapy outcomes for the treatment of unresectable intrahepatic and hilar cholangiocarcinoma: a retrospective analysis. Gastrointest Cancer Res 2011;4:155–60.
28. Lubner SJ, Mahoney MR, Kolesar JL, et al. Report of a multicenter phase II trial testing a combination of biweekly bevacizumab and daily erlotinib in patients with unresectable biliary cancer: a phase II Consortium study. J Clin Oncol 2010;28:3491–7.
29. Bengala C, Bertolini F, Malavasi N, et al. Sorafenib in patients with advanced biliary tract carcinoma: a phase II trial. Br J Cancer 2010;102:68–72.
30. El-Khoueiry AB, Rankin CJ, Ben-Josef E, et al. SWOG 0514: a phase II study of sorafenib in patients with unresectable or metastatic gallbladder carcinoma and cholangiocarcinoma. Invest New Drugs 2012;30:1646–51.
31. Ramanathan RK, Belani CP, Singh DA, et al. A phase II study of lapatinib in patients with advanced biliary tree and hepatocellular cancer. Cancer Chemother Pharmacol 2009;64:777–83.
32. Bekaii-Saab T, Phelps MA, Li X, et al. Multi-institutional phase II study of selumetinib in patients with metastatic biliary cancers. J Clin Oncol 2011;29:2357–63.
33. Philip PA, Mahoney MR, Allmer C, et al. Phase II study of erlotinib in patients with advanced biliary cancer. J Clin Oncol 2006;24:3069–74.
34. Jensen LH, Lindebjerg J, Ploen J, et al. Phase II marker-driven trial of panitumumab and chemotherapy in KRAS wild-type biliary tract cancer. Ann Oncol 2012; 23:2341–6.
35. Lee J, Park SH, Chang HM, et al. Gemcitabine and oxaliplatin with or without erlotinib in advanced biliary-tract cancer: a multicentre, open-label, randomised, phase 3 study. Lancet Oncol 2012;13:181–8.
36. Yi JH, Thongprasert S, Lee J, et al. A phase II study of sunitinib as a second-line treatment in advanced biliary tract carcinoma: a multicentre, multinational study. Eur J Cancer 2012;48:196–201.
37. Zhu AX, Meyerhardt JA, Blaszkowsky LS, et al. Efficacy and safety of gemcitabine, oxaliplatin, and bevacizumab in advanced biliary-tract cancers and correlation of changes in 18-fluorodeoxyglucose PET with clinical outcome: a phase 2 study. Lancet Oncol 2010;11:48–54.
38. Yoshikawa D, Ojima H, Iwasaki M, et al. Clinicopathological and prognostic significance of EGFR, VEGF, and HER2 expression in cholangiocarcinoma. Br J Cancer 2008;98:418–25.
39. Yoshikawa D, Ojima H, Kokubu A, et al. Vandetanib (ZD6474), an inhibitor of VEGFR and EGFR signalling, as a novel molecular-targeted therapy against cholangiocarcinoma. Br J Cancer 2009;100:1257–66.
40. Fingas CD, Mertens JC, Razumilava N, et al. Targeting PDGFR-beta in cholangiocarcinoma. Liver Int 2012;32:400–9.
41. Boonjaraspinyo S, Boonmars T, Wu Z, et al. Platelet-derived growth factor may be a potential diagnostic and prognostic marker for cholangiocarcinoma. Tumour Biol 2012;33:1785–802.

42. Fingas CD, Bronk SF, Werneburg NW, et al. Myofibroblast-derived PDGF-BB promotes Hedgehog survival signaling in cholangiocarcinoma cells. Hepatology 2011;54:2076–88.
43. Mertens JC, Fingas CD, Christensen JD, et al. Therapeutic effects of deleting cancer-associated fibroblasts in cholangiocarcinoma. Cancer Res 2013;73: 897–907.
44. Yoon JH, Werneburg NW, Higuchi H, et al. Bile acids inhibit Mcl-1 protein turn-over via an epidermal growth factor receptor/Raf-1-dependent mechanism. Cancer Res 2002;62:6500–5.
45. Jan YY, Yeh TS, Yeh JN, et al. Expression of epidermal growth factor receptor, apomucins, matrix metalloproteinases, and p53 in rat and human cholangiocarcinoma: appraisal of an animal model of cholangiocarcinoma. Ann Surg 2004; 240:89–94.
46. Terada T, Ashida K, Endo K, et al. c-erbB-2 protein is expressed in hepatolithiasis and cholangiocarcinoma. Histopathology 1998;33:325–31.
47. Lai GH, Zhang Z, Shen XN, et al. erbB-2/neu transformed rat cholangiocytes recapitulate key cellular and molecular features of human bile duct cancer. Gastroenterology 2005;129:2047–57.
48. Kiguchi K, Carbajal S, Chan K, et al. Constitutive expression of ErbB-2 in gall-bladder epithelium results in development of adenocarcinoma. Cancer Res 2001;61:6971–6.
49. Leone F, Cavalloni G, Pignochino Y, et al. Somatic mutations of epidermal growth factor receptor in bile duct and gallbladder carcinoma. Clin Cancer Res 2006;12:1680–5.
50. Zhang Z, Oyesanya RA, Campbell DJ, et al. Preclinical assessment of simultaneous targeting of epidermal growth factor receptor (ErbB1) and ErbB2 as a strategy for cholangiocarcinoma therapy. Hepatology 2010;52: 975–86.
51. Sirica AE, Lai GH, Endo K, et al. Cyclooxygenase-2 and ERBB-2 in cholangiocarcinoma: potential therapeutic targets. Semin Liver Dis 2002;22: 303–13.
52. Sirica AE, Lai GH, Zhang Z. Biliary cancer growth factor pathways, cyclooxygenase-2 and potential therapeutic strategies. J Gastroenterol Hepatol 2001;16:363–72.
53. Han C, Demetris AJ, Stolz DB, et al. Modulation of Stat3 activation by the cytosolic phospholipase A2alpha and cyclooxygenase-2-controlled prostaglandin E2 signaling pathway. J Biol Chem 2006;281:24831–46.
54. Han C, Wu T. Cyclooxygenase-2-derived prostaglandin E2 promotes human cholangiocarcinoma cell growth and invasion through EP1 receptor-mediated activation of the epidermal growth factor receptor and Akt. J Biol Chem 2005; 280:24053–63.
55. Zhang Z, Lai GH, Sirica AE. Celecoxib-induced apoptosis in rat cholangiocarcinoma cells mediated by Akt inactivation and Bax translocation. Hepatology 2004;39:1028–37.
56. Dobashi A, Imazu H, Tatsumi N, et al. Quantitative analysis of VEGF-C mRNA of extrahepatic cholangiocarcinoma with real-time PCR using samples obtained during endoscopic retrograde cholangiopancreatography. Scand J Gastroenterol 2013;48:848–55.
57. Benckert C, Jonas S, Cramer T, et al. Transforming growth factor beta 1 stimulates vascular endothelial growth factor gene transcription in human cholangiocellular carcinoma cells. Cancer Res 2003;63:1083–92.

58. Sugiyama H, Onuki K, Ishige K, et al. Potent in vitro and in vivo antitumor activity of sorafenib against human intrahepatic cholangiocarcinoma cells. J Gastroenterol 2011;46:779–89.

59. Wiedmann MW, Mossner J. Molecular targeted therapy of biliary tract cancer–results of the first clinical studies. Curr Drug Targets 2010;11:834–50.

60. Meng F, Yamagiwa Y, Taffetani S, et al. IL-6 activates serum and glucocorticoid kinase via p38alpha mitogen-activated protein kinase pathway. Am J Physiol Cell Physiol 2005;289:C971–81.

61. Tan FL, Ooi A, Huang D, et al. p38delta/MAPK13 as a diagnostic marker for cholangiocarcinoma and its involvement in cell motility and invasion. Int J Cancer 2010;126:2353–61.

62. Horiuchi H, Kawamata H, Furihata T, et al. A MEK inhibitor (U0126) markedly inhibits direct liver invasion of orthotopically inoculated human gallbladder cancer cells in nude mice. J Exp Clin Cancer Res 2004;23:599–606.

63. Horiuchi H, Kawamata H, Fujimori T, et al. A MEK inhibitor (U0126) prolongs survival in nude mice bearing human gallbladder cancer cells with K-ras mutation: analysis in a novel orthotopic inoculation model. Int J Oncol 2003;23:957–63.

64. Radaeva S, Ferreira-Gonzalez A, Sirica AE. Overexpression of C-NEU and C-MET during rat liver cholangiocarcinogenesis: a link between biliary intestinal metaplasia and mucin-producing cholangiocarcinoma. Hepatology 1999;29:1453–62.

65. Terada T, Nakanuma Y, Sirica AE. Immunohistochemical demonstration of MET overexpression in human intrahepatic cholangiocarcinoma and in hepatolithiasis. Hum Pathol 1998;29:175–80.

66. Socoteanu MP, Mott F, Alpini G, et al. c-Met targeted therapy of cholangiocarcinoma. World J Gastroenterol 2008;14:2990–4.

67. Ge X, Wang Y, Wang Y, et al. NK4 gene therapy inhibits HGF/Met-induced growth of human cholangiocarcinoma cells. Dig Dis Sci 2013;58:1636–43.

68. Sia D, Hoshida Y, Villanueva A, et al. Integrative molecular analysis of intrahepatic cholangiocarcinoma reveals 2 classes that have different outcomes. Gastroenterology 2013;144:829–40.

69. Andersen JB, Spee B, Blechacz BR, et al. Genomic and genetic characterization of cholangiocarcinoma identifies therapeutic targets for tyrosine kinase inhibitors. Gastroenterology 2012;142:1021–31.e15.

70. Tannapfel A, Sommerer F, Benicke M, et al. Mutations of the BRAF gene in cholangiocarcinoma but not in hepatocellular carcinoma. Gut 2003;52:706–12.

71. El Khatib M, Kalnytska A, Palagani V, et al. Inhibition of hedgehog signaling attenuates carcinogenesis in vitro and increases necrosis of cholangiocellular carcinoma. Hepatology 2013;57:1035–45.

72. Omenetti A, Diehl AM. Hedgehog signaling in cholangiocytes. Curr Opin Gastroenterol 2011;27:268–75.

73. Utispan K, Sonongbua J, Thuwajit P, et al. Periostin activates integrin alpha5-beta1 through a PI3K/AKTdependent pathway in invasion of cholangiocarcinoma. Int J Oncol 2012;41:1110–8.

74. Yeo W, Mok TS, Zee B, et al. A randomized phase III study of doxorubicin versus cisplatin/interferon alpha-2b/doxorubicin/fluorouracil (PIAF) combination chemotherapy for unresectable hepatocellular carcinoma. J Natl Cancer Inst 2005;97:1532–8.

75. Gish RG, Porta C, Lazar L, et al. Phase III randomized controlled trial comparing the survival of patients with unresectable hepatocellular carcinoma treated with nolatrexed or doxorubicin. J Clin Oncol 2007;25:3069–75.

76. Llovet JM, Ricci S, Mazzaferro V, et al. Sorafenib in advanced hepatocellular carcinoma. N Engl J Med 2008;359:378–90.
77. Cheng AL, Kang YK, Chen Z, et al. Efficacy and safety of sorafenib in patients in the Asia-Pacific region with advanced hepatocellular carcinoma: a phase III randomised, double-blind, placebo-controlled trial. Lancet Oncol 2009;10: 25–34.
78. Siegel AB, Cohen EI, Ocean A, et al. Phase II trial evaluating the clinical and biologic effects of bevacizumab in unresectable hepatocellular carcinoma. J Clin Oncol 2008;26:2992–8.
79. Thomas MB, Morris JS, Chadha R, et al. Phase II trial of the combination of bevacizumab and erlotinib in patients who have advanced hepatocellular carcinoma. J Clin Oncol 2009;27:843–50.
80. Kaseb AO, Garrett-Mayer E, Morris JS, et al. Efficacy of bevacizumab plus erlotinib for advanced hepatocellular carcinoma and predictors of outcome: final results of a phase II trial. Oncology 2012;82:67–74.
81. Boige V, Malka D, Bourredjem A, et al. Efficacy, safety, and biomarkers of single-agent bevacizumab therapy in patients with advanced hepatocellular carcinoma. Oncologist 2012;17:1063–72.
82. Thomas MB, Chadha R, Glover K, et al. Phase 2 study of erlotinib in patients with unresectable hepatocellular carcinoma. Cancer 2007;110:1059–67.
83. Bekaii-Saab T, Markowitz J, Prescott N, et al. A multi-institutional phase II study of the efficacy and tolerability of lapatinib in patients with advanced hepatocellular carcinomas. Clin Cancer Res 2009;15:5895–901.

Palliation

Treating Patients with Inoperable Biliary Tract and Primary Liver Tumors

Albert Amini, MD, T. Clark Gamblin, MD, MS*

KEYWORDS

- Palliation • Cholangiocarcinoma • Hepatocellular carcinoma • Systemic therapies
- Targeted therapies • Chemoembolization • Endoscopic therapies

KEY POINTS

- Hepatocellular carcinoma and cholangiocarcinoma are frequently unresectable because of advanced local disease.
- Patients with unresectable tumors may be amenable to ablation techniques administered through multiple routes and techniques of administration.
- Palliation should also include restoring biliary drainage, pain management, improving nutritional status and fat absorption, and improving pruritus.
- Systemic chemotherapy and sorafenib are palliative options used in conjunction with locoregional therapies or as sole therapeutic options.

Hepatocellular carcinoma (HCC) and cholangiocarcinoma (CCA) account for nearly all primary liver tumors.[1,2] Resection is the most effective therapy for both tumors but is frequently not possible, often because of advanced local disease.[3,4] Patients with unresectable tumors have a poor prognosis, with median survival often 3 to 6 months.[5] Although several treatment options exist, these are not curative approaches and rather palliative.

HCC is the most common primary liver tumor, representing 90% of primary liver cancers. Cirrhosis is associated with HCC in almost 90% of the cases.[6,7] Chronic hepatitis B virus and hepatitis C virus contribute to HCC development in approximately 80% of cases. The mean annual incidence of HCC in cirrhotic patients is 3% to 4%, and this figure increases proportionally with liver function impairment.[8] Less than 20% of these tumors are amenable to definitive surgical management,

Disclosures: No funding sources or conflicts of interests.
Division of Surgical Oncology, Department of Surgery, Medical College of Wisconsin, 9200 West Wisconsin Avenue, Milwaukee, WI 53226-3596, USA
* Corresponding author.
E-mail address: tcgamblin@mcw.edu

because of advanced intrahepatic disease or other medical conditions that prohibit major surgery. Locoregional therapies have been recommended in patients with HCC as a form of palliation.[9] Locoregional therapies include radiofrequency ablation (RFA), percutaneous ethanol injection (PEI), cryoablation, microwave ablation, transarterial chemoembolization (TACE), hepatic artery infusion (HAI), radioembolization (^{90}Y), and bland embolization.

CCA is the second most common primary liver cancer after HCC and comprises 10% of primary liver cancers. CCA can be subdivided into cancers affecting the intrahepatic, perihilar, and extrahepatic biliary tree. At presentation, most CCAs are perihilar (50%–60%), 20% are intrahepatic, 20% are distal extrahepatic, and 5% are multifocal.[10] Most patients with CCA have no known risk factors; however, there seems to be an association with chronic inflammation of the biliary epithelium and diseases such as primary sclerosing cholangitis, chronic infection with liver flukes, hepatolithiasis, and viral hepatitis.[11] Surgical resection offers the approach for long-term survival, but few patients are operative candidates.[12] Palliative strategies include surgical, percutaneous, and endoscopic techniques to decompress the biliary system and locoregional palliative therapies.

STRATEGY

The selection of the best treatment is dependent on the status of the underlying liver and the tumor stage. Although HCC is rare in a noncirrhotic liver, these patients are the most likely candidates for liver resection. In most cases in which cirrhosis underlies HCC, the degree of functional impairment often precludes safe surgery.[13] CCA develops in the background of cirrhosis in only 10% of patients; however, most CCA cases are deemed unresectable at presentation.

Most patients are not candidates for resection because of advanced tumors, tumor location near major intrahepatic vessels precluding a negative-margin resection, multifocal tumors, or poor hepatic functional reserve. Liver function is assessed through the Child-Turcotte-Pugh classification, and this is combined with a detailed evaluation of tumor extent. There are multiple staging systems for liver cancer, such as the TNM (Tumor, Node, Metastases), Okuda, CLIP (Cancer of the Liver Italian Program), and BCLC (Barcelona Clinic Liver Cancer) staging. These assessments examine the liver for characteristics such as multifocality, vascular invasion, and extrahepatic disease.[13,14] In addition, the general condition and performance status of the patient is assessed. Patients with high-risk tumors, multiple comorbid conditions and poor performance status may be candidates for palliative treatment alone.

Even in centers with extensive experience in hepatic resection, the resection rate for HCC is in the range of 10% to 37%.[15–17] In patients with unresectable HCC disease, liver transplantation should always be considered. Select patients may also be amenable to ablation techniques administered through multiple routes and techniques of administration. These options are reported to offer potential long-term benefit.[18] TACE and sorafenib administration are palliative approaches that have been shown to have a positive impact on survival.[19–21]

Treatment protocols for intrahepatic CCAs (ICCs) are not as common as those for HCC. Nevertheless, there is a clear role for hepatic resection when feasible, and chemoembolization has been used successfully in unresectable patients.[22,23] CCA is diagnosed at late stages in most patients and resection is possible in only 15% to 20% of cases.[24] If the disease is deemed unresectable, palliation should include restoring biliary drainage to reduce risk of cholangitis, pain management, improving nutritional status and fat absorption, and improving pruritus.[25]

TREATMENTS
Locoregional Therapy

RFA

If patients are not candidates for surgery, they are offered percutaneous ablation if focally confined disease exists.[14] RFA uses the energy of radiowaves for hyperthermic ablation of liver tumors. Several studies have reported complete tumor necrosis in 80% to 90% of HCCs smaller than 3 to 5 cm after a single session of RFA confirmed by contrast computed tomography.[26,27] The complete ablation rate for larger tumors is less favorable: a study of RFA for 126 HCCs 3.1 to 9.5 cm reported a complete necrosis rate of 48%.[28] The best results of ablation are achieved in solitary tumors smaller than 2 cm, in which these techniques may achieve complete necrosis, and recurrence rates are similar to resection in 90% of cases.[29,30] RFA is a safe procedure for treatment of HCC in carefully selected patients with cirrhosis. Because of the versatility of probe designs that allows quick ablation of large tumors and the safety reported, RFA has largely replaced cryoablation of liver tumors.[31]

Use of ablation for ICC management is increasing. In a study of 13 patients with ICC treated with RFA, local control was successful in 88% at a median follow-up of 19.5 months. The treatment failures occurred in the tumors more than 5 cm in diameter. The median overall survival after RFA was 38.5 months.[32] RFA may result in successful local tumor control in patients with intermediate (3–5 cm) or small (<3 cm) ICC. Tumor size more than 5 cm, tumor geometry, proximity to large intrahepatic vessels, or subcapsular location may result in insufficient ablations and are associated with poorer clinical outcomes.[33]

PEI

PEI can be used in the presence of contraindications for ablation such as tumor in a subcapsular location or in the vicinity of the gallbladder or heart. PEI induces tumor necrosis by cellular dehydration, protein denaturation, and thrombosis of small vessels. HCC is softer than the surrounding cirrhotic liver and is often encapsulated, thus allowing selective diffusion of ethanol within the tumor mass. Histopathologic studies have shown that PEI can induce complete tumor necrosis in about 70% of patients with HCCs smaller than 3 cm.[34,35] The extent of necrosis is closely related to the tumor size, with an almost 100% rate of complete necrosis in HCCs smaller than 2 cm.[36] PEI has been shown to be more cost effective than hepatic resection in patients with a single HCC smaller than 3 cm.[37]

Compared with PEI, necrosis induced by ablation is more predictable, and treatment by a single session is sufficient in most patients with small HCCs. A prospective nonrandomized study comparing ablation in 42 patients and PEI in 44 patients with HCCs 3 cm or smaller showed that ablation achieved a higher complete necrosis rate (90% vs 80%) with fewer treatment sessions (mean 1.2 vs 4.8 sessions) but was associated with a higher complication rate (12% vs 0%).[38]

Cryoablation

Cryoablation has been used for the treatment of liver tumors since the 1980s. Rapid freezing to subzero temperature leads to ice formation in the extracellular space and drawing of water from the cells, causing cellular damage by dehydration and destruction of the normal cellular architecture.[39] Although larger tumors can be treated, cryoablation is most effective for tumors smaller than 5 cm.[40] The largest series of cryoablation for HCC was performed by Zhou and Tang in China[41] and reported a 5-year survival rate of 37.9% among 191 patients with HCC and a 5-year survival of 53.1% in a subgroup of 56 patients with tumors smaller than 5 cm. Like other ablation techniques, complete necrosis of highly vascular tumors or tumors adjacent to large vessels may be impeded by the effects of blood flow.

RFA was compared with cryoablation in a meta-analysis involving 433 patients with HCC. The study showed that RFA resulted in fewer complications (odds ratio [OR]: 2.80, 95% confidence interval [CI]: 1.54–5.09) and less local recurrence (OR: 1.96; 95% CI: 1.12–3.42). There was no significant difference in mortality (OR: 2.21; 95% CI: 0.45–10.8).[42] Overall, current data suggest that cryoablation is an effective local ablative therapy for unresectable HCC.

Microwave ablation

Microwave ablation therapy is a form of thermoablative treatment in which tissue necrosis is induced by the heating effect of microwaves emitted from a needle electrode inserted into the tumor. The microwaves act mainly on the watery component of tissues, producing dielectric heat and tissue coagulation. Irreversible cellular damage from protein coagulation occurs at temperatures higher than 50°C. Compared with PEI, microwave ablation creates a more predictable and reproducible area of tissue necrosis, and it can ablate the tumor capsule as well as surrounding extracapsular invasion.[31] The percutaneous approach has the advantages of applicability to high-risk patients and repeatability, but it is most effective in HCC cases smaller than 3 cm.[43–45] Ohmoto and colleagues[45] studied the results of percutaneous microwave ablation in 17 tumor nodules and found complete ablation in 80% of tumors 2 cm or smaller, whereas 71% of tumors larger than 2 cm developed local recurrence. With a favorable safety profile and tumor ablation rate, microwave ablation seems to be a promising therapy for patients with unresectable HCC, especially those with small tumors associated with poor liver function.[46]

Regional Chemotherapy

HAI

HAI therapy represents another liver-directed treatment option.[47] Primary liver malignancies are predominately dependent on the hepatic artery for blood supply, whereas normal liver tissues are perfused primarily by the portal vein. HAI therapy allows delivery of increased local concentration of cytotoxic agents to hepatic malignancies not achievable by systemic administration, especially for drugs with high systemic clearance. The regional advantage of an agent given by HAI over an intravenous infusion is proportional to the systemic clearance and hepatic extraction of the drug. Fluorodeoxyuridine is an attractive agent for HAI therapy because of its high first-pass clearance and low toxicity. Gemcitabine is also reported to be a potential agent, with a favorable toxicity profile and proven effectiveness in primary liver cancers.[48] Unlike other locoregional therapies, HAI chemotherapy is not limited by tumor size, number, or proximity to major vasculatures, all of which are common contraindications to resection or ablation. A recently completed phase II study of HAI for patients with unresectable primary liver cancers reported positive findings. Sixteen of 34 evaluable patients (47%) had a partial response (15 of 26 with CCA and 2 of 8 with HCC). The median time to progression was 7.4 months, and overall survival was 29.5 months.[49]

Chemoembolization

TACE is a regional therapy widely used for unresectable HCC. Patients with more advanced disease (large or multifocal HCC) are candidates for TACE if liver function is preserved and performance status acceptable. Response to this locoregional approach is associated with improved survival, and it has a significant impact on outcome at this stage of the disease.[20] During the procedure, iodized poppyseed oil (lipiodol) and chemotherapeutic agents (doxorubicin, cisplatin, or mitomycin C) are administered through the feeding artery of the tumor, followed by arterial emboliza-tion.[31] Other regimens are also used and the method of TACE is often institutional specific. Because the blood supply to HCCs is predominantly derived from the hepatic artery, transarterial embolization can induce tumor necrosis in HCCs.[50,51] In a study of 100 patients with HCCs smaller than 4 cm treated by transarterial embolization alone, a complete necrosis rate of 64% and a 5-year survival rate of 53% were reported.[52] The combined use of a lipiodol-cytotoxic drug emulsion and embolization has some theoretic advantages over chemotherapy or embolization alone. The oil-based chemotherapy slurry is selectively retained in the tumor for weeks and therefore helps to concentrate the cytotoxic agents into the tumor. In addition, the necrotizing effect of the lipiodol-drug emulsion is further enhanced by an arterial embolization.[53] In a pro-spective trial, the 1-year survival rate after TACE was significantly better than survival after transarterial chemotherapy with a lipiodol-drug emulsion alone (86.3% vs 65.9%).[54]

A recent study comparing TACE with transcatheter arterial embolization (TAE) without chemotherapy and transcatheter arterial infusion (TAI) in HCC reported that TACE and TAE were more effective in reduction of tumor size than TAI, and although they were associated with more acute liver function damage, it was reversible.[55] How-ever, another study by Sumie and colleagues[56] comparing HAI chemotherapy using low-dose cisplatin and 5-fluorouracil with TACE found that HAI had a better antitumor effect than that of TACE, whereas the cumulative survival rates were comparable be-tween the 2 treatment groups. A randomized phase III trial comparing TACE with TAI using zinostatin stimalamar (SMANCS) showed that adding embolization did not in-crease survival over TAI in patients with HCC.[57] The ideal chemotherapeutic agent and whether embolization is necessary remain a point of debate.

The use of TACE for treating HCC is well established, with robust survival benefit outcomes.[58,59] Its use for CCA is less established. A recent study[60] randomized pa-tients with unresectable ICC to TACE (n = 72) or best supportive therapy alone (n = 83), and a strong survival benefit was observed. Those who underwent TACE survived a median of 12.2 months, and those who received supportive therapy, only 3.3 months. A study by Gusani and colleagues[23] showed that TACE with gemcitabine in combina-tion therapy (with oxaliplatin or cisplatin) offered better overall survival than gemcita-bine alone in unresectable CCA (13.8 vs 6.3 months). Kuhlman and colleagues[61] recently published promising data on the use of TACE using irinotecan-eluting beads (iDEB-TACE). Three independent trials were conducted, and 26 patients with ICC were treated with iDEB-TACE (200 mg irinotecan), 10 patients were treated with conven-tional TACE using 15 mg mitomycin C mixed with ionized oil (lipiodol) followed by gel foam embolization; and 31 patients were treated with systemic gemcitabine and oxaliplatin. Patients in the iDEB-TACE group had 6 months improved overall survival over the conventional TACE group.

Radioembolization

Transarterial internal radiotherapy for HCC is a targeted therapy, with a radioactive isotope carried in an agent that is selectively retained by the tumor. Intra-arterial iodine 131 injected with lipiodol produced a tumor response rate ranging from 40% to 52% in various studies, and it seems to be well tolerated.[62,63] Complete tumor necrosis has been shown with super selective high-dose therapy in patients with HCCs smaller than 5 cm.[64] A recent prospective randomized trial comparing transarterial iodine 131 (n = 65) and TACE (n = 64) showed no significant difference in tumor response rate (24% vs 25%) or 1-year survival rate (38% vs 42%), but the former treatment was better tolerated.[65]

Yttrium 90 delivered in glass microspheres is another form of transarterial radio-therapy that is approved by the US Food and Drug Administration under humanitarian use exemption. It has a higher radiation dose and thus a greater cytotoxic effect than iodine 131.[31] In a study of 71 patients with unresectable HCC treated with transarterial yttrium 90 microspheres, an overall response rate of 89% was reported and the me-dian survival was 9.4 months.[66] It remains unclear whether yttrium 90 has any advan-tage over iodine 131 treatment, because no comparable study has been reported.

Radioembolization is an established treatment of HCC but has not been commonly reported in the management of CCA. Radioembolization using yttrium 90 micro-spheres was assessed in 33 patients with unresectable ICC and appeared safe. Me-dian overall survival was 22 months and time to progression was 9.8 months.[67] Yttrium 90 radioembolization has been shown to have a minimal embolic effect and an accept-able safety profile in ICC as well.[68]

External-beam radiotherapy

The application of locoregional therapies is limited because of the size and number of tumors, liver function, portal hypertension, and the distribution or vascular supply of the tumor.[69–71] Stereotactic body radiosurgery (SBRT) has been shown to be effective by allowing the delivery of large doses of radiation to a precise location and sparing the surrounding normal tissues.[72] The use of SBRT for the treatment of primary liver tumors is emerging; however, one of the challenges is the low tolerance of the liver to irradiation. This factor is especially important when treating HCC, in which cirrhosis is frequently present, because radiation-induced liver disease occurs more frequently in patients with poor baseline liver function.[73]

A study by Ibarra and colleagues[74] was able to show comparable rates of freedom from local progression (FFLP) in patients treated with SBRT compared with other locoregional therapies. In this study, 21 patients with HCC and 11 patients with ICC were treated, and overall FFLP for advanced HCC was 63% at a median follow-up of 12.9 months. The median time to local progression was 6.3 months. The 1-year and 2-year overall survival rates were 87% and 55%, respectively. Patients with ICC had an overall FFLP of 55.5% at a median follow-up of 7.8 months. The median time to local progression was 4.2 months and the 6-month and 1-year overall survival rates were 75% and 45%, respectively. This finding compares favorably with other locoregional therapies. SBRT is a safe and effective option for the treatment of primary liver tumors. Small and nonmetastatic tumors have been shown to be associated with better responses and better long-term control.[75]

SBRT for advanced CCA has had promising results as well. A study by Barney and colleagues[76] had 10 patients with unresectable primary or recurrent CCA lesions who underwent abdominal SBRT. The median follow-up was 14 months. Local control, defined as freedom from progression within the SBRT field, was 100%, but 4 patients with treatment to intrahepatic sites experienced progression elsewhere in the liver. Estimates for freedom from distant progression at 6 and 12 months were 73% and 31%, respectively. Overall survival estimates for the cohort at 6 and 12 months were 83% and 73%, respectively. This study suggests that SBRT may affect patient survival in addition to local control in patients with CCA.

ENDOSCOPIC AND PERCUTANEOUS PALLIATION

The primary aim of palliation in a patient with unresectable CCA is to relieve the obstructive cholestasis and its associated morbidities, such as pruritus, cholangi-tis, and pain. Palliation of obstructive jaundice can be achieved successfully through 3 major routes: surgically, by the creation of a choledochojejunostomy, choledochoduodenostomy, or hepaticojejunostomy; percutaneously, via percutaneous transhepatic cholangiography (PTC) and stent placement; and endoscopically, via endoscopic retrograde cholangiopancreatography and stent placement. Photodynamic therapy (PDT) and intraluminal brachytherapy (ILBT) delivered by either the percutaneous or endoscopic route may be used in addition to stent placement.[25] In addition, a PTC may be the initial access to the biliary tree, which is then stented endoscopically (rendezvous procedure), or stents may be deployed via the PTC track.

Endoscopic therapy is the least invasive modality for achieving adequate symptom relief and perhaps may provide a survival benefit in these patients. Endoscopic stent placement has been shown to be as successful at restoring biliary flow and relieving obstructive jaundice as surgical hepaticojejunostomy or choledochojejunostomy.[77] A randomized trial of patients with low common bile duct obstruction compared surgical biliary bypass with endoscopic stent insertion, and 92% of patients in both groups achieved decompression, but there was a lower procedure-related mortality (3% vs 14%), major complication rate (11% vs 29%), and length of hospital stay (20 days vs 26 days) in the endoscopic group.[78] The decreased morbidity and mortality of endoscopic intervention to establish biliary drainage has significantly reduced the number of surgical interventions performed for biliary obstruction in malignancy.

Single or multiple biliary stents can be placed depending on the extent of the stricture. Single stents are adequate for strictures of the main bile duct below the confluence. However, for hilar strictures, debate exists as to whether single or double stents should be inserted. It is known that only 25% to 30% of the liver needs to be drained to achieve adequate palliation of obstructive jaundice.[79] Several studies have shown that a single stent achieves adequate drainage in 75% to 80% of cases; however, the necessity for 2 or more stents may be critical in the remaining 20% to 25%.[80,81] A prospective randomized controlled trial comparing unilateral versus bilateral stents found that unilateral stents achieved a higher success rate (81% vs 73%), with a lower early complication rate (19% vs 27%). There was no difference with respect to procedure-related mortality, late complications, or survival, suggesting that a unilateral stent is likely to suffice in most cases.[82]

A decision between metal versus plastic stents needs to be made with consideration to the long-term need of the stent. In patients surviving more than 6 months, metal stents, compared with plastic stents, are associated with fewer interventions, reduced hospital inpatient stay, and fewer overall complications than plastic stents.[10] Patency rates are higher with metal stents because of both larger diameter (10 mm when deployed) and material strength. Metal stents can also be revised with the placement of additional internal stents, allowing for long-term patency. Raju and colleagues[83] reported that metal stents for inoperable hilar CCA had a median patency time of 5.6 months, compared with 1.9 months for plastic stents, and were more cost effective, given the reduced need for salvage PTC and restenting. Plastic stents should therefore be reserved for temporary preoperative drainage in patients considered for curative resection. In those with advanced disease, in which palliation is necessary, plastic stents have limited use, because of their shorter and less predictable patency rates. Thus, metal stents are the treatment of choice in these situations.[84]

PDT has emerged as a promising new modality of treatment of patients who do not undergo resection. PDT involves the administration of a photosensitizing agent known to preferentially accumulate in tumor cells followed by the exposure of the target tissue to a light of the appropriate photoactivating wavelength. This process initiates a photochemical reaction with the generation of cytotoxic reactive oxygen species, resulting in apoptosis and necrosis of tumors cells.[85] In a prospective study, 39 patients with CCA were randomized to treatment with biliary stenting plus PDT or stenting alone. The PDT group had higher median survival (493 days vs 98 days), less cholestasis, better quality-of-life scores, and better stabilization of performance status than did the stenting group.[86] In a large retrospective study looking at patients with hilar CCAs treated with surgery, stenting alone or stenting with PDT, PDT and stenting resulted in longer median survival (12 months vs 6.4 months), lower serum bilirubin levels, and higher performance status compared with stenting alone.[87]

ILBT can be performed endoscopically or percutaneously. Iridium 192 seeds mounted on a catheter are placed directly across the stricture in the bile ducts. Several studies have evaluated ILBT for palliation of unresectable CCA.[88] Some studies have shown improved survival, whereas other studies have shown no benefit or an increased incidence of complications caused by cholangitis.[88,89]

Among patients with advanced HCC, jaundice occurs in 5% to 44% of patients.[90] Prognosis is worse in patients with unresectable HCC and obstructive jaundice.[91] TACE is not recommended in patients with a serum bilirubin level of more than 3 mg/dL, and systemic chemotherapy and radiotherapy are usually not well tolerated in patients with significant hyperbilirubinemia.[92] In patients who are not candidates for surgery, endoscopic and percutaneous biliary drainage are the 2 main nonsurgical treatment options, and they can provide palliation and allow for further adjuvant therapies. Endoscopy is usually the first-line treatment because of its low hemorrhagic risk and successful drainage rates. Mean stent patency time and mean survival range from 1 to 15.9 months and 2.8 to 12.3 months, respectively.[93] Choi and colleagues[90] compared endoscopic versus percutaneous biliary drainage in HCC and concluded that endoscopy had longer duration of drainage and higher rates of successful drainage. PDT can also be an effective treatment option for HCC with bile duct invasion. PDT has been shown to prolong survival in conjunction with biliary drainage in HCC.[91]

SYSTEMIC THERAPIES

Combination chemotherapy with gemcitabine and a platinum-based agent is regarded as a standard first-line treatment of advanced biliary tract cancer from the results from the ABC 01 and ABC 02 (Advanced Biliary Cancer phase 2 and phase 3) randomized trials.[94,95] In the phase 3 trial, median overall survival was 11.7 months in the gemcitabine plus cisplatin group and 8.1 months in the gemcitabine alone group. Results of several phase 2 studies have shown that the combination of gemcitabine and oxaliplatin has a similar antitumor activity against these cancers with a favorable toxic effect profile.[96–98] Similarly, results of a meta-analysis of 104 phase 2 and phase 3 trials including 2810 patients with biliary tract cancer showed that gemcitabine combined with platinum compounds such as cisplatin or oxaliplatin had a better response rate and survival when compared with gemcitabine alone.[99] Nevertheless, prognosis is still poor, and overall survival is less than 12 months when patients with locally advanced disease are included.[95]

In a study by Lee and colleagues,[100] 133 patients with metastatic biliary tract cancers were randomly assigned to chemotherapy alone and 135 to chemotherapy plus erlotinib. Median progression-free survival was 4.2 months in the chemotherapy alone group and 5.8 months in the chemotherapy plus erlotinib group. Significantly more patients had an objective response in the chemotherapy plus erlotinib group than in the chemotherapy alone group, but median overall survival was the same in both groups at 9.5 months. Subgroup analyses by primary site of disease showed that for patients with CCA, the addition of erlotinib to chemotherapy significantly prolonged median progression-free survival (5.9 months vs 3.0 months).

Sorafenib is an oral multikinase inhibitor with antiproliferative and antiangiogenic effects. In the SHARP (Sorafenib Hepatocellular Carcinoma Assessment Randomized Protocol) study (a multicenter, double-blind, randomized phase 3 trial), sorafenib was shown to be efficacious and well tolerated in Child A patients with advanced HCC. Patients with advanced HCC were randomly assigned to placebo (n = 303) or sorafenib 400 mg twice a day (n = 299). The primary end points of the study were overall survival and time to symptomatic progression (TTSP), with secondary end points including time to radiologic progression (TTP) and safety. Median overall survival was significantly longer in the sorafenib group (10.7 months) than in the placebo group (7.9 months); however, median TTSP did not differ significantly between the study groups (4.1 months vs 4.9 months). Median TTP was significantly longer in the sorafenib group (5.5 months) than in the placebo group (2.8 months).[101] Eighty-six patients (29%) of the sorafenib group and 90 patients (30%) of the placebo group who had previously received TACE were included in the SHARP study.

In a subgroup analysis of these patients, Galle and colleagues[102] reported that among the 176 patients after TACE, the overall survival and the time to progression were superior in the sorafenib group than in the placebo group (11.9 vs 9.9 months and 5.8 vs 4.0 months, respectively). These results suggest that sorafenib may be an effective treatment agent for patients with advanced HCC resistant to TACE. Furthermore, in another phase 3 randomized, double-blind, placebo-controlled trial, Cheng and colleagues[21] reported median overall survival of 6.5 months in patients treated with sorafenib, compared with 4.2 months in those who received placebo. Median TTP was 2.8 months in the sorafenib group compared with 1.4 months in the placebo group. As a result, sorafenib has recently been recommended for the treatment of patients with advanced HCC and extrahepatic metastasis or major vessel invasion with preserved liver function.[103]

SUMMARY

HCC and CCA account for nearly all primary liver tumors and are frequently unresectable because of advanced disease. Locoregional therapies including RFA, PEI, cryoablation, microwave ablation, TACE, HAI, bland embolization, radioembolization, and external-beam radiotherapy have all been recommended in patients with HCC and CCA as forms of palliation. Endoscopic and percutaneous techniques to decompress the biliary system are also frequently needed for obstructive jaundice. Systemic chemotherapy and sorafenib are palliative options used in conjunction with locoregional therapies or as sole therapeutic options.

REFERENCES

1. El-Serag HB, Mason AC. Rising incidence of hepatocellular carcinoma in the United States. N Engl J Med 1999;340:745–50.
2. Patel T. Increasing incidence of mortality of primary intrahepatic cholangiocarcinoma in the United States. Hepatology 2001;33:1353–7.
3. Endo I, Gonen M, Yopp AC, et al. Intrahepatic cholangiocarcinoma: rising frequency, improved survival, and determinants of outcomes after resection. Ann Surg 2008;248(1):1–13.
4. Altekruse SF, McGlynn KA, Reichman ME. Hepatocellular carcinoma incidence, mortality, and survival trends in the United States from 1975 to 2005. J Clin Oncol 2009;27:1485–91.
5. Cunningham SC, Choti MA, Bellavance EC, et al. Palliation of hepatic tumors. Surg Oncol 2007;16:277–91.

6. Bruix J, Boix L, Sala M, et al. Focus on hepatocellular carcinoma. Cancer Cell 2004;5:215–9.
7. Fattovich G, Stroffolini T, Zagni I, et al. Hepatocellular carcinoma in cirrhosis: incidence and risk factors. Gastroenterology 2004;127:S35–50.
8. Bolondi L, Sofia S, Siringo S, et al. Surveillance programme of cirrhotic patients for early diagnosis and treatment of hepatocellular carcinoma: a cost effectiveness analysis. Gut 2001;48:251–9.
9. Fuss M, Thomas CR. Stereotactic body radiation therapy: an ablative treatment option for primary and secondary liver tumors. Ann Surg Oncol 2004;11:130–8.
10. Khan SA, Davidson BR, Goldin RD, et al. Guidelines for the diagnosis and treatment of cholangiocarcinoma: an update. Gut 2012;61:1657–69.
11. Khan SA, Thomas HC, Davidson BR, et al. Cholangiocarcinoma. Lancet 2005; 366:1303–14.
12. Jarnagin WR. Cholangiocarcinoma of the extrahepatic bile ducts. Semin Surg Oncol 2000;19:156–76.
13. Llovet JM, Schwartz M, Mazzaferro V. Resection and liver transplantation for hepatocellular carcinoma. Semin Liver Dis 2005;25:181–200.
14. Forner A, Reig ME, de Lope CR, et al. Current strategy for staging and treatment: the BCLC update and future prospects. Semin Liver Dis 2010;30:61–74.
15. Fan ST, Lo CM, Liu CL, et al. Hepatectomy for hepatocellular carcinoma: toward zero hospital deaths. Ann Surg 1999;229:322–30.
16. Colella G, Bottelli R, De Carlis L, et al. Hepatocellular carcinoma: comparison between liver transplantation, respective surgery, ethanol injection and chemoembolization. Transpl Int 1998;11(1):S193–6.
17. Fong Y, Sun RL, Jarnagin W, et al. An analysis of 412 cases of hepatocellular carcinoma at a Western center. Ann Surg 1999;229:1669–77.
18. Groeschl RT, Gamblin TC, Turaga KK. Ablation for hepatocellular carcinoma: validating the 3-cm breakpoint. Ann Surg Oncol 2013;20:3591–5. http://dx.doi.org/10.1245/s10434-013-3031-5.
19. Forner A, Llovet JM, Bruix J. Hepatocellular carcinoma. Lancet 2012;379: 1245–55.
20. Llovet JM, Bruix J. Systematic review of randomized trials for unresectable hepatocellular carcinoma: chemoembolization improves survival. Hepatology 2003;37:429–42.
21. Cheng AL, Kang YK, Chen Z, et al. Efficacy and safety of Sorafenib in patients in the Asia-Pacific region with advanced hepatocellular carcinoma: a phase III randomized, double-blind, placebo-controlled trial. Lancet Oncol 2009;10:25–34.
22. Nguyen KT, Steel J, Vanounou T, et al. Initial presentation and management of hilar and peripheral cholangiocarcinoma: is a node-positive status or potential margin-positive result a contraindication to resection? Ann Surg Oncol 2009; 16:3308–15.
23. Gusani NJ, Balaa FK, Steel JL, et al. Treatment of unresectable cholangiocarcinoma with Gemcitabine-based transcatheter arterial chemoembolization (TACE): a single-institution experience. J Gastrointest Surg 2008;12:129–37.
24. Tan JC, Coburn NG, Baxter NN, et al. Surgical management of intrahepatic cholangiocarcinoma–a population-based study. Ann Surg Oncol 2008;15:600–8.
25. Chahal P, Baron TH. Endoscopic palliation of cholangiocarcinoma. Curr Opin Gastroenterol 2006;22:551–60.
26. Goletti O, Lencioni R, Armillotta N, et al. Laparoscopic radiofrequency thermal ablation of hepatocarcinoma: preliminary experience. Surg Laparosc Endosc Percutan Tech 2000;1:284–90.

27. Montorsi M, Santambrogio R, Bianchi P, et al. Radiofrequency interstitial thermal ablation of hepatocellular carcinoma in liver cirrhosis. Role of the laparoscopic approach. Surg Endosc 2001;15:141–5.
28. Livraghi T, Goldberg SN, Lazzaroni S, et al. Hepatocellular carcinoma: radiofrequency ablation of medium and large lesions. Radiology 2000;214:761–8.
29. Livraghi T, Meloni F, Di Stasi M, et al. Sustained complete response and complication rates after radiofrequency ablation of very early hepatocellular carcinoma in cirrhosis: is resection still the treatment of choice? Hepatology 2008;47:82–9.
30. Sala M, Llovet JM, Vilana R, et al. Initial response to percutaneous ablation predicts survival in patients with hepatocellular carcinoma. Hepatology 2004;40: 1352–60.
31. Poon RT, Fan ST, Tsang FH, et al. Locoregional therapies for hepatocellular carcinoma: a critical review from the surgeon's perspective. Ann Surg 2002;235(4): 466–86.
32. Kim JH, Won HJ, Shim YM, et al. Radiofrequency ablation for the treatment of primary intrahepatic cholangiocarcinoma. AJR Am J Roentgenol 2011;196:W205–9.
33. Kuhlman JB, Blum HE. Locoregional therapy for cholangiocarcinoma. Curr Opin Gastroenterol 2013;29:1–5.
34. Shina S, Tagawa K, Unuma T, et al. Percutaneous ethanol injection therapy for hepatocellular carcinoma. A histopathologic study. Cancer 1991;68:1524–30.
35. Livraghi T, Giorgio A, Marin G, et al. Hepatocellular carcinoma and cirrhosis in 746 patients: long-term results of percutaneous ethanol injection. Radiology 1995;197:101–8.
36. Vilana R, Bruix J, Bru C, et al. Tumor size determines the efficacy of percutaneous ethanol injection for the treatment of small hepatocellular carcinoma. Hepatology 1992;16:353–7.
37. Gournay J, Tchuenbou J, Richou C, et al. Percutaneous ethanol injection vs. resection in patients with small single hepatocellular carcinoma: a retrospective case-control study with cost analysis. Aliment Pharmacol Ther 2002;16: 1529–38.
38. Livraghi T, Goldberg SN, Lazzaroni S, et al. Small hepatocellular carcinoma; treatment with radiofrequency ablation versus percutaneous ethanol injection. Radiology 1999;210:655–61.
39. Ravikumar TS, Steele GD. Hepatic cryosurgery. Surg Clin North Am 1989;69: 433–40.
40. Cuschieri A, Crosthwaite G, Shimi S, et al. Hepatic cryotherapy for liver tumors. Development and clinical evaluation of a high-efficiency insulated multineedle probe system for open and laparoscopic use. Surg Endosc 1995;9:483–9.
41. Zhou XD, Tang ZY. Management of hepatocellular carcinoma: long-term outcome in 2639 cases. Gan To Kagaku Ryoho 1997;24:9–16.
42. Huang YZ, Zhou SC, Zhou H, et al. Radiofrequency ablation versus cryosurgery ablation for hepatocellular carcinoma: a meta-analysis. Hepatogastroenterology 2013;60. http://dx.doi.org/10.5754/hge121142.
43. Seki T, Wakabayashi M, Nakagawa T, et al. Ultrasonically guided percutaneous microwave coagulation therapy for small hepatocellular carcinoma. Cancer 1994;74:817–25.
44. Matsukawa T, Yamashita Y, Arakawa A, et al. Percutaneous microwave coagulation therapy in liver tumors. A 3-year experience. Acta Radiol 1997;38:410–5.
45. Ohmoto K, Miyake I, Tsuduki M, et al. Percutaneous microwave coagulation therapy for unresectable hepatocellular carcinoma. Hepatogastroenterology 1999; 46:2894–900.

46. Groeschl RT, Wong RK, Quebbeman EJ, et al. Recurrence after microwave ablation of liver malignancies: a single institution experience. HPB (Oxford) 2013;15:365–71.
47. Chung KY, Kemeny N. Regional and systemic chemotherapy for primary hepatobiliary cancers and for colorectal cancer metastatic to the liver. Semin Radiat Oncol 2005;15:284–98.
48. Tse AN, Wu N, Patel D, et al. A phase 1 study of gemcitabine given via intrahepatic pump for primary or metastatic hepatic malignancies. Cancer Chemother Pharmacol 2009;64:935–44.
49. Jarnagin W, Schwartz L, Gultekin DH, et al. Regional chemotherapy for unresectable primary liver cancer: results of a phase II clinical trial and assessment of DCE-MRI as a biomarker of survival. Ann Oncol 2009;20:1589–95.
50. Bhattacharya S, Davidson B, Dhillon AP. Blood supply of early hepatocellular carcinoma. Semin Liver Dis 1995;15:390–401.
51. Bruix J, Castells A, Montanya X, et al. Phase II study of transarterial embolization in European patients with hepatocellular carcinoma: need for controlled trials. Hepatology 1994;20:643–50.
52. Matsui O, Kadoya M, Yoshikawa J, et al. Subsegmental transcatheter arterial embolization for small hepatocellular carcinomas: local therapeutic effect and 5-year survival rate. Cancer Chemother Pharmacol 1994;33:S84–8.
53. Bhattacharya S, Novell JR, Winslet MC, et al. Iodized oil in the treatment of hepatocellular carcinoma. Br J Surg 1994;81:1563–71.
54. Hatanaka Y, Yamashita Y, Takahashi M, et al. Unresectable hepatocellular carcinoma: analysis of prognostic factors in transcatheter management. Radiology 1995;195:747–52.
55. Ma TC, Shao HB, Xu Y, et al. Three treatment methods via the hepatic artery for hepatocellular carcinoma–a retrospective study. Asian Pac J Cancer Prev 2013; 14:2491–4.
56. Sumie S, Yamashita F, Ando E, et al. Interventional radiology for advanced hepatocellular carcinoma: comparison of hepatic artery infusion chemotherapy and transcatheter arterial lipiodol chemoembolization. AJR Am J Roentgenol 2003;181:1327–34.
57. Okusaka T, Kasugai H, Shioyama Y, et al. Transarterial chemotherapy alone versus transarterial chemoembolization for hepatocellular carcinoma: a randomized phase III trial. J Hepatol 2009;51:1030–6.
58. Llovet JM, Real MI, Montana X, et al. Arterial embolization or chemoembolisation versus symptomatic treatment in patients with unresectable hepatocellular carcinoma: a randomised controlled trial. Lancet 2002;18:1734–9.
59. Lo CM, Ngan H, Tso WK, et al. Randomized controlled trial of transarterial lipiodol chemoembolization for unresectable hepatocellular carcinoma. Hepatology 2002;35:1164–71.
60. Park SY, Kim JH, Yoon HJ, et al. Transarterial chemoembolization versus supportive therapy in the palliative treatment of unresectable intrahepatic cholangiocarcinoma. Clin Radiol 2011;66:322–8.
61. Kuhlmann JB, Euringer W, Spangenberg HC, et al. Treatment of unresectable cholangiocarcinoma: conventional transarterial chemoembolization compared with drug eluting bead-transarterial chemoembolization and systemic chemotherapy. Eur J Gastroenterol Hepatol 2012;24:437–43.
62. Raoul JI, Bretagne JF, Caucanas JP, et al. Internal radiation therapy for hepatocellular carcinoma. Results of a French multicenter phase II trial of transarterial injection of iodine-131-labeled Lipiodol. Cancer 1992;9:346–52.

63. Leung WT, Lau WY, Ho S, et al. Selective internal radiation therapy with intra-arterial iodine-131-Lipiodol in inoperable hepatocellular carcinoma. J Nucl Med 1994;35:1313–8.
64. Yoo HS, Park CH, Lee JT, et al. Small hepatocellular carcinoma: high dose internal radiation therapy with superselective intra-arterial injection of I-131-labeled Lipiodol. Cancer Chemother Pharmacol 1994;33:S128–33.
65. Raoul JL, Guyader D, Bretagne JF, et al. Prospective randomized trial of chemoembolization versus intra-arterial injection of 131-1-labeled-iodized oil in the treatment of hepatocellular carcinoma. Hepatology 1997;26:1156–61.
66. Lau WY, Leung WT, Ho S, et al. Treatment of inoperable hepatocellular carcinoma with intrahepatic arterial yttrium-90 microspheres: a phase I and II study. Br J Cancer 1994;70:994–9.
67. Hoffman RT, Paprottka PM, Schon A, et al. Transarterial hepatic yttrium-90 radioembolization in patients with unresectable intrahepatic cholangiocarcinoma: factors associated with prolonged survival. Cardiovasc Intervent Radiol 2012; 35:106–16.
68. Saxena A, Bester L, Chua TC, et al. Yttrium-90 radiotherapy for unresectable intrahepatic cholangiocarcinoma: a preliminary assessment of this novel treatment option. Ann Surg Oncol 2010;17:484–91.
69. Minami Y, Kudo M. Radiofrequency ablation of hepatocellular carcinoma: a literature review. Int J Hepatol 2011;2011:104685.
70. Kuang M, Xie XY, Huang C, et al. Long-term outcome of percutaneous ablation in very early-stage hepatocellular carcinoma. J Gastrointest Surg 2011;15:2165–71.
71. Oliveri RS, Wetterslev J, Gluud C. Transarterial (chemo) embolization for unresectable hepatocellular carcinoma. Cochrane Database Syst Rev 2011;(3):CD004787.
72. Young RF. The role of the gamma knife in the treatment of malignant primary and metastatic brain tumors. CA Cancer J Clin 1998;48:177–88.
73. Lo SS, Dawson LA, Kim EY, et al. Stereotactic body radiation therapy for hepatocellular carcinoma. Discov Med 2010;9:404–10.
74. Ibarra RA, Rojas D, Snyder L, et al. Multicenter results of stereotactic body radiotherapy (SBRT) for non-resectable primary liver tumors. Acta Oncol 2012;51:575–83.
75. Kwon JH, Bae SH, Kim JY, et al. Long-term effect of stereotactic body radiation therapy for primary hepatocellular carcinoma ineligible for local ablation therapy or surgical resection. Stereotactic Radiotherapy Liver Cancer. BMC Cancer 2010;10:475.
76. Barney BM, Olivier KR, Miller RC, et al. Clinical outcomes and toxicity using stereotactic body radiotherapy for advanced cholangiocarcinoma. Radiat Oncol 2012;7:1–7.
77. Blechacz B, Gores GJ. Cholangiocarcinoma: advances in pathogenesis, diagnosis, and treatment. Hepatology 2008;48:308–21.
78. Smith AC, Dowsett JF, Russell RC, et al. Randomized trial of endoscopic stenting versus surgical bypass in malignant low bile duct obstruction. Lancet 1994; 344:1655–60.
79. Dowsett JF, Vaira D, Hatfield AR, et al. Endoscopic biliary therapy using the combined percutaneous and endoscopic technique. Gastroenterology 1989; 96:1180–6.
80. Hintze RE, Abou-Rebyeh H, Adler A, et al. Magnetic resonance cholangiopancreatography guided unilateral endoscopic stent placement for Klatskin tumors. Gastrointest Endosc 2001;53:40–6.

81. Freeman ML, Overby C. Selective MRCP and CT-targeted drainage of malignant hilar biliary obstruction with self-expanding metallic stents. Gastrointest Endosc 2003;58:41–9.

82. De Palma GD, Galloro G, Siciliano S, et al. Unilateral versus bilateral endoscopic hepatic duct drainage in patients with malignant hilar biliary obstruction: results of a prospective, randomized, and controlled study. Gastrointest Endosc 2001; 53:547–53.

83. Raju RP, Jaganmohan SR, Ross WA, et al. Optimum palliation of inoperable hilar cholangiocarcinoma: comparative assessment of the efficacy of plastic and self-expanding metal stents. Dig Dis Sci 2011;56:1557–64.

84. Shariff MI, Khan SA, Westaby D. The palliation of cholangiocarcinoma. Curr Opin Support Palliat Care 2013;7:1–7.

85. Ortner MA, Dorta G. Technology insight: photodynamic therapy for cholangiocarcinoma. Nat Clin Pract Gastroenterol Hepatol 2006;3:459–67.

86. Ortner ME, Caca K, Berr F, et al. Successful photodynamic therapy for non-resectable cholangiocarcinoma: a randomized prospective study. Gastroenterology 2003;125:1355–63.

87. Witzigmann H, Berr F, Ringel U, et al. Surgical and palliative management and outcome in 184 patients with hilar cholangiocarcinoma: palliative photodynamic therapy plus stenting is comparable to r1/r2 resection. Ann Surg 2006;244: 230–9.

88. Gerhards MF, van Gulik TM, Gonzalez Gonzalez D, et al. Results of postoperative radiotherapy for resectable hilar cholangiocarcinoma. World J Surg 2003;27:173–9.

89. Montemaggi P, Costamagna G, Dobelbower RR, et al. Intraluminal brachytherapy in the treatment of pancreas and bile duct carcinoma. Int J Radiat Oncol Biol Phys 1995;32:437–43.

90. Choi J, Ryu JK, Lee SH, et al. Biliary drainage for obstructive jaundice caused by unresectable hepatocellular carcinoma: the endoscopic versus percutaneous approach. Hepatobiliary Pancreat Dis Int 2012;11:636–42.

91. Bahng S, Yoo BC, Paik SW, et al. Photodynamic therapy for bile duct invasion of hepatocellular carcinoma. Photochem Photobiol Sci 2013;12:439–45.

92. Cho HC, Lee JK, Lee KH, et al. Are endoscopic or percutaneous biliary drainage effective for obstructive jaundice caused by hepatocellular carcinoma? Eur J Gastroenterol Hepatol 2011;23:224–31.

93. Minami Y, Kudo M. Hepatocellular carcinoma with obstructive jaundice: endoscopic and percutaneous biliary drainage. Dig Dis 2012;30:592–7.

94. Valle JW, Wasan H, Johnson P, et al. Gemcitabine alone or in combination with cisplatin in patients with advanced or metastatic cholangiocarcinomas or other biliary tract tumors: a multicenter randomized phase II study–the UK ABD-01 study. Br J Cancer 2009;101:621–7.

95. Valle J, Wasan H, Palmer DH, et al. Cisplatin plus gemcitabine versus gemcitabine for biliary tract cancer. N Engl J Med 2010;362:1273–81.

96. Andre T, Tournigand C, Rosmorduc O, et al. Gemcitabine combined with oxaliplatin (GEMOX) in advanced biliary tract adenocarcinoma: a GERCOR study. Ann Oncol 2004;15:1339–43.

97. Harder J, Riecken B, Kummer O, et al. Outpatient chemotherapy with gemcitabine and oxaliplatin in patients with biliary tract cancer. Br J Cancer 2006;95: 848–52.

98. Jang JS, Lim HY, Hwang IG, et al. Gemcitabine and oxaliplatin in patients with unresectable biliary cancer including gall bladder cancer: a Korean cancer study group phase II trial. Cancer Chemother Pharmacol 2010;65:641–7.

99. Eckel F, Schimd RM. Chemotherapy in advanced biliary tract carcinoma: a pooled analysis of clinic trials. Br J Cancer 2007;96:896–902.
100. Lee J, Park SH, Chang H, et al. Gemcitabine and oxaliplatin with or without erlotinib in advanced biliary-tract cancer: a multicenter, open-label, randomized, phase 3 study. Lancet Oncol 2012;13:181–8.
101. Llovet JM, Ricci S, Mazzaferro V, et al. Sorafenib in advanced hepatocellular carcinoma. N Engl J Med 2008;359:378–90.
102. Galle P, Blanc J, Van Laethem JL, et al. Efficacy and safety of Sorafenib in patients with advanced hepatocellular carcinoma and prior anti-tumor therapy: a subanalysis from the SHARP trial. J Hepatol 2008;48:s372.
103. Kudo M, Ueshima K. Positioning of a molecular-targeted agent, Sorafenib, in the treatment algorithm for hepatocellular carcinoma and implication of many complete remission cases in Japan. Oncology 2010;78:S154–66.

Index

Note: Page numbers of article titles are in **boldface** type.

Surg Oncol Clin N Am 23 (2014) 399–408
http://dx.doi.org/10.1016/S1055-3207(14)00009-X
1055-3207/14/$ – see front matter © 2014 Elsevier Inc. All rights reserved.

surgonc.theclinics.com

Moving?

Make sure your subscription moves with you!

To notify us of your new address, find your **Clinics Account Number** (located on your mailing label above your name), and contact customer service at:

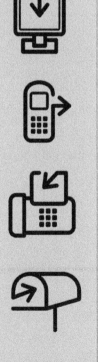

Email: journalscustomerservice-usa@elsevier.com

800-654-2452 (subscribers in the U.S. & Canada)
314-447-8871 (subscribers outside of the U.S. & Canada)

Fax number: 314-447-8029

Elsevier Health Sciences Division
Subscription Customer Service
3251 Riverport Lane
Maryland Heights, MO 63043

*To ensure uninterrupted delivery of your subscription, please notify us at least 4 weeks in advance of move.